Objective Structured Practical Examination (OSPE) Book Review in
OPHTHALMOLOGY

Get Video Contents Online at *emedicine360.com*

VIDEO CONTENTS

1. **VDO: 01:** Phacoemulsification
2. **VDO: 02:** Capsular tension ring (CTR)
3. **VDO: 03:** Capsulorhexis
4. **VDO: 04:** Hydrodissection
5. **VDO: 05:** Phacoemulsification: Femtosecond laser
6. **VDO: 06:** Phacoemulsification: Divide the nucleus
7. **VDO: 07:** Phacoemulsification: Sculpting of the lens
8. **VDO: 08:** LASIK (Laser in-situ keratomileusis)
9. **VDO: 09:** Continuous curvilinear capsulorhexis
10. **VDO: 10:** Cover test
11. **VDO: 11:** Alternate cover test
12. **VDO: 12:** Alternate prism cover test
13. **VDO: 13:** Trabeculectomy
14. **VDO: 14:** Endolaser photocoagulation
15. **VDO: 15:** Pars plana vitrectomy + scleral fixation IOL
16. **VDO: 16:** Optical coherence tomography (OCT) macula shows serous sensory detachment of the macula/PED/CSR
17. **VDO: 17:** Surge during phacoemulsification
18. **VDO: 18:** Fragmatome of dropped nucleus
19. **VDO: 19:** Put scleral buckle in RD surgery
20. **VDO: 20:** Small-gauge vitrectomy
21. **VDO: 21:** Manual small incision cataract surgery (MSICS)/SICS
22. **VDO: 22:** Nucleus delivery in MSICS/SICS
23. **VDO: 23:** Phacoemulsification with divide-and-conquer technique
24. **VDO: 24:** Intravitreal ranibizumab
25. **VDO: 25:** Pars plana vitrectomy
26. **VDO: 26:** Continuous curvilinear capsulorhexis in phacoemulsification
27. **VDO: 27:** Coaxial I/A handpiece
28. **VDO: 28:** Goniosynechialysis

Objective Structured Practical Examination (OSPE) Book Review in
OPHTHALMOLOGY

Second Edition

Md Anisur Rahman (Anjum)
MBBS (DMC) DO (DU) FCPS (Eye)
Professor and Head
Department of Ophthalmology
Dhaka Medical College
Dhaka, Bangladesh

Forewords
Dipak K Nag
Md Lutfor Rahman
Jalal Ahmed

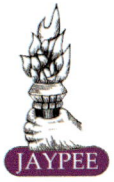

JAYPEE BROTHERS MEDICAL PUBLISHERS
The Health Sciences Publisher
New Delhi | London | Panama

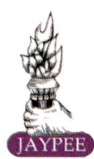

Jaypee Brothers Medical Publishers (P) Ltd

Headquarters
Jaypee Brothers Medical Publishers (P) Ltd
4838/24, Ansari Road, Daryaganj
New Delhi 110 002, India
Phone: +91-11-43574357
Fax: +91-11-43574314
Email: jaypee@jaypeebrothers.com

Overseas Offices
J.P. Medical Ltd
83 Victoria Street, London
SW1H 0HW (UK)
Phone: +44 20 3170 8910
Fax: +44 (0)20 3008 6180
Email: info@jpmedpub.com

Jaypee-Highlights Medical Publishers Inc
City of Knowledge, Bld. 235, 2nd Floor
Clayton, Panama City, Panama
Phone: +1 507-301-0496
Fax: +1 507-301-0499
Email: cservice@jphmedical.com

Jaypee Brothers Medical Publishers (P) Ltd
Bhotahity, Kathmandu, Nepal
Phone: +977-9741283608
Email: kathmandu@jaypeebrothers.com

Website: www.jaypeebrothers.com
Website: www.jaypeedigital.com

© 2019, Jaypee Brothers Medical Publishers

The views and opinions expressed in this book are solely those of the original contributor(s)/author(s) and do not necessarily represent those of editor(s) of the book.

All rights reserved. No part of this publication may be reproduced, stored or transmitted in any form or by any means, electronic, mechanical, photocopying, recording or otherwise, without the prior permission in writing of the publishers.

All brand names and product names used in this book are trade names, service marks, trademarks or registered trademarks of their respective owners. The publisher is not associated with any product or vendor mentioned in this book.

Medical knowledge and practice change constantly. This book is designed to provide accurate, authoritative information about the subject matter in question. However, readers are advised to check the most current information available on procedures included and check information from the manufacturer of each product to be administered, to verify the recommended dose, formula, method and duration of administration, adverse effects and contraindications. It is the responsibility of the practitioner to take all appropriate safety precautions. Neither the publisher nor the author(s)/editor(s) assume any liability for any injury and/or damage to persons or property arising from or related to use of material in this book.

This book is sold on the understanding that the publisher is not engaged in providing professional medical services. If such advice or services are required, the services of a competent medical professional should be sought.

Every effort has been made where necessary to contact holders of copyright to obtain permission to reproduce copyright material. If any have been inadvertently overlooked, the publisher will be pleased to make the necessary arrangements at the first opportunity. The **CD/DVD-ROM** (if any) provided in the sealed envelope with this book is complimentary and free of cost. **Not meant for sale.**

Inquiries for bulk sales may be solicited at: jaypee@jaypeebrothers.com

Objective Structured Practical Examination (OSPE) Book Review in Ophthalmology

First Edition: 2016
Second Edition: **2019**

ISBN 978-93-5270-971-7

Printed at Replika Press Pvt. Ltd.

Dedicated to
*My teacher, guide and mentor
Professor Syed Modasser Ali.*

Foreword

Book that will help you on the way to reach your goal....

Objective Structured Practical Examination (OSPE) Book Review in Ophthalmology by Md Anisur Rahman (Anjum) has recently come out in our hands with lots of possibilities. Objective Structured Practical Examination (OSPE) has become an integral part both in undergraduate and postgraduate examinations. The aim of adopting such a procedure is to make the examination valid and reliable, so that each student would be assessed on the keypoint knowledge with equal opportunity. The conventional way of answering the question is somehow descriptive, and this basic difference made OSPE difficult for the students during their examination. As such, special knowledge and techniques are required for doing good in OSPE. Unfortunately, book, particularly focused on OSPE is very limited if not at all absent in our surroundings. In this regard, I would say, Anisur Rahman has taken a time demanding initiative to fill-up such a lacking in the field of medical examination.

Additionally, Anisur Rahman has quite a long experience in OSPE from his active participation in teaching and evaluating students in various examinations. He tried to cover all the aspects of OSPE, e.g. questioning pattern, answering technique, OSPE on examining procedure, OSPE on counseling, OSPE on history taking, etc. I hope students will be immensely benefited by reading this book.

On top of that, for the faculties who are involved in examining students in the field of ophthalmology and the ophthalmologists who want pinpoint knowledge on the common ophthalmic situations would boost up their ability by going through this book.

Last but not least, I would like to thank Md Anisur Rahman (Anjum) for all his efforts bringing an invisible segment into light in a simpler manner.

Dipak K Nag
MBBS MSc (Epid, UK) MSc (CEH, UK) FCPS (BD) FRF (India)
Fellow, Retina Foundation
Ahmedabad, Gujarat, India
Professor and Head, Vitreo-retina
National Institute of Ophthalmology and Hospital
Sher-E-Bangla Nagar, Dhaka, Bangladesh

Foreword

Objective Structured Practical Examination (OSPE) Book Review in Ophthalmology is a new entity. This book reflects the vast experience of one of the renowned ophthalmologist Md Anisur Rahman (Anjum), who has devoted his knowledge and skills in teaching ophthalmic students. He is also an executive editor of the Bangladesh Ophthalmic Journal; he is also engaged in different activities of the Ophthalmological Society of Bangladesh (OSB), Bangladesh Academy of the Ophthalmology (BAO), and National Institute of Ophthalmology. I have thoroughly gone through the book. It is my realization that the book is very helpful for the postgraduate ophthalmic students like FCPS, MS, MCPS, and DO. The book reflects the guidelines for the postgraduate ophthalmic students in preparing and answering the OSPE questionnaires. There is no such type of book in Bangladesh. Postgraduate ophthalmic students are seeking to such type of books for a long time. I think the book can fulfill the demand of the students. So, I sincerely want success of the book.

Md Lutfor Rahman
FCPS, Fellowship in Neuro-ophthalmology
Associate Professor and Head
Department of Neuro-ophthalmology
National Institute of Ophthalmology and Hospital
Sher-E-Bangle Nagar, Dhaka, Bangladesh

Foreword

Medical writing skills are crucial for clinicians, educators, and researchers alike. Whether you work in a busy practice or in an academic setting, Md Anisur Rahman (Anjum) has done this hard job in an easy way. Objective Structured Practical Examination (OSPE) is not a very new concept in medical examination. It is an important component for both undergraduate and postgraduate examination. But it is a very funny thing that there is not a single book on OSPE in the market. Why not OSPE? Most probably to make an OSPE station is very crucial and takes a lot of time to make a station. To write a book with more than 250 stations!! Unbelievable!! But Md Anisur Rahman has done this unbelieving job. I hope he will publish the subsequent edition of the book and it will be a continuous process. Last of all, demand of our students for an OSPE book has fulfilled by Professor Md Anisur Rahman (Anjum). I hope students will collect the book and help to better circulation of the book.

Best wishes

Jalal Ahmed
MBBS (DMC) FCPS (Eye)
Ex-Director cum Professor
National Institute of Ophthalmology and Hospital
Sher-E-Bangle Nagar, Dhaka, Bangladesh

Preface to the Second Edition

By the demand of students, I decided to publish the second edition of *Objective Structured Practical Examination (OSPE) Book Review in Ophthalmology*. This edition has some differences from the first edition, such as the under grade chapters have been omitted.

In previous edition, the answers of the OSPE were given at the end of the book and it was a problem for the readers because they needed to search the answers at last page haphazardly, but now we have added the answers at the end of each chapter.

Though we have discarded the MBBS chapter from the book, but the total number of the OSPE has been increased. And many new ideas have been applied. In the first edition, there were 276 OSPE questions and answers, but now total questions and answers are 390 and we have added a new chapter (VIDEO station). There are 28 video clips online at *emedicine360.com* and answers are in the book.

I hope, postgraduate students will be benefited from this new edition.

Md Anisur Rahman (Anjum)

Preface to the First Edition

For the last 3 years at my institute (National Institute of Ophthalmology, Dhaka, Bangladesh) in addition to my regular lecture class with postgraduate students I was taking a class of objective structured practical examination (OSPE). From my experience, I can say most of the students know the answer of the question, but with a limited period of time (each station for 5 minutes) they cannot answer properly of the question, so most of the students fail in final examination just for OSPE. So, I try to make them accustomed with the new pattern of the examination. In July 2014, I had uploaded some OSPE in Google (if you want to visit it write "OSPE Dr Md Anisur Rahman" in Google). Many people have visited those from home and abroad. These inspire me to compile my lectures in a book. This book is divided into two parts. Part A which contains the questionnaire of the station. There are 14 chapters in Part A. Chapter 1 is composed of 24 questions; these are for undergraduate students. The last chapter, Chapter 14, is SCA (Structured/Short Clinical Answer) which is for MS student. But SCA and OSPE have very limited difference; if you know the fact about your question then answer becomes easy whatever it may be OSPE/SCA. Part B of the book is a checklist and answer section. It contains 14 chapters. In the final part of FCPS (Fellow of College of Physicians and Surgeons) examination, previously there was one station for examination procedure of a simulated person. But BCPS (Bangladesh College of Physicians and Surgeons) has come to a conclusion that examination procedure is a part of long case and short case. So faculty of ophthalmology decided to give up that station from OSPE examination and increased the optics question. In this book, the answer has been given in a bit descriptive way, but during the examination (each station for 5 minutes) you should write the answer shortly, such as a scenario has given and you made the diagnosis, it is a case of "Eale's disease" and the next question is what the hallmark of the disease is? You know the answer is "Recurrent vitreous hemorrhage". You should only write the keywords, no need to write "Recurrent vitreous hemorrhage is the hallmark of this disease", because time is constrain. But in this book I have written a bit descriptive way such as I have written here "Recurrent vitreous hemorrhage is the hallmark of this disease". And some answers are a bit bigger than the examination answer because to maintain the pace of the answers. When answer is controversial I try to give the explanation of the answer. In this book, I have tried to maintain the answer mainly from the Jack J Kanski (7th edition) first and then American Academy of Ophthalmology (AAO). Not a single answer is from experience, because in OSPE station there is no scope to answer by gazing. To the point answer is the key to success. If answer or checklist is contradicted with the latest edition of Kanski or AAO you follow the latest edition for your answer.

Md Anisur Rahman (Anjum)

Acknowledgments

I acknowledge following persons for their valuable efforts for the book:
1. Professor Dr Dipak K Nag, FCPS, Fellow, vitreo-retina, National Institute of Ophthalmology, Dhaka
2. Dr Ishtiaque Anwar, FCPS, ICO, Consultant, Bangladesh Eye Hospital, Dhaka
3. Dr Sharah Rahman, FCPS, ICO, Consultant, Bangladesh Eye Hospital, Dhaka
4. Dr Mukti Rani Mitra, FCPS, Assistant Professor, Dhaka Medical College, Dhaka
5. Dr Soheli Nasrin, FCPS, Dhaka Medical College, Dhaka
6. Dr Jamsed Faridi, DO, Dhaka Medical College, Dhaka
7. Dr Murtuza Nuruddin, Chittagong Eye Infirmary and Training Complex, Chittagong
8. Dr Soma Rani Roy, Chittagong Eye Infirmary and Training Complex, Chittagong
9. Dr Shams Md Noman, FCPS, Chittagong Eye Infirmary and Training Complex, Chittagong
10. Dr Bipul Kumer De Sarker, FCPS, Islamia Eye Institute and Hospital, Dhaka
11. Dr Ruhi Mannan, FCPS, BIRDEM, General Hospital, Dhaka
12. Dr Sabrina Rahmatullah, FCPS, Lions Eye, Hospital, Dhaka
13. Dr Md Basirul Azam, Chuadanga Eye Care Hospital, Chudanga
14. Asif Iqbal Joarder, FCPS, Dr Sirajal Islam Medical College and Hospital, Dhaka, Bangladesh.

Lastly, I would like to thank Shri Jitendar P Vij (Group Chairman), Mr Ankit Vij (Managing Director), Ms Chetna Malhotra Vohra (Associate Director-Content Strategy) of M/s Jaypee Brothers Medical Publishers (P) Ltd, New Delhi, India, for their untiring support.

Contents

1. Optics — 1
2. Scenarios Based — 22
3. Retina and Uveal Tissue — 63
4. Glaucoma — 114
5. Neuro-ophthalmology — 133
6. Lens and Cataract — 144
7. Oculoplasty — 155
8. Cornea — 167
9. Drug Preparation — 176
10. Procedure — 181
11. Examination Procedures — 191
12. History Taking — 198
13. Counseling — 207
14. Radiology — 226
15. Miscellaneous — 245
16. Video Station — 263

CHAPTER 1

Optics

QUESTIONS

OSPE: 01
What will be the reading glass prescription when addition is +2.0 D and interpupillary distance (IPD) is 64 mm for the following? (Write the reading glass after addition of +2.0 D).
OD: +1.00 −1.25 × 180°
OS: +1.25 −1.00 × 175°

OSPE: 02
OD: −1.00 Dsph/ −1.25 Dcyl 180°
OS: −1.25 Dsph/ −1.00 Dcyl 175°
IPD: 65 mm
Mr "X", 40-year-old, is using the above glass and he is quite satisfied with his glass for watching TV, driving, etc. But he is now facing problem during reading. He is not comfortable with bifocal glass, which was prescribed elsewhere.
Now he came to you only for the reading glass. Write down his reading glass prescription.

OSPE: 03
Do the simple transposition of the following prescription:
OD: −0.50 Dsph/ +1.00 Dcyl 145°
OS: +1.00 Dsph/ −0.50 Dcyl 35°

OSPE: 04
Do the simple transposition of the following prescription:
OD: +1.75 Dsph/ +2.50 Dcyl 130°
OS: Plano/ −1.50 Dcyl 140°

OSPE: 05
Calculate the spherical equivalent of the following prescription:
A. +2.00/ −1.00 × 80°
B. −3.00/ +2.00 × 90°
C. +1.50/ −3.50 × 45°
D. Plano/ −1.50 × 90°

OSPE: 06
Following are the retinoscopy findings (assuming the working distance is 1 meter).
Convert them into spectacle with minus cylinder notation.

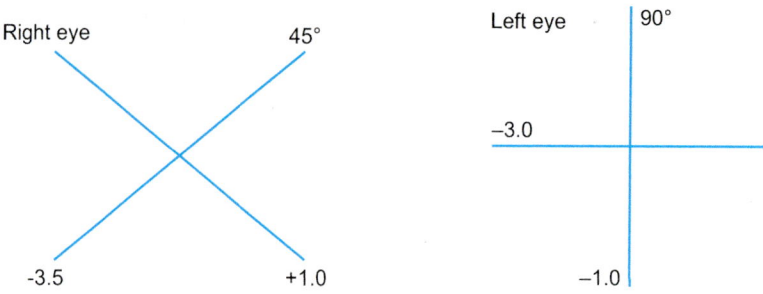

OSPE: 07
Following patients are selected for phacoemulsification with posterior chamber intraocular lens (PC IOL) implantation. They have the following refractive errors.
- Patient A: K reading 43.00/46.00 axis 90°. Refraction: –1.00 Dsph/ –3.00 Dcyl 175°
- Patient B: K reading 44.25/44.50 axis 160°. Refraction: –0.75 Dsph/ +2.25 Dcyl 170°

Do you think both patients are fit for astigmatic keratotomy during cataract surgery?

OSPE: 08
A patient needs +2.50 D to see distance clearly. However, he can tolerate up to +4.00 D without getting blurred distance vision. His cycloplegic refraction is +5.00 D sphere. What will be the following values?

A. Total hypermetropia
B. Latent hypermetropia
C. Facultative hypermetropia
D. Manifest hypermetropia
E. Absolute hypermetropia

OSPE: 09
Do the toric transposition of:

$$\frac{+4.0}{+2.0 \text{ axis } 90°}$$

Base curve –6.0 D

OSPE: 10
Following are the retinoscopy findings (assuming the working distance is 67 cm). Convert them into spectacle with plus cylinder notation.

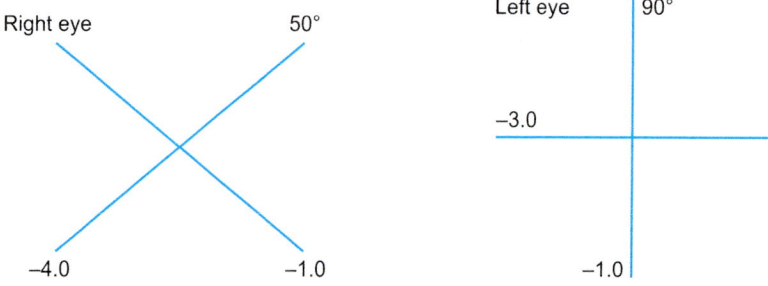

OSPE: 11
Do the simple transposition and state the type of astigmatism, which is present in each.
A. −4.00 Dsph/ −1.50 Dcyl 70°
B. +1.25 Dsph/ +3.00 Dcyl 90°
C. Plano/ +1.50 Dcyl 40°
D. −1.00 Dsph/ +1.00 Dcyl 50°
E. −1.75 Dsph/ +2.00 Dcyl 135°

OSPE: 12
A patient is selected for cataract surgery, whose axial length and keratometric readings are as below:
- Axial length—24.00 mm
- K1—43.00 DS   K2—44.00 DS
- A-constant of the lens to be used—118.0

A. Calculate the lens power needed to achieve emmetropic
B. During the operation, there is posterior capsular tear and decided to implant the lens in sulcus. Would you use a lens (same A-constant) with a higher or lower power compared to the bag implantation?

OSPE: 13
An aphakia patient is using glass with good vision, but she has some problems so she desires for a soft contact lens what will be the power of soft contact lens, when his glass power is +10, back vertex distance is 15 mm. Now:
A. Find the power of the contact lens.
B. Now what others information you need to fit the contact lens?
C. Mention three problems with aphakic glass.

OSPE: 14
Write down the following image characters of a concave mirror when object is placed at:
- In front of focal point
- Between focal point and center of curvature
    i. Location of the image
    ii. Orientation (either upright or inverted)
    iii. Size of the image (magnified, minified, or same)
    iv. Type of image (either real or virtual).

OSPE: 15
1. An object is kept in between two mirrors at right angle; how many images of the object will be formed?
2. Another object is kept in between two mirrors at 60°, how many images of the object will be formed?
3. Where this property of mirror is used?

OSPE: 16
A junior resident did the refraction of a 45-year-old man (working distance: 1 meter). His retinoscopic findings and glass prescription is as follows. If his retinoscopic finding is correct

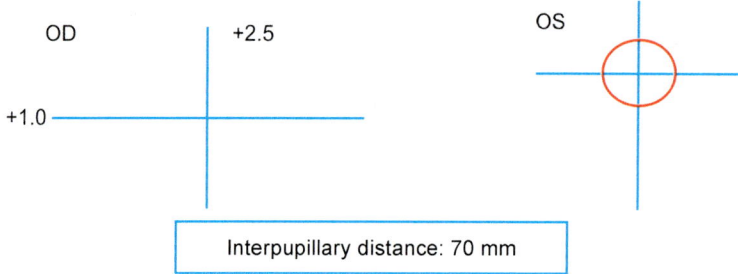

He wrote the prescription:

	OD			OS			
	sph	cyl	ax	sph	cyl	ax	
Dis		+1.50	90°	Plano			
Near	+1.75	+1.50	90°	+1.75			
IPD: 70 mm							

A. How many mistakes he had committed?
B. And what are the mistakes?

OSPE: 17
When performing cycloplegic retinoscopy on an anxious 7-year-old boy, you notice that the central reflex shows with movement while the peripheral reflex shows against movement.
1. What is the most likely physiological cause?
2. Why there are different central and peripheral reflexes?
3. If it is physiological, how will you overcome of it?
4. What is the most likely pathological cause?

OSPE: 18
What will be the prism position to correct?
  i. Convergence
 ii. Divergence
iii. Hypermetropia in right eye.

OSPE: 19
Calculate the binocular prismatic effects of the following:
A. Right eye 7 prism diopter, base-out
   Left eye 4 prism diopter, base-out
B. Right eye 5 prism diopter, base-out
   Left eye 7 prism diopter, base-in
C. Right eye 5 prism diopter, base-up
   Left eye 2 prism diopter, base-down
D. Right eye 2 prism diopter, base-up
   Left eye 3 prism diopter, base-up

OSPE: 20
A patient who is 60-year-old came to you for cataract surgery, he has history of vitrectomy with silicon oil.
A. Now what will the effect of silicon oil on the eye?
B. When you will go for A-scan, what will be the problem?
C. Mention two complications of silicon oil on ocular tissue.

Optics

OSPE: 21
A girl of 20 years came to you for soft contact lens, her glass prescription is –10 D (B/E) and her back vertex distance is 14 mm.
A. Calculate the power of the soft contact lens.
B. What other information you have to know to fit the contact lens?

OSPE: 22
Few months after ECCE with PC IOL implantation surgery following keratometric reading was recorded by keratometer:
42.00 @60
45.00 @120
A. What is the power and axis of cylinder required to correct the postoperative astigmatism?
B. If a tight radial placed suture is present, in which meridian would you most likely find it?

OSPE: 23
This is the prescription of a spectacle.
OD: +1.0 Dsph/ +1.0 Dcyl 180°
OS: +1.0 Dsph/ +2.0 Dcyl 180°
Draw the retinoscopy findings of the above spectacle from 1-meter distance.

OSPE: 24
This is the prescription of a spectacle.
OD: –2.0 Dsph/ +3.0 Dcyl 40°
OS: +2.0 Dsph/ +0.5 Dcyl 140°
Draw the retinoscopy findings of the above spectacle from 67 cm distance.

OSPE: 25
A resident performs biometry of your cataract unit, but 60% of his biometry is overcorrected.
A. What may be the problem?
B. Which is the better technique of IOL power management?

OSPE: 26
A 20-year-old lady came to you for soft lens, she is using spectacle R/E: –2.0 Dsph/ –1.0 Dcyl 90° and L/E: –1.25 Dsph/–1.50 Dcyl 90°; in this case toric soft lens is ideal, but you have no such lens so you do the spherical conversion and prescribe –2.50 Dsph in R/E, and –2.0 Dsph in L/E.
A. What problem she will face? Mention two problems.
B. Which contact lens will be better for her? Why?
C. What is alternative she can prefer?

OSPE: 27
What will be the prism position to correct?
A. Convergence
B. Divergence
C. Hypertropia in right eye.

OSPE: 28
Calculate the binocular prismatic effects of the following:
A. Right eye 4 prism diopter, base-out
   Left eye 5 prism diopter, base-out
B. Right eye 5 prism diopter, base-out
   Left eye 8 prism diopter, base-in
C. Right eye 3 prism diopter, base-up
   Left eye 6 prism diopter, base-down
D. Right eye 2 prism diopter, base-up
   Left eye 5 prism diopter, base-up

OSPE: 29

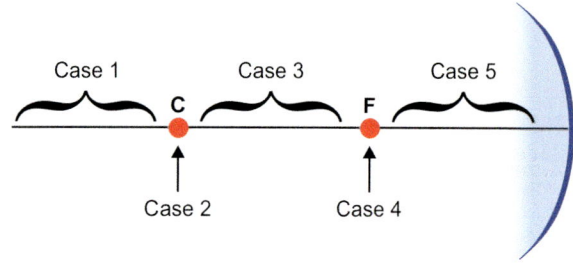

This is a concave mirror, five objects are placed in five different locations.
1. Write down the location of the images.
2. Write down where it will be real and virtual.

OSPE: 30
Do the:
- Simple transposition,
- Spherical equivalent, and
- Type of astigmatism for the following prescription:

OD: −0.50 Dsph/ +1.00 Dcyl 145°
OS: +1.00 Dsph/ −0.50 Dcyl 35°

OSPE: 31

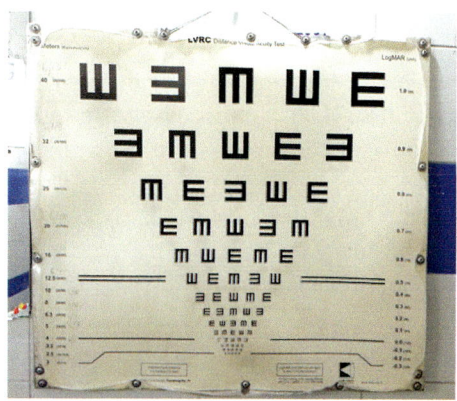

(*Image courtesy:* Dr Jamshed Faridi. DMC)

A. What is the name of the above chart?
B. What it stands for?

Optics

C. Where it is mainly used?
D. An observer who can resolve details as small as 1 minute of visual angle, what is his log value?
E. What is the distance between the two letters in each row?
F. What is the distance between adjacent rows of letters?
G. What is the LogMAR value for a visual acuity of:
   i. 6/60   ii. 6/6

OSPE: 32

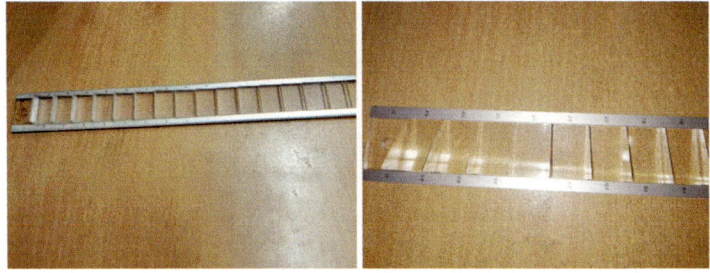

(*Image courtesy:* Dr Jamshed Faridi, DMC)

A. What is the name of the above instrument?
B. What is diagnosed by left instrument, in which orientation?
C. What is diagnosed by right instrument, in which orientation?
D. Is it an objective and subject measurement?
E. What types of squint cannot be measured with this instrument?

OSPE: 33

A. What is the name of this image?   B. What is the indication of this investigation?
C. Which formula is used here?   D. When this formula is used?

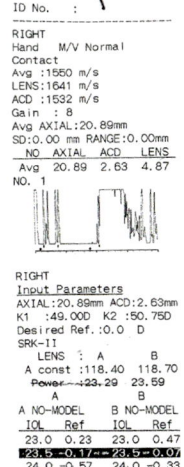

(*Image courtesy:* Dr Jamshed Faridi, DMC)

OSPE: 34

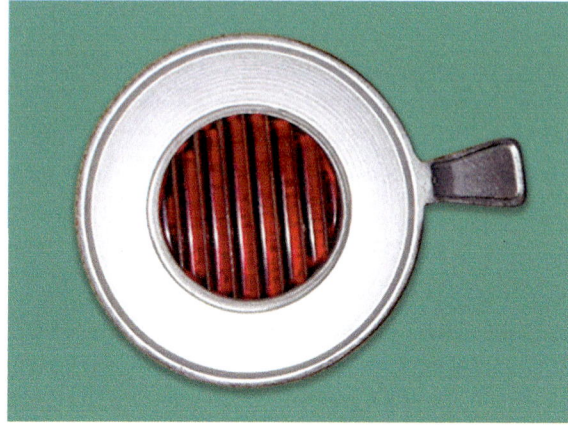

(*Image courtesy:* Dr Jamshed Faridi, DMC)

A. What is the name of the above instrument?
B. What are the indications of its uses? Mention two indications.
C. Is this a subjective or objective test?
D. What is the disadvantage?

OSPE: 35

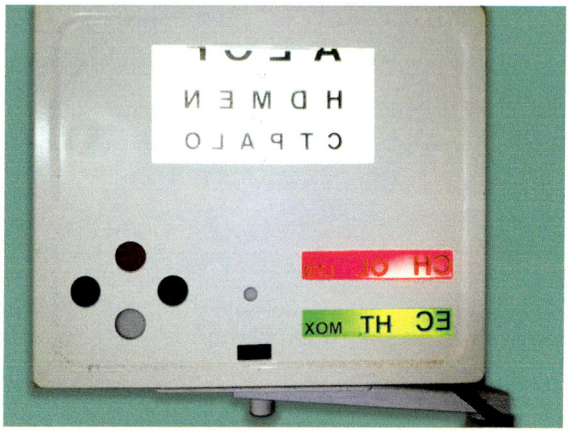

(*Image courtesy:* Dr Jamshed Faridi, DMC)

A. What test can be done with the red and green color of this chart?
B. What is the basis of this test?
C. Who will see the red color better?
D. Who will see the green color better?
E. Is this test valid for color blind person?
F. Mention one reason for your comment regarding question E.

OSPE: 36

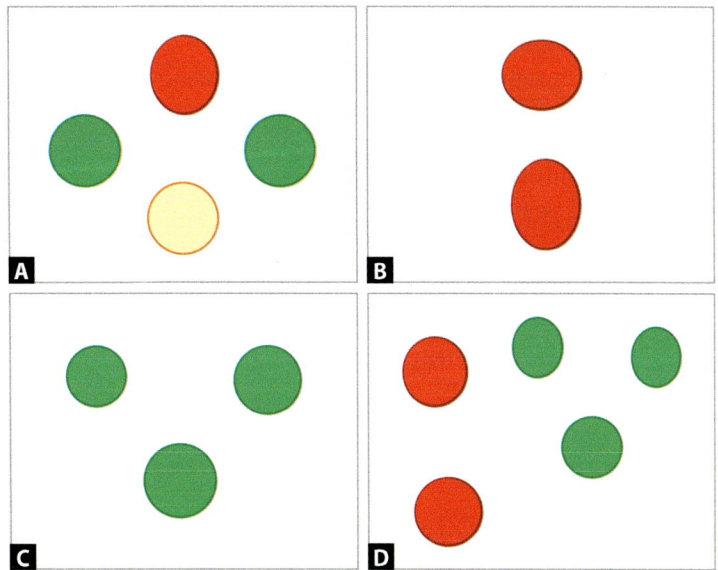

During this test, your patient wears green glass on right eye and red glass on left eye. Figure A is normal.
A. What is the name of the test?
B. What type of test is this?
C. What is your diagnosis in case of B, C, and D?

OSPE: 37

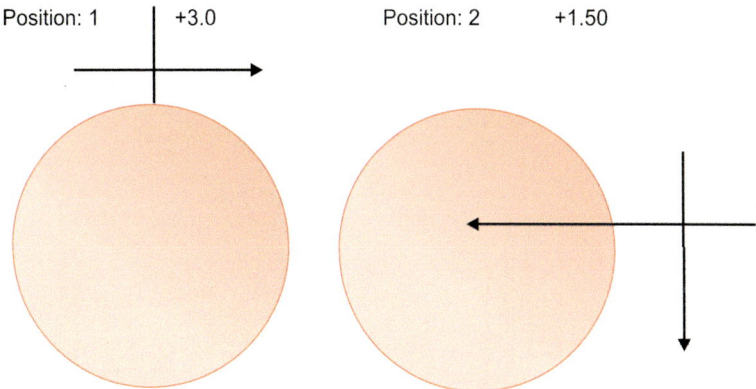

A stenopic slit showed above is used to test the eye of a patient with astigmatism. When the slit is held at position "1", the patient requires a +3.00 D sphere to see clearly and when the slit is held at position "2", the patient requires a +1.50 D sphere to see clearly.
A. Draw the power cross for this patient.
B. What is the prescription needed to correct this patient's vision?

OSPE: 38

This is the auto refractometer reading of a patient of 14 years old came to defective vision for last 8 years when he admitted at school

A. What is your diagnosis in right eye and left eye, respectively?
B. Do you think spectacle will work for this condition?
C. If you give full correction, what may be the problem?
D. What are the other options to treat? Mention one option.
E. Do you think vision will be 6/6 (B/E) now?

```
----------4153---------
NAME                           M/F
       29/MAR/2019   06:00 PM
VD=12.00mm
WD=40cm

<R>      S       C        A
      - 6.00 - 1.25   171   9
      - 5.75 - 1.25   171   9
      - 5.75 - 1.25   172   9
      <- 5.75 - 1.25  171>

<L>      S       C        A
      + 3.25 + 0.25    55   9
      + 3.25 + 0.00     0   7
      + 3.25 + 0.25   105   7
      <+ 3.25 + 0.25   80>

PD 64                    N 60

              NIDEK    ARK-1
        FASHION EYE HOSPITAL LTD
```

OSPE: 39

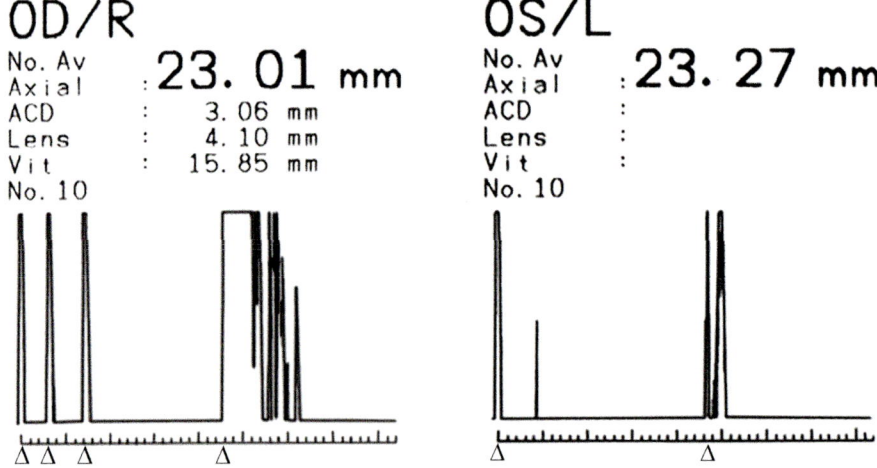

(*Image courtesy:* Dr Jamshed Faridi, DMC)

Optics | 11

This is the biometry of a patient both eyes. The OD shows three spikes subsequently, in OS it shows only one spike is there, the smaller one in OS is an artifact.
A. What it indicates three spikes in OD and one spike in OS?
B. What is your diagnosis in both cases?
C. What is treatment of choice if patient desires for cataract surgery? Mention three options and its advantages and disadvantages?

OSPE: 40

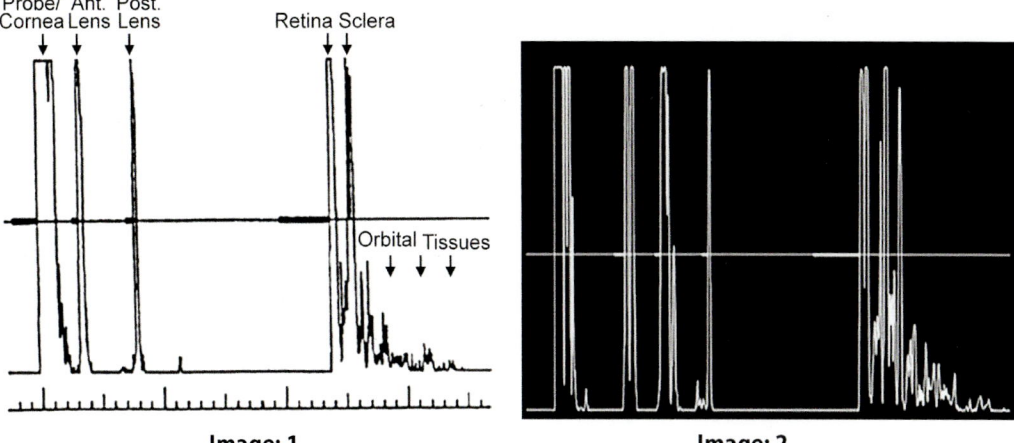

Image: 1   Image: 2

(Image courtesy: Dr Jamshed Faridi, DMC)

This is the A-scan biometry of two patients.
A. What is the technique difference between 1 and 2 images?
B. Why there is one more spike in image 2?
C. Which is more accurate? And why?

ANSWERS

OSPE: 01. Prescription of reading glass
OSPE: 02. Prescription of reading glass
OSPE: 03. Simple transposition
OSPE: 04. Simple transposition
OSPE: 05. Calculate the spherical equivalent
OSPE: 06. Retinoscopy findings given convert them into spectacle with minus cylinder notation
OSPE: 07. Who is fit for astigmatic keratotomy during cataract surgery?
OSPE: 08. Types of hypermetropia
OSPE: 09. Toric transposition
OSPE: 10. Retinoscopy findings given, convert them into spectacle with minus cylinder notation
OSPE: 11. Do the simple transposition and state the type of astigmatism
OSPE: 12. Calculate the IOL power
OSPE: 13. Calculate the power of soft contact lens when BVD of glass is 15 mm
OSPE: 14. Write down the image character of a concave mirror when object is placed at......
OSPE: 15. How many images of the object will be formed by two plain mirrors?
OSPE: 16. Find out the mistake of a spectacle prescribe by a junior resident.
OSPE: 17. Cycloplegic retinoscopy.
OSPE: 18. What will be the prism position to correct?
OSPE: 19. Calculate the binocular prismatic effects.
OSPE: 20. Effects of silicon oil.
OSPE: 21. Prescription of a soft contact lens when glass power is –10.0 D.
OSPE: 22. K reading has been given. Find the power and axis of cylinder.
OSPE: 23. Draw the retinoscopy finding from 1 m of spectacle when the power of spectacle is known.
OSPE: 24. Draw the retinoscopy finding from 67 cm of spectacle when the power of spectacle is known.
OSPE: 25. A resident perform biometry, and 60% of his biometry is overcorrected.
OSPE: 26. What will be the problem when using contact lens of wrong power?
OSPE: 27. What will be the prism position to correct?
OSPE: 28. Calculate the binocular prismatic effects.
OSPE: 29. Five objects are placed in five different locations from a concave mirror.
OSPE: 30. Do the simple transposition. Calculate spherical equivalent and mention the type of astigmatism in each.
OSPE: 31. LogMAR chart.
OSPE: 32. Vertical and horizontal prism bar.
OSPE: 33. Biometry results.
OSPE: 34. Maddox rod.
OSPE: 35. Duochrome test.
OSPE: 36. Worth four-dot test.
OSPE: 37. Stenopic slit.
OSPE: 38. Types of astigmatism.
OSPE: 39. Biometry.
OSPE: 40. Biometry.

Optics

ANS: 01
OD: +3.00 Dsph/ −1.25 Dcyl 180°	4
OS: + 3.25 Dsph/ −1.00 Dcyl 175°	4
IPD: 60 mm	2
TOTAL	***10***

(Explanation: Addition should be given only with the spherical power of the distance. The cylinder and axis will be as usual. Near IPD usually is 4–5 mm less than the distance IPD, but most of the ophthalmologists like to deduct 4 mm from the distance IPD)

ANS: 02
OD: −1.25 Dcyl 180°	4
OS: −0.25 Dsph/ −1.00 Dcyl 175°	4
IPD: 61 mm	2
TOTAL	***10***

(Explanation: Here patient is 40 years old, so, add + 1.00 Dsph with the distance correction. Remember, the rule of thumb for the presbyopia which is +1.00 for 40 years. +1.50 for 45 years + 2.00 for 50 years and +2.50 for 55-year-old person)

ANS: 03
OD: + 0.50 Dsph/ −1.00 Dcyl 55°	5
OS: + 0.50 Dsph/ +0.50 Dcyl 125°	5
TOTAL	***10***

ANS: 04
OD: +4.25 Dsph/ −2.50 Dcyl 40°	5
OS: −1.50 Dsph/ +1.50 Dcyl 50°	5
TOTAL	***10***

Explanation: 3 steps for simple transposition.

Step 1: Add cylinder power to the sphere power (algebraically!); this becomes your new sphere power.

Step 2: Change the cylinder sign: if its plus (+), make it minus (-), or vice-versa.

Step 3: Change the axis by 90° (can't go over 180!).

ANS: 05
A.	+1.50	2.5
B.	−2.00	2.5
C.	+ 0.25-	2.5
D.	−0.75	2.5
TOTAL		***10***

Explanation: Rule of spherical equivalent power calculation:
Divide cylinder power by 2 and add this cylinder power with the spherical power.

ANS: 06
R/E → −4.50 Dcyl 135°	5.0
L/E → −2.0 Dsph / −2.0 Dcyl 90°	5.0

Explanation: First, we have to deduct 1.0 from the retinoscopy finding (distance is 1 meter)

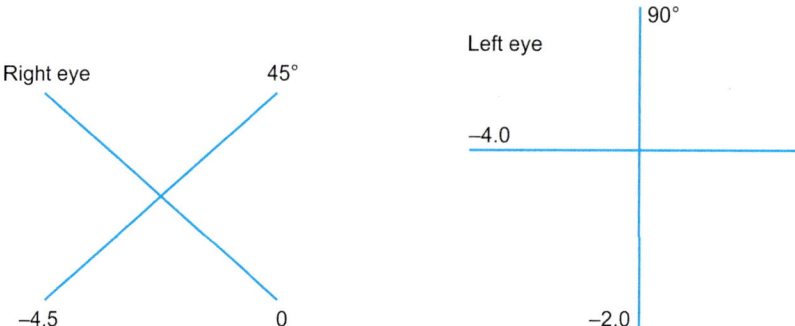

Now, if you want to make the prescription into minus cylinder, take common of the lower minus in right eye, take 0 and –4.50 will be in 135°
In left eye, take common –2.0
So, prescription will be:
R/E → –4.50 × 135
L/E → –2.0/ –2.0 × 90

ANS: 07
Both the patients are not fit for astigmatic keratotomy during cataract surgery, only patient A is fit for astigmatic keratotomy during cataract surgery.
In patient A, the astigmatism is corneal origin, and 5.0
In patient B, it is not corneal origin may be lenticular origin 5.0
TOTAL *10*

ANS: 08
A. *Total hypermetropia means highest correction after cycloplegia. Here it is +5 D* ....
B. *Absolute hypermetropia is the least amount of plus lens for clear distance vision. Here it is + 2.50 D*
C. *Manifest hypermetropia is defined as without cycloplegia, the most plus correction that can be tolerated without blurring of vision here it is +4.0 D*
D. *Facultative hypermetropia is defined as the difference between absolute and manifest hypermetropia (+4.00 D) – (+2.50 D) = +1.50 D*
E. *Latent hypermetropia is defined as the difference between total hypermetropia and manifest hypermetropia.*

ANS: 09
Step: A
Transpose the prescription so that the cylinder and the base curve are of the same sign, for example:

$$\frac{+6.0 \, DS}{-2.0 \, DC \, axis \, 180°}$$

Base curve –6 D

Optics

Step: B
Calculate the required power of the spherical surface (the numerator of the final formula). This is obtained by subtracting the base curve power from the spherical power:
$$+6.0 - (-6.0) = +12.0$$

Step: C
Specify the axis of the base curve. As this is the weaker principal meridian of the toric surface, its axis is at 90° to the axis of the required cylinder. That is:
$$-6.0 \text{ axis } 90°$$

Step: D
Add the required cylinder to the base curve power:
$$-6 + (-2.0) = -8.0 \text{ axis } 180°$$

The complete toric formula is thus:

$$\frac{+12.0 \text{ DS}}{-6.\text{DS axis } 90°/-8.0 \text{ DC axis } 180°}$$

ANS: 10

R/E → −5.50 Dsph/ +3.0 × 130° 5.0
L/E → 4.5 Dsph/ +2.0 Dcyl 180° 5.0

Explanation: First, we have to deduct 1.5 from the retinoscopy finding (distance is 67 cm)

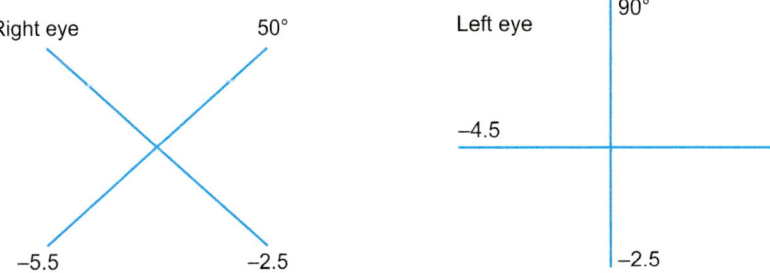

Now, *if you want to make the prescription into plus cylinder, take common of the lower plus or higher minus)*
In right eye, take common −5.5 so it will be R/E → −5.50 Dsph/ + 3.0 × 130°
In left eye take common −4.5 it will be in L/E −4.5 Dsph/ +2.0 Dcyl 180°
So, prescription will be:
R/E → −5.50 Dsph/ +3.0 × 130°
L/E → −2.0 / −2.0 × 90

ANS: 11

A. −5.50 Dsph/ +1.50 Dcyl 160°   Compound myopic astigmatism
B. + 4.25 Dsph/ −3.00 Dcyl 180°   Mixed astigmatism
C. +1.50 Dsph/ −1.50 Dcyl 130°   Simple hypermetropic
D. −.0 1400 Ds Dcyl 140°   Simple hypermetropic astigmatism
E. +0.25/ −2.00 Dcyl 45°   Compound myopic astigmatism

16 Objective Structured Practical Examination (OSPE) Book Review in Ophthalmology

ANS: 12
A. Using the IOL formula
   A −2.5 [(axial length) −0.9 (average K reading)]
   118 − 2.5 (24) − 0.9 (43.5)
   118 − (60 + 39) = 118 − 99 = 19.0
B. Moving the lens forward increases the power of the lens and therefore a weaker lens is needed. This is usually 0.5 D less than in the bag IOL.

ANS: 13
A. Required power of contact lens = $F2 = \dfrac{F1}{1-dF1}$

$$= \dfrac{10}{1-(0.015 \times 10)}$$

$$= \dfrac{10}{1-0.15} = \dfrac{10}{0.85} = +11.75$$

B. Base curve and diameter
C.
   i. Ring scotoma
   ii. Pincushion effect
   iii. Excessive magnification
   iv. Altered depth perception
   v. Weight of the glasses.

ANS: 14
- At focal point:
   i. *Location of the image*: Behind the mirror
   ii. *Orientation*: Upright image
   iii. *Size of the image*: Magnified
   iv. *Type of image*: Virtual.
- Between focal point and center of curvature:
   i. *Location of the image*: Beyond center of curvature
   ii. *Orientation*: Inverted
   iii. *Size of the image*: Magnified
   iv. *Type of image:* Real

ANS: 15
1. 3..4
2. 5..4
3. To manufacture kaleidoscopes 2

ANS: 16
A. Four mistakes are there.
B.
   - In right axis will be 180°
   - In left eye power will be −1.0 Dsph
   - Addition will be +1.50
   - IPD: 70/66 mm

Optics

ANS: 17
1. Spherical aberration
2. The periphery of the human lens is more curved than the center, so the incoming light rays show increased refraction compared with the light rays that strike the central lens. In retinoscopy, this can result in the appearance of different central and peripheral reflexes.
3. Concentrate on the central light reflex when performing retinoscopy
4. Keratoconus.

ANS: 18
i. To correct convergence, the prisms must be base-out, e.g. 8 D base-out R and L
ii. To correct divergence, the prisms must be base-in, e.g. 6 D base-in R and L
iii. To correct vertical deviation, the orientation of the prisms is opposite for the two eyes, e.g. 2D base-down in right eye and 2D base-up in left eye for right hypertropia.

ANS: 19
A. The resultant prism is found by adding the powers of the two prisms = 11 prism diopter, base-out.. 2.5
B. The resultant prism is found by subtracting the power of weaker prism from the power of stronger prism = 2 prism diopter, base-in 2.5
C. The resultant prism is found by addition of two prisms power = 7 prism diopter, base-down 2.5
D. The resultant prism is found by subtracting the weaker prism from the stronger prism = 1 prism diopter, base-up.. 2.5

ANS: 20
A. Hypermetropic shift

   (Explanation: Silicone oil has a higher refractive index than the crystalline lens and causes the posterior surface of the lens to become a diverging rather than a converging interface. As a result, a hypermetropic shift occurs).
B. Longer than expected

   (Explanation: Silicone oil reduces the speed of ultrasound and will therefore give an erroneously longer axial length)
C. Band keratopathy and glaucoma are known complications of silicone oil.

ANS: 21
A. We know the power of contact lens = $F2 = \dfrac{-10}{1-(0.014) \times (-10)}$

$$= \dfrac{-10}{1-(-0.14)}$$

$$= \dfrac{-10}{1.14}$$

$$= -8.75$$

B. Base curve and diameter of the lens.

ANS: 22

A. There are 3.0 differences between the two meridians. Therefore, the required cylinder correction is either: –3.00 × 60 or + 3.00 × 120° 5
B. The tight suture is at 60° and need to be removed 5

ANS: 23

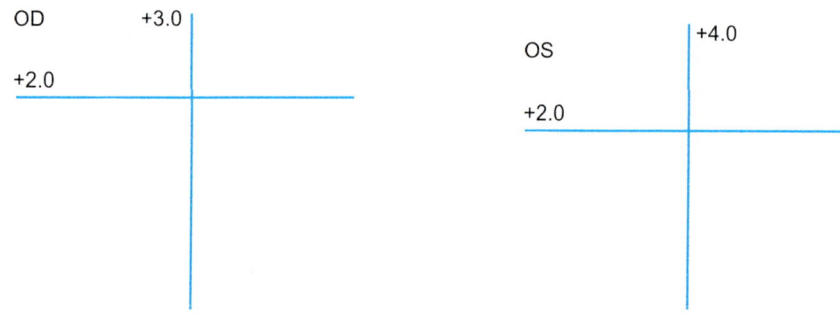

ANS: 24

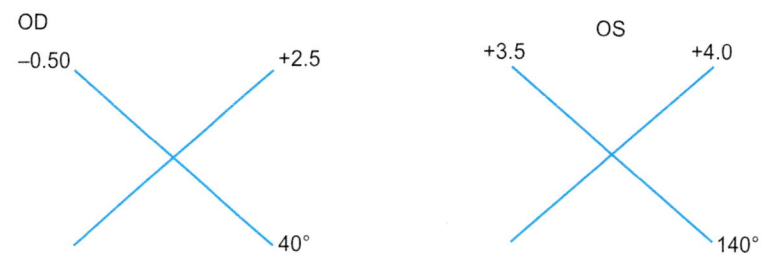

ANS: 25

A. The resident causes more indentation in the cornea so there is false reading and the axial length is less than the actual length, so calculated power will be overestimated.
B. Immersion technique is the better.

ANS: 26

A. i. Vision will not be clear
    ii. Headache (headache is due to no cylinder correction is there)
B. Rigid gas permeable (RGP) contact lens will be better because it corrects astigmatism by its curvature (in soft lens there is no space between lens and cornea but in RGP there is precorneal tear layer, so it corrects astigmatism)
C. Lasik.

ANS: 27

A. To correct convergence, the prisms must be base-out, e.g. 8 D base-out R and L
B. To correct divergence, the prisms must be base-in, e.g. 6 D base-in R and L
C. To correct vertical deviation, the orientation of the prisms is opposite for the two eyes, e.g. 2D base-down in right eye and 2D base-up in left eye for right hypertropia.

ANS: 28

A. The resultant prism is found by adding the powers of the two prisms 4 + 5 = 9 prism diopter base-out
B. The resultant prism is found by subtracting the weaker prism from the stronger prism = 8 − 5 = 3 prism diopter, base-in
C. The resultant prism is found by adding the powers of the two prisms 3 + 6 = 9 prism diopter, base-down
D. The resultant prism is found by subtracting the weaker prism from the stronger prism = 3 prism diopter, base-up..

TOTAL 10

ANS: 29

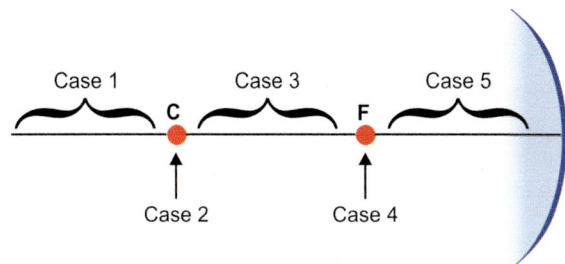

Case 1: Between C and F. REAL IMAGE..2
Case 2: Image will be at C. REAL IMAGE...2
Case 3: Image will be beyond C. REAL IMAGE 2
Case 4: No image will be form 2
Case 5: The image will always be located somewhere on the opposite side of the mirror. It will be virtual image..2

ANS: 30

Simple transposition:
OD: +0.5 Dsph/ −1.00 Dcyl 55°..2
OS: + 0.5 Dsph/ + 0.5 Dcyl 125° 2

Spherical equivalent:
OD: Plano 1
OS: + 0.75 Dsph 1

Type of astigmatism:
OD: Mixed astigmatism 2
OS: Compound Hypermetropic 2

TOTAL 10

ANS: 31

A. LogMar chart. It is also called the Bailey-Lovie chart..2
B. Logarithm of the minimum angle of resolution..2

C. It is mainly used in research purpose 1
D. His log value is 0 1
E. The distance between the letters in each row is equal to one letter width of the same row 1
F. The distance between adjacent row is equal to the height of the letters in the smaller row, i.e. the letters below 1
G. i. For 6/60 and 1
    ii. 0 for 6/6 1
TOTAL **10**

ANS: 32
A. Vertical and horizontal prism bar
B. In vertical prism bar (left instrument) apex either up or down and used to see the hyper- and hypotrophia
C. Horizontal prism bar (right instrument) apex is laterally placed (right or left side) to see the exo and esodeviation.
D. It is an objective test
E. (a) Cyclotropias or torsional deviations
    (b) Patients with eccentric fixation.

ANS: 33
A. Biometry results
B. To calculate the power of the implanted lens in cataract surgery
C. SRK/T formula
D. When the eyeball is too long

ANS: 34
A. Maddox rod
B. Can be used to detect and measure a latent, manifest, horizontal, or vertical strabismus for near and distance
C. It is a subjective test
D. i. Cannot differentiate between tropias and phorias
    ii. Not suitable for the measurement of large deviations, nor for accommodation deviation as accommodation cannot be controlled with this test
    iii. Cannot be done when there are sensory anomalies present
    iv. Cannot be performed, if a patient has suppression as they are unable to see the light

ANS: 35
A. Duo chrome test 2.0
B. Chromatic aberration 2.0
C. Myopes 1.5
D. Hypermetrope 1.5
E. Yes 1.0
F. Color blindness does not invalidate the test because it depends on the position of the image with respect to the retina 2.0
TOTAL **10**

ANS: 36
A. Worth four-dot test.
B. Dissociation test.
C. i. Diagnosis in B   ii. Diagnosis in C   iii. Diagnosis in D.

ANS: 37
A.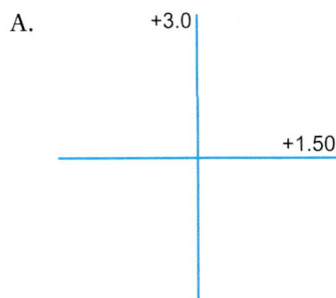

B. Glass prescription is: + 1.50/ +1.50 Dcyl 180°
(Remember that the power is 90° from the axis, when writing the power cross, the power is placed 90° to the axis)

ANS: 38
A.
- Compound myopic (Right eye) 2
- Compound hypermetropic (Left eye) 2

B. No 2
C. Double vision 2
D. Contact lens 2
E. No. There is certainly amblyopia in hypermetropic eye

ANS: 39
A. In OD there are three spikes subsequently meaning of the first spike in OD is cornea and the other two is for lens. But in OS, the one spike is for cornea.
B. *Upper one:* Aphakia. Lower one: Phakic eye
C. Treatment will depend upon the choice of patient, we can only have asked him for the options and its advantages and disadvantages
   i. Phaco with PCIOL implantation in right eye
   ii. SICS with PCIOL implantation in right eye
   iii. If we do any of these two in right eye there will be mono vision. If patient desires for binocular vision, second eye will go for secondary Intraocular lens implantation.

ANS: 40
A. *Image* 1 is contact technique and image 2 is immersion technique
B. In image 2, the first spike is the probe spike
C. Immersion technique is more accurate. In contact technique there is chance of indentation by probe so there is more chance of false axial length (smaller than the actual size)

CHAPTER 2

Scenarios Based

QUESTIONS

OSPE: 01

A patient of 75-year-old came to you with the complaint of vertigo accompanied by double vision, graying of vision, and blurred vision. The patient gave history of suddenly becoming weak at the knee and crumple to fall that lead to significant head injury. There was no disk edema.

A. What may be the probable cause?
B. Mention two differential diagnosis.
C. Mention one clinical examination and one laboratory investigation to rule out the diagnosis, beyond eye.
D. Two hematological investigations.
E. Two radiological investigations.

OSPE: 02

A lady of 50-year-old came to you with the complaints of double vision, which is sometimes horizontal and sometimes vertical. On examination, you got no positive findings of double vision. Pupillary reaction was also normal, both direct and consensual. After taking history you came to a conclusion that there is variability of the double vision which is usually marked after physical exertion and at evening. There is no history of eye pain, headache, neurologic symptoms, dysphagia, and viral infection or recent trauma.

A. What is your probable diagnosis?
B. Mention two differential diagnoses?
C. Mention one clinical test for diagnosis and one investigation to rule out other pathology

OSPE: 03

A lady of 30-year-old (not diabetic or hypertensive), but taking oral contraceptive for last 6–7 years came to you with the complaints of sudden loss of vision in left eye. On examination, you got visual acuity 6/24 (R/E), normal pupillary reaction. On examination of ocular fundus, you got retinal hemorrhage, soft exudates, and macular edema.

A. What is your probable diagnosis?
B. What is the most common site for this scenario?
C. Mention three risk factors?
D. What may be the cause of persistent poor vision?

OSPE: 04
2 years earlier, a 75-year-old man came to you with gradual loss of vision due to senile mature cataract and was advised for surgery at that time, but he did not come for surgery. After 2 years he came to you with sudden loss of vision, raised intraocular pressure (IOP), with painful red eye with photophobia, and severe conjunctival hyperemia. On slit-lamp examination, there was presence of cells and flare without keratic precipitates, pseudohypopyon, deep anterior chamber, and an open anterior chamber angle was there.
A. What is the most likely diagnosis?
B. The lack of keratic precipitates helps to distinguish what?
C. Treatment: (i) Immediate and (ii) Definitive treatment.
D. Why pseudohypopyon is there?
E. Lens-induced glaucoma may cause open angle or close angle glaucoma. Mention the name of two open angle and one close angle glaucoma.

OSPE: 05
A man of 30-year-old came to you with acute periorbital redness, swelling, and pain in right eye. On examination, you found congestive proptosis and ophthalmoplegia. CT shows ill-defined orbital opacifications and loss of definition of contents.
A. What may be diagnosis?
B. Write three differential diagnoses.
C. When it may be unilateral or bilateral?
D. Which tissue of the orbit is involved in this disease?

OSPE: 06
A man of 25-year-old (normotensive, non-diabetic, non smoker and non-alcoholic) came to you with the complaint of sudden loss of vision. He has also gave history of repeated attacks of dimness of vision at morning and recovers it after a short time. But this time vision loss is persisting.
A. What is your diagnosis?
B. What is the hallmark of the disease?
C. Write three causes of vision loss.
D. In fundus fluorescein angiography (FFA), how will you differentiate active and chronic phase?
E. Write three differential diagnoses. (On the basis of FFA report) (FFA not supplied).

OSPE: 07
- A 66-year-old patient complains of episodic headaches and transient bilateral visual loss, the attacks always occur on the same side and visual symptoms follow rather than precede the onset of headache.

A. Which two lesions have to rule out?
B. What two investigations you have to do?
C. What may be the other diagnosis? Mention two.

OSPE: 08
A 25-year-lady came to you with the complaint of transient visual obscurations lasting only a few seconds and characterized by a "graying out" or "darkening" of vision in one or both eyes, often precipitated by changes in posture.

A. What is your diagnosis?
B. Write two D/D.
C. Mention two investigations.

OSPE: 09

A 60-year-old patient is presented with sudden loss of vision, headache, and jaw claudication.
A. What is your clinical diagnosis?
B. Name three investigations for diagnosis.
C. Mention one common treatment.

OSPE: 10

A middle-aged female referred to neuro-ophthalmology clinic by an ophthalmologist who noted mild papilledema both eyes with recent onset of severe headache which was not relieved by any analgesics, a month of treatment with adequate acemox tablets, and repeated lumbar puncture, prior to which CT scan and MRI revealed nothing except ventriculomegaly [gave no impression of intracranial space occupying lesion (ICSOL) or duct stenosis].
A. What might be the possibilities? Mention two.
B. What else investigations do you want to do? Mention three.
C. What may be the treatment? Mention two.

Explanation: The clinical features mimic this is a case of idiopathic intracranial hypertension (HTN) but it denies when not responding to any of its treatments. Again, it denies ICSOL or aqueduct stenosis since CT scan and MRI revealed nothing except ventriculomegaly, in case of idiopathic intracranial hypertension (IIH), the ventricles become slit-like but never dilate. The dilemma in diagnosis of such cases of middle-aged women with nonresponding headache commonly present with cerebral venous sinus thrombosis which is confirmed by MRV (magnetic resonance venogram) that shows segmentation of blood column in cerebral sinuses. The treatment is by low-molecular weight heparin or warfarin. Another possibility in the context of our country is obstructive hydrocephalus following TB meningitis.

(Courtesy: Dr Hasanuzzaman. Long-term fellow: Oculoplastic).

OSPE: 11

It is an idiopathic multisystem disorder. One of the most common systemic associations of uveitis. It can affect essentially any organ system. It more frequently (10:1) affects patients of black than white ethnicity but is more common in colder climates. Females are more commonly affected than males; peak age is 20–50 years.
A. What is the name of the disease?
B. Name the three major organs it affects.
C. Write two anterior segment findings.
D. Write three posterior segment findings.

OSPE: 12

Go through the scenario carefully and answer the following questions: A patient complains of bilateral floaters, distortion of central vision, which is wax and wane over many months. The external eye is often white and uninflamed.
A. What is your diagnosis?
B. What are the systemic diseases associated? Mention two.

C. What findings will you get? Mention three.
D. What ocular investigation will you do? Mention two.
E. What are the causes of vision loss? Mention two.

OSPE: 13
It is the most common painful orbital mass in the adult population, and is associated with proptosis. It is a non-neoplastic, non-infective, space occupying orbital infiltration with inflammatory features. It has a varied clinical presentation depending on the involved tissue. Sometimes, clinically we are confused with dysthyroid ophthalmopathy.
A. What is the diagnosis?
B. How can you differentiate it from dysthyroid ophthalmopathy by MRI?
C. It is usually unilateral, but may be bilateral. When?
D. What feature will you get in CT scan?
E. What is the natural course? Mention three.

OSPE: 14
It is a recurrent bilateral disorder of conjunctiva, and sometimes cornea also, in which both IgE- and cell-mediated immune mechanisms play important roles. It primarily affects boys and onset is generally from about the age of 5 years onward (mean age 7 years). 95% of cases remit by the late teens although many of the remainder develops a topic.
A. What is the diagnosis?
B. How many types of this disease? Name them.
C. Which one effects cornea more?
D. When is the incidence high?
E. Do you need any investigation?
F. It has rarely one corneal association. Mention it.

OSPE: 15
A 10-year-old boy came to you along with his father with the complaints of swelling at upper nasal quadrant of the right orbit which is as it is for the last couple of years. But he gave the history, when he was playing with his friends, one of them was trying to strangulate him, and suddenly the eye became bulged and everybody was frightened to see that.
A. What may be the cause?
B. Why there was proptosis?
C. And why it was reversible?
D. What may be the complication?
E. What is the indication of surgery?

OSPE: 16
Histologically, it is crack-like dehiscence in brittle thickened and calcified Bruch membrane, associated with atrophy of the overlying retinal pigment epithelium (RPE), with optic disc drusen.
A. What is the name of the disease?
B. What are the causes of loss of vision? Mention three.
C. Mention one systemic association with this ocular finding.
D. What is the usual prognosis of this condition?

OSPE: 17

A patient came to you with the complaints of diplopia (vertical). But the diplopia goes on when he tilts his head and worsens on looking down. When you asked him about the onset, he told probably it is sudden but he cannot recognize when it started. On examination you found that pupillary reaction is normal, and there is no ptosis.

A. What is the probable diagnosis?
B. What are the causes for this sort of abnormality?
C. Which history you would have to know from the patient? Mention one.
D. What clinical tests you should do for diagnosis? Mention two.

OSPE: 18

Transmission of this disease may also occur by contaminated blood or needle. It targets CD4+ T cells, a steady decline in the absolute number of CD4+ T cells therefore occurs, and cell-mediated immunity declines.

A. What is the name of the disease?
B. How you measure the disease progression? In spite of systemic organ, it involves ocular structure, from eyelid to posterior segment. Mention:
   - Two eyelid findings
   - Three anterior segment findings
   - Three posterior segment findings.

OSPE: 19

A 63-year-old man presented to you with complaints of sudden dimness of vision in his left eye. He also gave the history that he has severe nausea and yellow coloration of his sclera for last 1 month.

A. What should be the diagnosis?
B. What might be the cause of his reduced vision? Mention three.
C. Why jaundice is there?
D. What investigations do you suggest to reach the diagnosis and management? Mention three.

OSPE: 20

A medicine specialist referred a 70-year-old patient to an ophthalmologist with severe headache and sudden onset of profound visual loss in one eye. On examination, it was found that mild ptosis and adduction deficit in the same eye. He had high ESR and high platelet count.

A. What is the most likely diagnosis?
B. Why ptosis and adduction deficit are there?
C. What specific investigations do you suggest to reach the diagnosis? Mention two.

OSPE: 21

You received a call from obstetrics emergency ward to see a hypertensive 40-year-old lady pregnant for last 7 months who gave history of repeated convulsions followed by loss of vision. You found visual acuity—only perception of light (both eyes), fundus and pupil reactions are normal in B/E.

A. What is the possibility?

B. What might be the underlying causes? Mention two.
C. What investigations you suggest? Mention four.

OSPE: 22
The disease probably has an autoimmune basis, and may be precipitated by exposure to an infectious agent with subsequent cross-reaction. The disease typically affects patients from the ancient "Silk Road" route. There are no specific tests to confirm a diagnosis. The diagnosis is based on clinical criteria. Tumor necrosis factor (TNF) thought to be an important

A. Mention the name of the disease.
B. Which systemic structures it involves? Mention three.
C. Which ocular structures it involves? Mention three.

OSPE: 23
A 70-year-old lady came to you with the complaints flushing of lightning-like arc induced by eye or head movement, in the temporal periphery and is more noticeable in dim illumination. She denied any "shades" or "curtains" in her temporal vision. On examination, you found a ring-like appearance in front of the disk.

A. What is name of the ring?
B. What is your probable diagnosis?
C. What is the importance of the history of "She denied any 'shades' or 'curtains' in her peripheral vision"?
D. Mention three risk factors?

OSPE: 24
It is an uncommon idiopathic multisystem autoimmune disease featuring inflammation of melanocyte-containing tissues; predominantly affects pigmented individuals. The disease is divided into two components; one is skin changes and anterior uveitis and other in which neurological features and exudative retinal detachments predominate.

A. What is the name of the disease?
B. Which ethnic group sufferers more?
C. In chronic stage it has a similar immunopathogenesis, with another disease, what is the name of that disease?
D. What is the name of the disease when there are skin changes and anterior uveitis?
E. What is the name of the disease when neurological features and exudative retinal detachments predominate?
F. How many people are suffering from auditory problem?

OSPE: 25
A man came to you with some photographs of his baby (2-year-old). You carefully observed these and found in some pictures the face turned laterally. In some, the eyeball looked normal and in some it looked smaller.

A. What may be the diagnosis?
B. Can you predict in which direction the eyeball looks normal?
C. Why the eyeball looks normal?
D. Why the eyeball looks smaller?
E. Mention two other nonocular congenital defects?

OSPE: 26

A 25-year-old male came to you with complaint of red, painful, photophobic eye, with some decrease in visual acuity. He also complains unilateral "headlight in the fog". On funduscopy, you got lesion with multiple surrounding healed chorioretinal scars.

A. What may be the diagnosis?
B. It appears that polymerase chain reaction (PCR) is typically positive early in the acute infection, when does it becomes negative?
C. If there is associated pars planitis, it broadens the consideration of other disease. Mention two diseases.
D. Congenital infection is associated with a classic triad. What is the triad?

OSPE: 27

Patient with transient visual loss:

A. What is the maximum time limit of transient visual loss?
B. Onset of visual loss within seconds and duration of symptoms between one and 10 minutes were associated with-----What?
C. Transient visual loss (monocular or binocular) lasting seconds and often precipitated by a change in posture (called "transient obscurations of vision") is common in patient with-----What?
D. Visual loss may last from seconds to an hour and may be accompanied by positive visual phenomena such as flashes, sparkles, or heat waves, and is due to-----What?
E. The typical binocular scintillating scotoma lasts for 20–30 minutes and is due to-----What?

OSPE: 28

A 50-year-old male patient came to you with the complaints of pulsatile proptosis, conjunctival chemosis, and a humming sound within the skull 10 days after head injury. On examination, visual acuity of right eye was 6/18 and left eye 6/6. IOP of right eye was 35 mm Hg and left eye 15 mm Hg. On gonioscopy, there was blood in the right trabecular meshwork. Fundus was within normal limit. The proptosis was pulsatile but non-tender and it goes on if pressing over the carotid artery.

A. What is your most likely diagnosis?
B. What may be the other cause?
C. What is the reason for humming sound within the skull?
D. Why IOP is raised?
E. Here it is ipsilateral, can it be bilateral or contralateral in the same injury?

OSPE: 29

A 45-year-old man, otherwise healthy, non-diabetic, and normotensive, suffers from sudden attack of ipsilateral headache and complete third nerve palsy with pupil involvement.

A. What may be the diagnosis?
B. Where is the lesion?
C. When there is no pain but progressive visual loss?
D. When there is associated ocular and forehead pain?

OSPE: 30
A patient with bilateral anterior and intermediate uveitis is suspected of having sarcoidosis. There is no conjunctival or eyelid granuloma. Chest X-ray shows no abnormalities. Serum angiotensin-converting enzyme (ACE) level is normal.
A. Which investigation will confirm the diagnosis?
B. Which is the best single screening test for sarcoidosis?
C. What is the characteristic of Heerfordt syndrome (uveoparotid fever)?

OSPE: 31
A newborn baby came to you with central corneal opacity present at birth, iridocorneal adhesions, cataract, elevated IOP, and cardiac abnormalities.
A. What may be the possible diagnosis?
B. What are the differential diagnoses? Mention two.
C. Is the condition usually bilateral or unilateral?

OSPE: 32
Neither the patient nor the physician could see anything.
A. What may be the cause? Mention three.
B. Which is the systemic disease you think? Mention one.
C. Which radiological investigation you will go for? Mention one.

OSPE: 33
A 16-year-old boy has referred to you with the complaints of severe itching of both eyes since childhood and it was diagnosed a case of vernal keratoconjunctivitis (VKC). At present, the boy is complaining gradual dimness of vision of both eyes which is not corrected by spectacles, and sometimes "ghost" image. You thought it may be a case of steroid-induced glaucoma (history of injudicious use of steroid is present), so you measured the IOP which was 8 mm Hg and 10 mm Hg in right and left eye, respectively. So you done the ophthalmoscopy, retinoscopy, and slit-lamp examination.
A. What findings will you get with ophthalmoscope? Mention one.
B. What findings will you get with retinoscopy? Mention one.
C. What findings will you get with slit-lamp biomicroscope? Mention two.
D. What investigations will your advice for diagnosis? Mention one.

OSPE: 34
A 35-year-old patient came to you with the complaints of reduced visual acuity for distance and near. He is also suffering from impairment of color vision, which mainly affects red and green. On examination, you find relative afferent pupillary defect (RAPD). You have done visual field analysis, and got central scotoma.
A. What may be the probable diagnosis?
B. In this scenario, what are the differential diagnoses of central scotoma? Mention three.
C. Mention one radiological investigation?
D. In this scenario, what will happen to light brightness sensitivity and contrast sensitivity?

OSPE: 35
A 15-year-old SSC examinee came to you along with his father. On examination, you find orthophoria for distance but a large exophoria for near.
A. What it indicates?
B. What are the symptoms? Mention three.
C. What are the treatments? Mention two.

OSPE: 36
A 60-year-old lady suffering from dry eye and using artificial tear drop for last 4 years now develops recurrent allergic conjunctivitis.
A. What may be the possible cause?
B. How will you overcome it?
C. Who is the more sufferer of dry eye male/female?
D. Which test measures the stability of the tear film?

OSPE: 37
It is an immune-mediated inflammation of the stroma sparing the epithelium and endothelium of the cornea. It may be congenital or acquired. In congenital, presentation is usually between 5 years and 25 years. The initial symptom is acute anterior uveitis with marked dimness of vision.
A. What may be the possible cause?
B. When is it usually unilateral and bilateral?
C. What type of uveitis you may get?
D. What other ocular features you may get? Mention four.
E. Mention three points on healed stage.

OSPE: 38
It is a chronic, autoimmune, multisystem disease, ocular involvement in one-third of cases. Sometimes potentially blinding disease
A. What is the systemic disease?
B. What is the other name of the disease?
C. Which part of the eye it affects more?
D. What is the most common ocular symptom?
E. Sometimes patient may present with severe ache' or 'boring' pain with sight threatening and requires urgent assessment by an ophthalmologist. What may be the ocular diagnosis?

OSPE: 39
It is a rare disease. Male to female ratio is 1:9. It occurs most commonly in childbearing age. Immune complex formation is thought to be an important mechanism of tissue damage in active disease, leading to vasculitis and organ damage. The most common ocular symptom is dry eye (mainly aqueous layer deficiency). In addition to that, treatment of this disease with systemic medication may cause ocular toxicity.
A. Name the disease.
B. Name the medicine which causes ocular toxicity?
C. What type of medicine is this?
D. What are the toxicities? Mention two.

Scenarios Based

OSPE: 40
It is an anticonvulsant, also used in the treatment of migraine. It can cause acute angle-closure glaucoma with associated myopia due to ciliochoroidal effusion.
- A. Name the medicine.
- B. After how long the complication may arise?
- C. What are the presenting symptoms? Mention three.
- D. What are the signs? Mention two.
- E. What is the treatment? Mention two points.
- F. What is the prognosis?

OSPE: 41
A 45-year-old man came to you with the complaints of headaches and nose bleeds. His blood pressure is 180/120 mm Hg. On dilated fundus examination, you found numerous exudates, flame-shaped hemorrhages, cotton-wool spots, and severe attenuation of the arterioles. You do not find arteriovenous (A/V) crossing changes and the arteriolar light reflex is normal.
- A. What type of hypertension the patient is suffering from?
- B. Is it acute or chronic hypertension?
- C. Mention two points from above findings in favor of your comment.
- D. You have to refer the patient to internist, if internist is not available, to whom will you refer the patient?
- E. In spite of blood sugar and lipid profile, what will be the next blood test?
- F. Is it a medical emergency?

OSPE: 42
A patient referred to you by an internist. He reports feeling especially tired lately, becoming fatigued after only moderate activity. He is also concerned about his vision; everything seems "dingy" or "yellow" to him. He is not sure when his visual symptoms started. The patient has a history of heart disease for which he takes cardiac medications. Systemic examination reveals no health problems, other than his heart condition, which appears stable. Ocular examination reveals only hypertensive retinopathy grade 1.
- A. What may be cause of his vision problem?
- B. Is the visual symptom reversible or irreversible?
- C. If you have the option to ask a question to patient, what should you ask first?
- D. In this condition, is it always "yellow"; is it possible to becomes green, blue, red or brown vision?

OSPE: 43
A 70-year-old man is suffering from age-related cataract and he likes to go for cataract surgery. He is taking medication (but cannot remember the name of medicine) for his urine flow?
- A. What medicine that you think can cause surgery difficult?
- B. Which syndrome is associated with this medicine?
- C. What difficulties you may face during surgery? Mention three.
- D. How can you overcome them? Mention four.

OSPE: 44

A 32-year-old HIV-positive man visits your clinic with complaints of decreased vision and floaters in his left eye for the past 2 weeks. On examination, you note retinal hemorrhages but no vasculitis and areas of white retinal opacifications.

A. What is your diagnosis?
B. Mention two D/Ds.
C. How you measure the progression of AIDS?
D. Nowadays, this sort of ocular involvement is reduced in AIDS patients. Why?

OSPE: 45

It is a systemic disease in 30% cases, it comes with ocular presentation. Usual range of presentation is 20–50 years of age, mean age is 30 years. Patient may complain phosphene and ocular pain during eye movements mainly in upper gaze. On examination, visual acuity is 6/18 – 6/60 not improve with pin hole. On visual field examination, there is diffused depression of sensitivity in central 30° field.

A. What may be the probable diagnosis?
B. Why the ocular pain mainly in upper gaze?
C. In visual field analysis, in spite of sensitivity what is the other change you may get?
D. You examine the other eye and observed temporal disc pallor. What may be the cause of this feature?
E. What is the early and late natural course of the disease?

OSPE: 46

A 30-year-old man came to you with complains of visual loss for last 3 days accompanied by tiny white or colored flashes or sparkles. Discomfort or pain in or around the eye, which is exacerbated by ocular movements. There is also frontal headache and tenderness of the globe.

On examination:

- VAR: 6/60; VAL: 6/6.
- Ocular motility: Full in all gazes.
- Optic disc: Nothing abnormality detected temporal disc pallor in the fellow eye.
- Visual field shows diffused depression of sensitivity in the entire central 30°.

A. What is your diagnosis?
B. What may be the systemic cause?
C. Mention two non-ocular investigations.
D. What other field defect you may observe in this disease? Mention two.

OSPE: 47

A 55-year-old patient came to you and apart from gradual reducing visual acuity, also complains of impaired contrast sensitivity, difficulties with glare, and monocular diplopia. On history, you found that you have done phacoemulsification with posterior chamber intraocular lens (PC IOL) 2 years back; the lens was +20.D and made of poly (methyl methacrylate) (PMMA). The surgery was uneventful.

A. What may be the cause?
B. Who is more prone to develop this complication?
C. Write three precautions you should take during surgery to avoid this complication?
D. How will you manage it?

OSPE: 48
A healthy 48-year-old man complains of seeing "floating black dots" in the field of vision of his right eye for 2 days, associated with the sensation of brief flashing lights in the periphery of his visual field. He states that he has a disturbance in the temporal field of vision of his right eye, "like a curtain coming down." His visual acuity is 6/60. Pupils are normal. Confrontation visual field examination shows mild temporal visual field loss in the right eye only.
A. What may be the probable cause?
B. What it indicates if the VA is less than 6/60?
C. What it indicates when there is cessation of flashing of lights? Mention two indications.

OSPE: 49
Bilateral proptosis is the most common ocular presentation of this disease usually by contiguous spread from the paranasal sinuses or nasopharynx. Primary orbital involvement is less common.
A. What is the probable diagnosis?
B. Mention two D/Ds.
C. Mention two coexistent ocular involvements.
D. Mention one important serological test for diagnosis.

OSPE: 50
A 70-year-old man has noted visual distortion over the past week. His concern increased when he discovered that the distortion was in the right eye only. Straight lines viewed through his left eye remained straight, but they appeared too deep down in the center when viewed with his right eye only. Visual acuity testing revealed OD 6/18, OS 6/6.
A. What further tests will help determine the source of the patient's visual loss?
B. What is your diagnosis?
C. What are the risk factors of this disease? Mention three.

OSPE: 51
A 70-year-old woman came to you with recent onset of headache; it was not associated with nausea or vomiting. There was pain in the jaw when taking food but her teeth had no caries or pain. There was scalp tenderness when she was combing his hair. She also gave some nonspecific symptoms such as fever, night sweats, malaise, and weight loss.
A. What is your diagnosis?
B. What type disease is this?
C. At elderly, new onset of headache indicates ICSOL. How will you differentiate it from history and from one investigation?
D. What are the independent risk factors? Mention two.
E. What ocular complication is common? Mention one.

OSPE: 52
A 90-year-old woman has recently noticed visual loss OD, along with a persistent right-sided headache, generalized fatigue, and a 10-pound weight loss. Examination reveals visual acuity of OD 6/24 and OS 6/9. There is a right relative afferent pupillary defect. Confrontation visual field assessment shows inferior visual field loss in the right eye; the left eye is normal. On dilated retinal examination, the right optic disc was swollen and there were flame-shaped hemorrhages around the disc.
A. What is your diagnosis?

B. What primary disease can cause this?
C. Mention two blood tests and one special test to confirm the diagnosis

OSPE: 53
Rapidly progressive unilateral proptosis is usual, and average age of onset is 7 years. The tumor is derived from undifferentiated mesenchymal cells. Various genetic predispositions have been identified, including variants of the *RB1* gene.
A. What is the probable diagnosis?
B. What is the most common site in the orbit?
C. Which type is the worse prognosis?
D. Which is the most confirmatory diagnosis?

OSPE: 54
A 30-year-old man, jobless (smoker and alcohol abuser) came to you with the complains of painless, progressive, and bilateral loss of vision. On examination, you got visual acuity of 6/36 (R/E) and 6/24 (L/E), reduced color vision, and temporal disc pallor. On visual field examination, you observed bilateral cecocentral scotoma.
A. What may be the diagnosis in this case?
B. What are the precipitating factors?
C. In this scenario, if the disc is swollen what should you think?
D. In spite of neuro-ophthalmologist, to whom you can refer the man?
E. Mention two drugs which can give this scenario?

OSPE: 55
It is rare autoimmune corneal diseases, usually affecting older people but sometimes younger people can get affected, and diagnosed as a disease of exclusion. There is a progressive circumferential peripheral stromal ulceration with later central spread. Symptoms include severe pain, photophobia, and blurred vision.
A. What may be the probable diagnosis?
B. When it is unilateral and bilateral?
C. Which one has the worst prognosis?
D. The statement "Limbitis may be present but not scleritis" differentiate it with which diseases?
E. What are the characteristics of healing stage?

OSPE: 56
The pathology of the disease is analog to that of syphilitic interstitial keratitis (IK). It is characterized by disc-shaped central gray stromal opacity. There is fold in Descemet's membrane.
A. What may be diagnosis?
B. What is about vision?
C. What is about corneal sensation?
D. Mention two drugs to treat and route of administration
E. Which organism is commonly responsible for the involvement?

OSPE: 57
A 70-year-old lady, nondiabetic but hypertensive, came to you with the complains of black or gray dots lines, cobwebs, or blobs like objects moving in front of her right eye which

increases when she stares at a bright, plain surface, such as the sky, a reflective object, or blank paper.
A. What may be the cause?
B. What is the pathology?
C. Who suffers more, male or female?
D. What is the treatment?
E. When they are alarming? Mention three points.

OSPE: 58

It is a rare chronic inflammatory disease of the superior bulbar conjunctiva, limbus, and upper cornea of unknown etiology. But there may be history of contact lens wear, and previous eyelid surgery or trauma.

Females are more commonly affected than males. Usually it may be associated with abnormal thyroid function.
A. What may be probable diagnosis?
B. What is the main pathogenesis? Mention one.
C. Mention four symptoms.
D. Though it is an adnexal disease, but it involves the structure proper of the eye. Mention one structure.
E. Mention name of four eye drops for treatment.

OSPE: 59

A 70-year-old man complains of generalized headache. He also complains of scalp tenderness during combing hair (though he has few hair). There is also neck pain, weight loss, fever, night sweats, and malaise. You refer the patient to Internist. But after a few days the patient came to you with loss of vision OD.
A. What may be the diagnosis?
B. What investigation you have to do?
C. What is the confirmatory investigation?
D. Blindness of sudden onset with minimal systemic upset is uncommon, but it may happen. Then it is called_____.

OSPE: 60

A parent came to you with his 4-year-old child with the complains of defective vision. On examination, you got his visual acuity less than 6/60; both eyes bilateral healed chorioretinal scars with satellite lesion. After taking full history, you did not get a single clue such as family history, birth injury, and consanguinity of marriage. Only mother gave history of flu-like symptoms at third trimester.
A. What may be the cause of defective vision?
B. In spite of ocular symptoms, what other signs you may get? Mention four.
C. Which is the gold standard serological test for diagnosis of this patient?

OSPE: 61

It is a disease of unknown etiology and obese young adult women are the most commonly affected group. Women are affected about 20 times more often than men. The most common symptom is headache. It is characteristically worse in the morning, generalized in character,

and throbbing in nature. It may be associated with nausea and vomiting. So, you go for MRI of the brain to exclude ICSOL, there was no ICSOL.
A. What is your diagnosis?
B. What history should you have asked to patient?
C. What findings you may get in MRI.
D. What other investigation you have to do and why?
E. What are the precipitating factors?
F. What are the roles of an ophthalmologist in this case?

OSPE: 62

A 43-year-old man came to you with sudden onset of vertical diplopia in the absence of ptosis, combined with head tilt.
A. What is the pathology?
B. What may be the cause? Mention three.
C. When there is contralateral superior oblique weakness?
D. Mention two special clinical tests to diagnosis.
E. Do you think any routine radiological test is needed?
F. Why head tilt is there?

OSPE: 63

A 14-year-old boy is referred to you from pediatric nephrology department for blurring of vision, who admitted with complains of hematuria and ankle edema.

On urine R/M, proteinuria present. On slit-lamp examination, there is bilateral anterior lenticonus. He also complains of hearing loss.
A. What is your most probable diagnosis?
B. What type of disease it is?
C. What other ocular features you may expect?
D. What type of hearing loss occurs?

OSPE: 64

A 10-year-old boy came to you with rapid swelling of the right eye associated with pain exacerbated by eye movement, visual impairment, and double vision. He has also given history of flu-like symptoms for the last 5 days.

On examination:

Tender, firm, erythematous, and warm eyelids, with periocular and conjunctival (chemosis) edema. There is also reduced VA and impairment of color vision.
A. What is your provisional diagnosis?
B. What might be the cause? Mention three.
C. Mention three D/D.
D. Why is the impairment of color vision?

OSPE: 65

It is a disease of diagnosis of exclusion and should be investigated fully. Orbital and periorbital region is affected. Presentation is with ipsilateral periorbital or hemicranial pain, and diplopia due to one or more ocular motor paresis, with pupillary and eyelid involvement in many cases. Proptosis, if present, is usually mild.
A. What is your probable diagnosis?

B. What type of disease is this?
C. What is the line of treatment? Mention two.
D. What is the prognosis?

OSPE: 66
Pain that persists for more than 1 month after other signs and symptoms disappears.
A. What is the probable diagnosis?
B. Which age group suffers more?
C. What are the characteristics of pain? Mention three.
D. Why some of the patients suffered from depression?
E. What is the most devastating life-threatening condition?
F. What are the local treatments? Mention two.

OSPE: 67
Which of the following series correctly depicts the relative duration of drug action?
A. Atropine>homatropine>scopolamine>cyclopentolate>tropicamide
B. Atropine>scopolamine>homatropine>cyclopentolate>tropicamide
C. Cyclopentolate>tropicamide>scopolamine>homatropine>atropine
D. Homatropine>cyclopentolate>tropicamide>scopolamine>atropine
E. Homatropine>atropine>scopolamine>cyclopentolate>tropicamide

OSPE: 68
A 70-year-old patient came to you with age-related cataract (both eyes) R>L for surgery. He came with some medicine which he is taking for last 5–7 years for his different systemic diseases. You found the medicines are metformin (500 mg) twice daily, adrenergic antagonists 0.8 mg once daily, and blood thinner.
A. Now what precaution (preoperative) should you take for cataract surgery?
B. What complication may arise during surgery?
C. How will you overcome of it?

OSPE: 69
It is noninflammatory, mostly sporadic or autosomal dominant (occasionally), disease of the cornea. There is gradually decreasing vision particularly in the morning, sometimes associated with pain. Onset is usually in middle age or later. On slit-lamp examination, specular reflection shows "beaten metal" appearance of the endothelium.
A. What is the name of the diseases?
B. Why there is blurring of vision at morning?
C. Why sometimes pain at there?
D. Why "beaten metal" appearance is there in specular reflection?
E. What other signs you may get by slit-lamp examination?
F. What is the definitive treatment to restore vision?

OSPE: 70
It is the most common cause of unilateral and bilateral internuclear ophthalmoplegia in young people. Lesions in the visual pathways occur in 50% of cases.
A. What may be the probable cause?
B. What radiological test will you perform?
C. What finding is the most important in radiological investigation?

D. What may be the size of the lesion?
E. What is the most common ophthalmic finding in this disease?

OSPE: 71

It is a unilateral chronic non-granulomatous condition of the uveal tissue (mainly iris and ciliary body). There is no racial or gender predilection. Commonly presented with gradual dimness of vision, it is due to cataract. There is also persistent floaters and heterochromia.

A. What is the name of the disease?
B. In which condition, the affected eye is hypochromic and hyperchromic?
C. What type of cataract is seen initially (morphologically)?
D. What are the possibilities of complications of cataract surgery?

OSPE: 72

It is the most common soft tissue tumor of childhood; average age of onset is 7 years. The tumor is derived from undifferentiated mesenchymal cells. It may mimic an inflammatory condition such as orbital cellulitis.

A. What is the name of the tumor?
B. How many subtypes are there? Name them.
C. Which one is the most common?
D. Which is the most common site?

OSPE: 73

It is a systemic autoimmune disorder most commonly affecting women of childbearing age. As a multisystem disease, it can involve almost every ocular and periocular structure. Approximately 3–10% of patients will have retinal disease ranging from asymptomatic cotton-wool spots and intraretinal hemorrhages to blinding vaso-occlusive disease. Choroidopathy is less common and presents as multifocal serous elevations of the neurosensory retina and RPE.

A. What is the most likely diagnosis?
B. Do you need any treatment of cotton wool spot?
C. What it indicates?
D. How it causes retinal venous occlusive disease?
E. Though it is a systematic disease, you have talk to other specialist. Can you mention which specialist?

OSPE: 74

Both the systematic diseases have affection to ocular structure and they cause retinal vasculitis. In one case, only veins are affected in a segmental manner and rarely occlusive. In contrast, in other case, it usually affects both arteries and veins, is diffuse, frequently occlusive, and is associated with vitritis.

A. Mention the name of both diseases.
B. In which case only veins are affected?
C. Where both arteries and veins are affected?
D. How you differentiate these from viral retinitis?

OSPE: 75

Uveitis is a frequent and early feature. More than 80% of cases manifested before or within 1 year after the onset of systemic disease.

A. What is the name of the systemic disease?

B. What type of uveitis is the most common?
C. What is the most common cause of vision loss?
D. When there is hormonal abnormality?
E. It causes retinal periphlebitis and has a specific name. Mention the name.

OSPE: 76
A father came to you along with his 2-year-old child. According to his statement, the vision of the child is very limited since birth, and it is diminishing day-by-day, but during birth his eyeball was normal in shape and size, day-by-day eyeballs became smaller may be due to constant rubbing of the eyeball. He has also complained about squinting. On examination, there is no pupillary light reflex, On EUA, you observed that there is cataract and hypermetropia. Fundus is near to normal, only arteriolar attenuation and macular pigmentation.
A. What is your probable diagnosis?
B. Why the eyeball is becoming smaller?
C. What may be the electroretinogram (ERG) findings?
D. What are the systemic associations? Mention three.

OSPE: 77
A 40-year-old patient, myopic, came to you with the complains of sudden loss of vision (R/E) for last 5 days, she also complains that waking in the morning vision is better than night. She said, before vision loss, she had feeling of flashing lights and floater and all of a sudden a curtain came to her periphery of visual field.
   On examination, you got VAR: 3/60. VAL: 6/9 with glass (not improve with pin hole). RAPD: present and IOP: 5 mm Hg. Iritis is present.
A. What is your diagnosis?
B. Why IOP is 5 mm Hg?
C. Why vision became better at morning?
D. Has myopia any correlation with her suffering?
E. Iritis should be differentiated from which syndrome?

OSPE: 78
They are extracellular deposits located at the interface between the RPE and Bruch membrane. They are derived from immune-mediated and metabolic processes in the RPE. They are rare before the age of 40, but are common by the sixth decade.
A. What is name of the deposits?
B. In which disease you found it more?
C. What positive finding will you get in OCT?
D. What positive finding will you get in FFA?

OSPE: 79
Inheritance is autosomal dominant with variable penetrance and expressivity. It has five stages:
Stage 1: Subnormal EOG in an asymptomatic infant or child with a normal fundus.
Stage 2: Develops in infancy or early childhood and does not usually impair vision. A round, sharply delineated macular lesion is seen.
Stage 3: Pseudohypopyon may occur when part of the lesion regresses often at puberty.
Stage 4: The lesion breaks up and visual acuity drops.
Stage 5: Atrophic stage.

Now, answer the following questions:
A. What is your probable diagnosis?
B. What will be findings in following investigations?
   (a) OCT
   (b) FFA
   (c) EOG

OSPE: 80

Any patient dying of an undiagnosed neurological disorder is suspected to have prion disease and the organs of the deceased, such as eyes, kidney, liver, etc. cannot be used for transplantation.

A. What is prion disease?
B. What is prion?
C. How they transmit?
D. Name two prion diseases.
E. What are the general symptoms? Mention four.
F. What are the neurological symptoms? Mention three.
G. Mention four ocular symptoms.
H. How the contamination can be sterilized?

ANSWERS

OSPE: 01. Vertebrobasilar artery insufficiency
OSPE: 02. Ocular myasthenia
OSPE: 03. CMO
OSPE: 04. Phacolytic glaucoma
OSPE: 05. Idiopathic orbital inflammatory disease (IOID)
OSPE: 06. Vasculitis retinae/Eales' disease
OSPE: 07. Occipital arteriovenous malformation
OSPE: 08. Papilledema
OSPE: 09. Superficial temporal arteritis (giant cell arteritis)
OSPE: 10. Cerebral venous sinus thrombosis
OSPE: 11. Sarcoidosis
OSPE: 12. An intermediate uveitis/pars planitis
OSPE: 13. Idiopathic orbital inflammatory disease (IOID)
OSPE: 14. VKC
OSPE: 15. Orbital varies
OSPE: 16. Angioid streaks
OSPE: 17. Bilateral 4th nerve palsy
OSPE: 18. AIDS
OSPE: 19. Choroidal melanoma
OSPE: 20. Giant cell arteritis with (3rd nerve palsy)
OSPE: 21. Cortical blindness
OSPE: 22. Bchçet's disease
OSPE: 23. PVD
OSPE: 24. VKH
OSPE: 25. Duane retraction syndrome
OSPE: 26. Toxoplasmic chorioretinitis
OSPE: 27. Transient visual loss
OSPE: 28. Direct carotid cavernous fistula (CCF)
OSPE: 29. Rupture of the aneurysm
OSPE: 30. Sarcoidosis
OSPE: 31. Peters anomaly
OSPE: 32. RBN
OSPE: 33. Keratoconus
OSPE: 34. Optic neuritis
OSPE: 35. Convergence insufficiency
OSPE: 36. Artificial tear
OSPE: 37. Interstitial keratitis (IK)
OSPE: 38. SLE
OSPE: 39. SLE
OSPE: 40. Topiramate
OSPE: 41. Secondary hypertension
OSPE: 42. Digitalis intoxication

OSPE: 43. Tamsulosin
OSPE: 44. Cytomegalovirus retinitis
OSPE: 45. Demyelinating optic neuritis
OSPE: 46. Optic neuritis
OSPE: 47. PCO
OSPE: 48. RD
OSPE: 49. Wegener granulomatosis
OSPE: 50. Amsler grid test
OSPE: 51. Giant cell arteritis
OSPE: 52. AION
OSPE: 53. Rhabdomyosarcoma
OSPE: 54. Optic atrophy
OSPE: 55. Mooren ulcer
OSPE: 56. Disciform keratitis
OSPE: 57. Asteroid hyalosis (Benson disease)
OSPE: 58. Superior limbic keratoconjunctivitis
OSPE: 59. Arteritic anterior ischemic optic neuropathy (AAION)
OSPE: 60. Congenital Toxoplasmosis
OSPE: 61. Idiopathic intracranial hypertension
OSPE: 62. Trochlear nerve
OSPE: 63. Alport syndrome
OSPE: 64. Bacterial orbital cellulitis
OSPE: 65. Tolosa-Hunt syndrome
OSPE: 66. Post-herpetic neuralgia
OSPE: 67. Duration of action of drugs
OSPE: 68. Precaution (preoperative) for cataract surgery
OSPE: 69. Fuchs endothelial corneal dystrophy
OSPE: 70. MS
OSPE: 71. Fuchs uveitis syndrome (FUS)
OSPE: 72. Rhabdomyosarcoma
OSPE: 73. SLE
OSPE: 74. Sarcoidosis
OSPE: 75. Sarcoidosis
OSPE: 76. Leber congenital amaurosis
OSPE: 77. Rhegmatogenous RD
OSPE: 78. Drusen
OSPE: 79. Best Vitelliform macular dystrophy
OSPE: 80. Prion disease

ANS: 01

A. Vertebrobasilar artery insufficiency 2
B. Any two (1 × 2) 2
    (a) Giant cell arteritis (GCA)
    (b) Ischemic optic neuropathy

Scenarios Based 43

    (c) Central retinal artery/vein occlusion
    (d) Migraine with aura
C. (a) Blood pressure in each arm to rule out subclavian steal syndrome...........................1
   (b) ECG/24 hours Holter monitor to rule out dysrhythmia...1
D. (a) CBC 1
   (b) Serum cholesterol 1
E. (a) MRA 1
   (b) Transcranial/vertebral artery Doppler 1
TOTAL..**10**

ANS: 02
A. Ocular myasthenia..4
B. (a) Chronic progressive external ophthalmoplegia 2
   (b) Multiple sclerosis 2
C. (a) Tensilon test...1
   (b) MRI..1
TOTAL..**10**

ANS: 03
A. BRVO..3
B. Supratemporal quadrant 2
C. ....1 × 3...3
   (a) Age
   (b) Hypertension
   (c) Hyperlipidemia
   (d) DM
D. Chronic macular edema 2
TOTAL..**10**

ANS: 04
A. Phacolytic glaucoma..2
B. The lack of KP helps distinguish phacolytic glaucoma from phacoantigenic glaucoma...1
C. Medications to control IOP should be used immediately, definitive therapy requires cataract extraction...2
D. There may be large floating white particles in the AC, consisting of lens protein and protein-containing macrophages which may impart a milky appearance to the aqueous if very dense and can form a pseudohypopyon 2
E. Lens-induced glaucomas
   • Open-angle (any 2)..1 × 2 2
     i. Phacolytic glaucoma
     ii. Lens particle glaucoma
     iii. Phacoantigenic glaucoma
   • Angle-closure
     i. Phacomorphic glaucoma 1
TOTAL..**10**

ANS: 05

A. Idiopathic orbital inflammatory disease (IOID), previously known to as orbital pseudotumor 3
B. ....(Any 3) ....3 × 1... 3
    (a) Bacterial orbital cellulites
    (b) Severe acute TED (Thyroid eye disease)
    (c) Systemic disorders (Wegener granulomatosis, polyarteritis nodosa)
    (d) Malignant orbital tumors, particularly metastatic
    (e) Ruptured dermoid cyst
C. It is unilateral in adult and bilateral in children 2
D. It may involve any tissue of the orbit 2
TOTAL **10**

ANS: 06

A. Vasculitis retinae/Eales' disease 2
B. Recurrent vitreous hemorrhage 1
C. (a) Vitreous hemorrhage; (b) Macular ischemia; and (c) Traction macular detachment.. .... 1 × 3 3
D. Early: Staining of the vein. Late: Extravasations of dye 1
E. Any 3: (a) Coat's disease; (b) PDR; (c) Sickle cell retinopathy; (d) Ischemic CRVO; (e) Syphilitic neuroretinitis ....

ANS: 07

A. Occipital arteriovenous malformation 2.0
    Tumor 2.0
B. (a) MRI 1.5
    (b) Cerebral angiography 1.5
C. Any two
    (a) Migraine 1.5
    (b) Occipital ischemia 1.5
    (c) Occipital seizure 1.0
TOTAL **10**

ANS: 08

A. Papilledema 2
B. (a) IIH (Idiopathic intracranial hypertension) 2
    (b) ICSOL 2
C. (a) MRI of the brain 2
    (b) LP (Lumber puncture) 2
TOTAL **10**

ANS: 09

A. Superficial temporal arteritis (giant cell arteritis) 3.0
B. Investigations (any 3) ....1.5 × 3 .... 4.5
    (a) High ESR
    (b) Raised C-reactive protein
    (c) Thrombocytosis

(d) Superficial temporal artery biopsy.
C. Rx, Systemic steroid, 1-2-year duration 2.5
TOTAL *10*

ANS: 10
A. Possibilities are:
   (a) Cerebral venous sinus thrombosis 2.0
   (b) Obstructive hydrocephalus following TB meningitis 2.0
B. Other investigations (any 3) .... 3 × 1 .... 3.0
   (a) MRV
   (b) CSF study
   (c) MT test
   (d) CBC with ESR
C. Treatment (any 2) .... 1.5 × 2 .... 3.0
   (a) Refer to neurologist
   (b) Heparin or warfare therapy
   (c) Anti-TB drug 9-month regimen with steroid, sometimes shunt surgery may be required in difficult cases
TOTAL *10*

Explanation: The clinical features mimics this is a case of idiopathic intracranial HTN, but it denies when not responding to any of its treatments. Again it denies ICSOL or aqueduct stenosis since CT scan and MRI revealed nothing except ventriculomegaly, in case of IIH the ventricles become slit like but never dilated. The dilemma in diagnosis of such case of middle-aged woman with nonresponding headache commonly present with cerebral venous sinus thrombosis which is confirmed by MRV (magnetic resonance venogram) that shows segmentation of blood column in cerebral sinuses. The treatment is by low molecular weight heparin or warfarin. Another possibility in the context of our country is obstructive hydrocephalus following TB meningitis.

ANS: 11
A. Sarcoidosis 2.0
B. .... 3 × 1 .... 3.0
   (a) Lung
   (b) Skin
   (c) Eye.
C. Any two .... 2 × 1 .... 2.0
   (a) Conjunctival granuloma
   (b) Lacrimal gland involvement/dry eye
   (c) Acute or chronic uveitis
D. Any 3 .... 3 × 1 .... 3.0
   (a) Periphlebitis
   (b) Choroidal infiltrates
   (c) Multifocal choroiditis
   (d) Retinal granuloma
   (e) Peripheral retinal neovascularization
   (f) Optic nerve involvement.
TOTAL *10*

ANS: 12

A. An intermediate uveitis/pars planitis 1.0
B.
   - MS 1.0
   - Sarcoidosis 1.0
C. (Any 3)
   - Vitreous cell 1.0
   - Vitreous snow ball 1.0
   - Vitreous snow banking 1.0
   - Peripheral periphlebitis 0.5
D.
   - FA 1.0
   - OCT (macula protocol) .... (0.5 + 0.5) 1.0
E. (Any 2)
   - Chronic CME 1.0
   - Macular hole formation 1.0
   - Neovascularization 0.5

TOTAL 10

ANS: 13

A. Idiopathic orbital inflammatory disease (IOID) 2
B. In MRI, the tendon of extraocular muscle is involved but in dysthyroid ophthalmopathy it will spare 2
C. In systemic condition/In case of children 1
D. CT shows ill-defined orbital opacifications and loss of definition of contents 2
E. Course. This follows one of the following patterns: .... 1 × 3 3
   - Spontaneous remission after a few weeks without sequelae.
   - Intermittent episodes of activity with eventual remission.
   - Severe prolonged inflammation eventually leading to progressive fibrosis of orbital tissues, resulting in a 'frozen orbit'

TOTAL 10

ANS: 14

A. Vernal keratoconjunctivitis (VKC) 2
B. 3 types 3
   - Palpebral VKC
   - Limbal
   - Mixed VKC
C. Palpebral VKC 1
D. Peak incidence over late spring and summer 1
E. No 1
F. Corneal ectasia 1

TOTAL 10

ANS: 15

A. Orbital varices 2
B. It was due to external compression over the jugular vein 2

C. As the orbital veins are devoid of valves 2
D. Acute hemorrhage and thrombosis .... 1 + 1 2
E. Indications include .... 0.5 × 4 2
    (a) Recurrent thrombosis
    (b) Pain
    (c) Severe proptosis
    (d) Optic nerve compression.
TOTAL *10*

ANS: 16

A. Angioid streaks 2.0
B .... 1.5 × 3 .... 4.5
- CNV
- Choroidal rupture
- Foveal involvement by a streak.

C. Pseudoxanthoma elasticum 1.5
D. The prognosis is guarded in 70% of cases .... 1 + 1 .... 2.0
TOTAL *10*

ANS: 17

A. Bilateral 4th nerve palsy 3
B .... 3 × 1 3
    (a) Congenital
    (b) Traumatic
    (c) Vascular
C. History of trauma 2
D .... 2 × 1 2
    (a) Parks-Bielschowsky 3-step test
    (b) Double Maddox rod test
TOTAL *10*

ANS: 18

A. AIDS 1
B. CD4+ T 1
- Eyelid findings (any 2) .... 2 × 1 2
    (a) Blepharitis
    (b) Kaposi sarcoma
    (c) Multiple moll scum lesions
- Anterior segment: (Any 3) .... 3 × 1 3
    (a) Conjunctival Kaposi sarcoma
    (b) Squamous cell carcinoma and microangiopathy
    (c) Keratitis due to microsporidia
    (d) Herpes simplex and
    (e) Herpes zoster

- Posterior segment (Any 3).................................3 × 1 3
  - (a) HIV microangiopathy
  - (b) HIV retinitis
  - (c) Cytomegalovirus retinitis
  - (d) Progressive outer retinal necrosis
  - (e) Choroidal pneumocystosis
  - (f) Toxoplasmosis, frequently atypical.

TOTAL 10

ANS: 19

A. This might be choroidal melanoma 2
B. Causes are .... 3 × 1 3
  - (a) Hemorrhage
  - (b) Retinal detachment
  - (c) Secondary glaucoma
C. Melanoma metastasized to liver compromising its function producing jaundice 2
D. Investigations:........................... any 3 .... 3 × 1 3
  - (a) B-scan USG
  - (b) FFA (ICGA preferable)
  - (c) Biopsy (needle aspiration/vitrectomy)
  - (d) USG of hepatobiliary system to see the liver metastasis

TOTAL 10

ANS: 20

A. It is giant cell arteritis with (3rd nerve palsy) 3
   Visual loss is due to Arteritic anterior ischemic optic neuropathy (involvement of ophthalmic, posterior ciliary artery often combined with central retinal artery)
B. Ptosis and adduction deficit due to 3rd nerve palsy 3
C. Temporal artery biopsy and C-reactive protein 4

TOTAL 10

ANS: 21

A. Cortical blindness 3.0
B. Causes
  - (a) Eclampsia leading to occipital infraction 1.5
  - (b) Hypertensive aneurismal rupture leading to occipital hemorrhage 1.5
C. The investigations .... 1 × 4 .... 4.0
  - (a) CT scan of brain .... for hemorrhage
  - (b) MRI of brain .... for infraction
  - (c) Urinary protein .... for eclampsia
  - (d) Total platelet counts and or FDP (fibrin degradation product) .... for DIC (platelet count will be decrease & FDP will increase)

TOTAL 10

(Explanation: The lady has eclampsia attack leading to disseminated intravascular coagulation (DIC) or hypertensive aneurismal rupture causing occipital infraction or hemorrhage, respectively)

ANS: 22

A. Behçet's disease 4
B. (Any 3)
    (a) Vascular system 1
    (b) Joint 1
    (c) GIT/Mouth 1
    (d) Skin 1
    (e) Kidney 0.5
C. (a) Uveal tissue 1
    (b) Retina 1
    (c) Vitreous 1
TOTAL 10

(Note: In spite of uveal tissue if any one writes iris, ciliary body, choroid he will get 1. If she/he writes one component, he will get 0.33)

ANS: 23

A. Weiss ring 3
B. PVD 2
C. At present there is no RD 2
D. Risk factors are (any 3) .... 1 × 3 3
- Older age
- Myopia
- Intraocular inflammation
- Trauma

TOTAL 10

ANS: 24

A. Vogt-Koyanagi-Harada syndrome 3
B. Darkly pigmented ethnic groups (Asians, Asian Indians, Hispanic individuals, Native Americans, and Middle Easterners) 2
C. Sympathetic ophthalmitis 2
D. Vogt-Koyanagi 1
E. Harada disease
F. Auditory problems are observed in 75% of patients 1

TOTAL 10

ANS: 25

A. Duane retraction syndrome 2.0
B. On abduction 1.0
C. On attempted abduction, the palpebral fissure opens and the globe assumes its normal position 1.5
D. On adduction as a result of co-contraction of the medial and lateral recti with resultant narrowing of the palpebral fissure 1.5
E. Perceptive deafness and speech disorder 2.0

TOTAL 10

ANS: 26
A. Toxoplasmic chorioretinitis..3
B. Becomes negative as antibody response begins 2
C. Lyme disease, as well as other diseases, such as multiple sclerosis...................2
D. A classic triad is chorioretinitis, calcifications (intracranial) and convulsion (3C).........3
TOTAL 10

ANS: 27
A. 24 hours 2.5
B. Ipsilateral internal carotid artery stenosis of 70–99% 1.5
C. (a) .... Optic disc drusen.......................................1.5
   (b) Papilledema..1.5
D. Vasospasm or migraine 1.5
E. Migraine 1.5
TOTAL 10

ANS: 28
A. Direct carotid cavernous fistula (CCF) due to head injury...............................3.0
B. (a) Surgical injury 1.0
   (b) Rupture of an intracavernous aneurysm, or in......................................1.0
   (c) Association with connective tissue disorders.......................................0.5
   (d) Vascular diseases and 0.5
   (e) Dural fistulas 0.5
C. Humming sound within the skull due to high blood flow through the arteriovenous fistula 1.5
D. It is due to raised episcleral venous pressure 1.0
E. It may be bilateral, or even contralateral, because of midline connections between the two cavernous sinuses 1.0
TOTAL 10

ANS: 29
A. Rupture of the aneurysm..3
B. Aneurysms at the junction of the internal carotid and posterior communicating arteries...3
C. When not ruptures but gradually increase in size 2
D. When they are confined by the walls of the cavernous sinus 2
TOTAL 10

ANS: 30
A. High-resolution computed tomographic scan of the chest.............................3
B. X-ray chest..3
C. Heerfordt syndrome (uveoparotid fever), is characterized by:
   (a) Uveitis 1
   (b) Parotitis 1
   (c) Fever, and..1
   (d) Facial nerve palsy 1
TOTAL 10

Explanation: The definitive diagnosis of sarcoidosis relies on histologic confirmation of non-caseating granulomata. A chest radiograph is probably the best single screening test for sarcoidosis, as it reveals abnormal results in approximately 90% of the patients with active disease. Thin-cut spiral CT imaging is a more sensitive imaging modality and may be particularly valuable in the patient with a normal-appearing chest radiograph in whom there remains a high clinical suspicion for disease. In such cases, parenchymal, mediastinal, and hilar structures with distinctive CT patterns highly suggestive for sarcoidosis may lead to the diagnosis. Although serum ACE and lysozyme levels may be abnormally elevated neither is diagnostic nor specific.

ANS: 31

A. Peters anomaly 4
B. Any 2 4
    (a) Congenital hereditary endothelial dystrophy (CHED)
    (b) Congenital glaucoma
    (c) Peters plus
C. About 80% of the case is bilateral 2
TOTAL *10*

ANS: 32

A. (a) RBN 2
    (b) Malingering 2
    (c) Cortical blindness 2
B. MS 2
C. MRI 2
TOTALS *10*

ANS: 33

A. Oil droplet 2
B. Scissor reflex 2
C. Vogt's striae. (i) Prominent corneal nerve. (ii) Fleischer ring and (iii) Rizutti's sign ....
    (any 2) .... 2 × 2 4
D. Corneal topography 2
TOTAL *10*

ANS: 34

A. Optic neuritis 3.0
B. (Any 3)
    (a) Demyelination 1.0
    (b) Toxic and nutritional 1.0
    (c) Compression 1.0
    (d) Leber hereditary optic neuropathy 0.5
C. MRI 1.0
D. Both will diminish .... 1.5 + 1.5 .... 3.0
TOTAL *10*

ANS: 35

A. Convergence insufficiency 3
B. (a) Asymptomatic 1
   (b) Headache/eye-strain after close work......................1+1 2
   (c) Blurry vision while reading...1+1 2
C. (a) Convergence exercise 1
   (b) Use of base-in prism 1
TOTAL **10**

ANS: 36

A. Preservative of the tear drop (Usually BAK) 2.5
B. Preservative free artificial tear drop... 2.5
C. Female 2.5
D. TBUT.. 2.5
TOTAL **10**

ANS: 37

A. Interstitial keratitis (IK) 2.5
B. It is bilateral when congenital and unilateral when acquired............................. 2.0
C. Granulomatous anterior uveitis. 2.0
D. Ocular features...0.5 × 3 .... 1.5
   i. dislocated/sublimated lens,
   ii. cataract,
   iii. optic atrophy,
   iv. salt and pepper pigmentary retinopathy and
   v. Argyll Robertson pupils.
E. The healed stage is characterized by................................0.5 × 3 .... 1.5
   i. ghost vessels,
   ii. feathery deep stromal scarring
   iii. band keratopathy.
TOTAL **10**

ANS: 38

A. SLE 2
B. Discoid lupus erythematosus... 2
C. Lacrimal gland 2
D. Dry eye.. 2
E. Scleritis 2
TOTAL **10**

ANS: 39

A. SLE 2
B. Chloroquine/Hydroxychloroquine.. 2
C. Melanotropic... 2
D. (a) Chloroquine retinopathy 2
   (b) Vortex keratopathy (cornea verticillata) 2
TOTAL **10**

ANS: 40

A.	Topiramate	2.0
B.	Usually within a month of starting treatment	1.5
C.	Any 3 .... 3 × 0.5	1.5
	• Blurred vision	
	• Haloes	
	• Ocular pain	
	• Redness	
D.	• Shallowing of the anterior chamber and	1.0
	• Raised intraocular pressure	1.0
E.	• Reducing the intraocular pressure and	1.0
	• Stopping the drug	1.0
F.	It is usually good provided the complication is recognized	1.0
TOTAL		***10***

ANS: 41

A.	Secondary hypertension	2
B.	Acute	1
C.	Absence of A/V crossing and normal arteriolar light reflex	2
D.	Nephrologists	2
E.	Serum creatinine	2
F.	Yes	1
TOTAL		***10***

ANS: 42

A.	Digitalis intoxication	5
B.	Reversible	2
C.	Name of the medicine, he is using	2
D.	Yes	1
TOTAL		***10***

(Digitalis intoxication with this widely used cardiovascular drug almost always produces blurred vision or abnormally colored vision (chromatopsia). Classically, normal objects appear yellow with the over dosage of digitalis; but green, red, brown, or blue vision can occur. White halos may be perceived on dark objects or objects may seem frosted in appearance. Usually, fatigue and weakness develop concomitantly with digitalis intoxication, but the visual disturbances often dominate the patient's complaints)

ANS: 43

A.	Tamsulosin (Flomax) and other adrenergic antagonists	3
B.	Intraoperative, floppy iris syndrome (IF IS)	2
C.	.... 3 × 1	3
	• Pupil that may not dilate fully and may constrict during cataract surgery	
	• The iris may billow and prolapsed through the incision	
	• The risk of capsule rupture and vitreous loss is increased.	

D. ....(Any 4) .... 4 × 0.5................................ 2
- Use of Healon
- Preoperative pupillary dilatation with atropine
- Intracameral epinephrine
- Iris hooks, and
- Low aspiration flow rates

TOTAL **10**

ANS: 44

A. Cytomegalovirus retinitis 2
B. Toxoplasmosis and Candida retinitis 2+2 4
C. By measure CD4+ T cells 2
D. Treatment with 'highly active antiretroviral therapy' (HAART), reduces ocular involvement 2

TOTAL **10**

(Ref: Basic Ophthalmology, 9th Edition. Richard A. Harper, MD. Executive Editor. American Academy of Ophthalmology Page 181)

ANS: 45

A. Demyelinating optic neuritis 3.0
B. Because the superior rectus muscle is originating from the optic nerve sheath mainly 2.0
C. Altitudinal/arcuate defect 1.5
D. Previous optic neuritis 1.5
E. (a) Vision worsens over several days to 2 weeks 1.0
   (b) Then begins to improve 1.0

TOTAL **10**

ANS: 46

A. Optic neuritis 2
B. Multiple sclerosis 2
C. (a) Lumbar puncture 1
   (b) MRI 1
D. Any two .... 2 + 1 2
   (a) Altitudinal/arcuate defects and then by focal
   (b) Central/centrocecal scotoma
   (c) Superimposed generalized depression.
   (d) Vision worsens over several days to 2 weeks and then begins to improve .... 1 + 1 2

TOTAL **10**

(Source: Kanski Neuro Ophthalmology)

ANS: 47

A. PCO 2.5
B. Younger patient has more chance to develop it 2.5
C. (a) *Surgery technique:* The incidence of PCO is reduced when the capsulorhexis opening is in complete contact with the anterior surface of the IOL 2.0

(b) *Lens material:* Silicon or acrylic 1.0
  (c) *Lens design:* Square edge to the optic appears to inhibit PCO 1.0
D. YAG Laser capsulotomy... 1.5
TOTAL..*10*

PCO is actually a misnomer, because it not the capsule opacifies.... rather an opaque membrane develops over the PC. Types of PCO Soemmering ring. Elschning pearl capsular fibrosis.

ANS: 48

A. RD 3
B. Macula off 3
C. (a) Either separation of the adhesion or... 2
  (b) Complete tearing away of a piece of retina (operculum) 2
TOTAL..*10*

ANS: 49

A. Wegener granulomatosis.. 2.0
B. (a) Thyroid eye disease.. 2.0
  (b) Orbital cellulitis 2.0
C. (a) Scleritis 1.0
  (b) Peripheral ulcerative keratitis 1.0
D. The antineutrophil cytoplasmic antibody (cANCA) is a useful serological test............. 2.0
TOTAL..*10*

ANS: 50

A. Amsler grid test 3.5
B. ARMD 3.5
C. Risk factor
  (a) Age 1.0
  (b) Race 1.0
  (c) Heredity 1.0
  (d) Smoking 0.5
  (e) Hypertension.. 0.5
TOTAL..*10*

(Ref: Basic Ophthalmology, 9th Edition. Richard A. Harper, MD. Executive Editor. American Academy of Ophthalmology Page 69)

ANS: 51

A. Giant cell arteritis.. 3.0
B. It is a granulomatous necrotizing arteritis... 2.5
C. There was no morning nausea and vomiting. MRI of the brain................... 1 + 1
   .... 2.0
D. The independent risk factors are (any 2)............. 0.5 × 2..................................... 1.0
   • Smoking,
   • Low body mass index and
   • Early menopause
E. Arteritic anterior ischaemic optic neuropathy (AAION) 1.5
TOTAL..*10*

ANS: 52
A. AION 4
B. Giant cell arteritis 2
C. ESR & C-reactive protein test. Temporal artery biopsy 1+ 1 + 2 4
TOTAL **10**

ANS: 53
A. Rhabdomyosarcoma 3
B. Most commonly superonasal or superior orbit 3
C. Alveolar 2
D. Incisional biopsy followed by histopathology 2
TOTAL **10**

(Reference: Kanski 8th edition p 109)

ANS: 54
A. Optic atrophy 2.0
B. (a) Tobacco abuse 1.0
   (b) Alcohol abuse 1.0
C. Leber hereditary optic neuropathy 2.0
D. Internist 2.0
E. (a) Chloramphenicol 1.0
   (b) ethambutol 1.0
   (c) isoniazid 0.5
   (d) streptomycin 0.5
TOTAL **10**

(Reference: The Wills Eye Manual 6th edition. Chapter 10.20 Miscellaneous optic neuropathies)

ANS: 55
A. Mooren's ulcer 3.0
B. In case of older patient it is unilateral, and in younger it is bilateral 2.0
C. Bilateral 2.0
D. Peripheral ulcerative keratitis (PUK) associated with systemic autoimmune disease .. 1.5
E. Thinning, vascularisation and scarring 1.5
TOTAL **10**

ANS: 56
A. Disciform keratitis 2.5
B. Vision is impaired 2.0
C. Loss of sensation 1.5
D. • Corticosteroid: local administration 1.0
   • Acyclovir: topical or systemic 1.0
E. Herpes simplex 2.0
TOTAL **10**

ANS: 57
A. Asteroid hyalosis (Benson disease) 2.0
B. Vitreous 2.0
C. Male 2.0
D. Assurance/Counseling 2.0
E. .... 0.5 × 4 .... 2.0
   (a) If they begin occurring more frequently
   (b) When also see flashes of light
   (c) When lose your peripheral (side) vision
   (d) When develop eye pain
   Combined with eye floaters, these symptoms may be a sign of more dangerous conditions.
TOTAL *10*

ANS: 58
A. Superior limbic keratoconjunctivitis 2.0
B. Blink-related trauma between the upper lid and the superior bulbar conjunctiva 2.0
C. .... any 4 .... 0.5 × 4 .... 2.0
   (a) Foreign body sensation,
   (b) Burning,
   (c) Mild photophobia,
   (d) Mucoid discharge and
   (e) Frequent blinking.
D. Cornea 2.0
E. .... any 4 .... 0.5 × 4 .... 2.0
   (a) Lubricants
   (b) Acetylcysteine
   (c) Mast cell stabilizers
   (d) Ciclosporin
   (e) Autologous serum
TOTAL *10*

ANS: 59
A. Arteritic anterior ischemic optic neuropathy (AAION) is caused by giant cell arteritis .....
   .... 3.0
B. ESR, Platelet count, C-reactive protein, temporal artery biopsy. 2.0
C. Temporal artery biopsy. 2.0
D. Occult arteritis 3.0
TOTAL *10*
(Source: Kanski. Chapter: 19. Optic nerve)

ANS: 60
A. Congenital toxoplasmosis 4
B. If it occurs during late pregnancy it may result in 4
   i. Convulsions,

  ii. Paralysis,
  iii. Hydrocephalus and
  iv. Visceral involvement
C. Dye test (Sabin-Feldman) 2
TOTAL **10**

(Sabin-Feldman test: utilizes live organisms which are exposed to the patient's serum complement. The cell membranes of the organisms are lysed in the presence of the specific anti-Toxoplasmic IgG, and as consequence the organisms fail to stain with methylene blue dye. This test remains the gold standard for the diagnosis of toxoplasmosis)

ANS: 61

A. Idiopathic intracranial hypertension (IIH) 2.5
B. Drug history 2.0
C. MRI:
  (a) Empty sella sign. 1.0
  (b) Slit like ventricle. 1.0
D. MRV is usually carried out to exclude cerebral venous sinus thrombosis or stenosis ... 1.0
E. (a) Over weight.. 0.5
  (b) Some medicine: contraceptive pill, steroid, tetracycline......................... 0.5
F. Role of ophthalmologist is usually confined to diagnosis and the monitoring of..............
  0.5 × 3 .... 1.5
  (a) Visual function with VA
  (b) Colour vision and fields, and
  (c) Optic nerve appearance/photography
TOTAL **10**

ANS: 62

A. Trochlear nerve.. 2.0
B. i. Idiopathic 1.0
  ii. Trauma.. 1.0
  iii. Microvascular lesion 0.5
C. When there is nuclear palsies 1.5
D. (a) Parks three step test/Bielschowsky head tilt test.................................. 1.0
  (b) Double Maddox rod test 1.0
E. No.. 1.0
F. To compensate the diplopia 1.0
TOTAL **10**

ANS: 63

A. Alport syndrome 3
B. (a) Genetic... 2
  (b) Inheritance AD and X-linked... 1
C. (a) Corneal dystrophy... 1
  (b) Retinal flecks 1
  (c) Cataract... 1
D. Sensory neural deafness... 1
TOTAL **10**

ANS: 64
A. Bacterial orbital cellulitis 3.0
B. Any 3 .... 3 × 1 .... 3.0
    i. *Streptococcus pneumoniae*
    ii. *Staphylococcus aureus*
    iii. *Streptococcus pyogenes*
    iv. *Haemophilus influenzae*
C. .... 3 × 1 .... 3.0
    i. Fungal orbital infection
    ii. Acute dacryocystitis
    iii. Acute orbital hemorrhage.
D. Due to compression of optic nerve 1.0
TOTAL ***10***

ANS: 65
A. Tolosa-Hunt syndrome 3
B. Granulomatous disease 3
C. Systemic steroids and other immunosuppressant's as necessary 2
D. The clinical course is characterized by remissions and recurrences 2
TOTAL ***10***

ANS: 66
A. Post-herpetic neuralgia 2.5
B. Above 70 years 1.5
C. Pain may be constant or intermittent, worse at night and aggravated by minor stimuli, touch and heat
D. Neuralgia can impair the Quality of Life (QOL), and may lead to depression
E. Patient may commit suicide
F.   i. Local cold compresses
    ii. Topical capsaicin 0.075%
    iii. Lidocaine 5% patches

ANS: 67
B. The duration of action of atropine is 7–14 days, scopolamine is 4–7 days, homatropine is 3 days, cyclopentolate is 2 days, and tropicamide is 4–6 hours.
(Source: AAO Vol: 2. Page: 413)

ANS: 68
A. (a) Control DM 2.0
    (b) Stop blood thinner 3–5 days before surgery 1.0
    (c) Maximum dilatation of the pupil as far as can even with atropine 1% eye drop 1.0
B. (a) Pupil may constrict during cataract surgery. 1.0
    (b) The iris may billow and prolapsed through the incision 1.0
    (c) The risk of capsule rupture and vitreous loss is increased 1.0
C. Strategies for management include the
    (a) Use of Healon 5 .... 0.5
    (b) Preoperative pupillary dilatation with atropine 0.5

(c) Intracameral epinephrine 0.5
(d) Iris hooks, and 1.0
(e) Low aspiration flow rates 0.5
TOTAL ***10***

ANS: 69
A. Fuchs endothelial corneal dystrophy 3.0
B. Due to corneal edema... 1.5
C. Rupture of the corneal bullae... 1.5
D. In specular reflection, there is tiny dark spots caused by disruption of the regular endothelial mosaic and it shows like a beaten metal appearance................................... 2.0
E. Cornea guttata... 1.0
F. Keratoplasty: may be posterior lamellar or PKP 1.0
TOTAL ***10***
(Name of the posterior lamellar keratoplasty: Descemet's Stripping Endothelial Keratoplasty (DSEK) or Descemet's Stripping Automated Endothelial Keratoplasty (DSAEK).

ANS: 70
A. MS... 2
B. MRI 2
C. Plaques 2
D. 1 mm to several cm 2
E. Optic neuritis 2
TOTAL ***10***
(Parsons' diseases of the eye 21st edition. P: 510)

ANS: 71
A. Fuchs uveitis syndrome (FUS) 3.0
B. (a) In brown eyes it becomes hypochromic 1.0
   (b) And in blue eyes it becomes hyperchromic... 1.0
C. Posterior subcapsular cataract (PSC) 2.0
D. Complications includes:
   (a) Poor mydriasis... 1.0
   (b) Postoperative hyphemia 1.0
   (c) Increased inflammation 0.5
   (d) Zonular dehiscence... 0.5
TOTAL ***10***

ANS: 72
A. Rhabdomyosarcoma... 4
B. 4 subtypes
   • Embryonal, Alveolar, Botyroid, Pleomorphic 2
C. Most common type is the embryonal 2
D. The tumor is most commonly superonasal or superior 2
TOTAL ***10***

ANS: 73

A. SLE 3
B. No 1
C. It indicates activeness of disease Systemic lupus erythematosus (SLE) 2
D. Lupus anticoagulant and antiphospholipid antibodies (Kanski) 2
E. Though it's a systematic disease rheumatologist should be included. 2
TOTAL 10

(*Source:* AAO 190)

ANS: 74

A.   i. Sarcoidosis 2
     ii. Behçet's syndrome 2
B. Sarcoidosis 2
C. Behçet's syndrome 2
D. In viral retinitis the infiltrates eventually coalesce 2
TOTAL 10

ANS: 75

A. Sarcoidosis 2.0
B. Granulomatous anterior uveitis 2.0
C. CMO 2.0
D. When there is pituitary gland involvement 2.0
E. Candle wax dripping 2.0
TOTAL 10

ANS: 76

A. Leber congenital amaurosis 3.0
B. Due to constant rubbing it causes orbital fat atrophy and enophthalmos ... 2.0
C. ERG is usually non-recordable 2.0
D. Any 3 .... 1 × 3 .... 3.0
   (a) Mental handicap
   (b) Deafness
   (c) Epilepsy
   (d) Skeletal malformation
TOTAL 10

ANS: 77

A. Rhegmatogenous RD 2
B. Choroidal detachment is associated with RD 2
C. Spontaneous absorption of SRF while inactive overnight 2
D. Myopic patient has greater chance to developed RD 2
E. Schwartz–Matsuo syndrome 2
TOTAL 10

ANS: 78

A.	Drusen	3.0
B.	ARMD	3.0
C.	Hyper-reflective irregular nodules beneath the RPE	2.0
D.	Window defect	2.0
	TOTAL	**10**

ANS: 79

A.	Best Vitelliform macular dystrophy		3
B.	(a)	OCT shows material beneath, above and within the RPE	3
	(b)	Hypofluorescent	2
	(c)	Severely subnormal	2
	TOTAL		**10**

ANS: 80

A. A group of slowly degenerative diseases of the nervous system 1.5
B. Infectious protein is called prion 1.0
C. Transmission by ingesting infected meat of affected animals 1.0
D.   i. Creutzfeldt–Jacob diseases (CJD) 1.0
    ii. Madcow diseases 1.0
E. Any 4 .... 0.5 × 4 .... 2.0
    (a) Fatigue
    (b) Malaise
    (c) Loss of weight
    (d) Headache
    (e) Disturbed sleep
F. .... 0.25 × 4 .... 1.0
    (a) Seizures
    (b) Cerebellar ataxia
    (c) Parkinsonism like symptoms
    (d) Progressive dementia
G. .... 0.5 × 2 .... 1.0
    i. Loss of vision
    ii. Supranuclear gaze palsy
H. 132°C for 5 hours 0.5
    TOTAL **10**

Retina and Uveal Tissue

CHAPTER 3

QUESTIONS

OSPE: 01

A patient having diabetes and hypertension for last 20 years presented to you with visual acuity 6/24 and with following fundus picture:

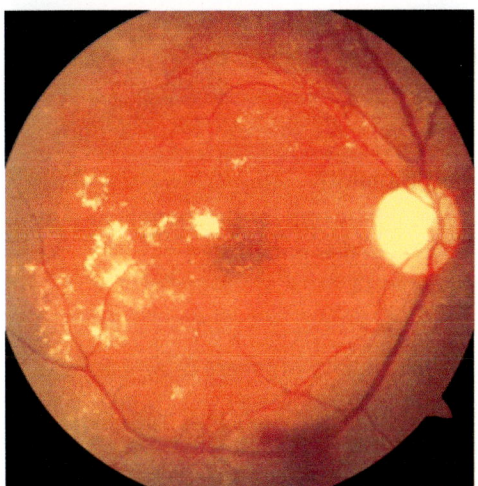

(Image courtesy: Prof. Dipak Kumar Nag, National Institute of Ophthalmology)

A. What are the positive findings? Mention two.
B. What is your diagnosis?
C. What is the possible cause of vision loss of this patient? Mention one.
D. What are the laboratory investigations need to do for this patient? Mention 3.
E. Name two appropriate diagnostic tools for this patient and why?
F. What treatment options to manage such retinopathy? Mention two.

OSPE: 02

A 70 year-old, nondiabetic but hypertensive, patient came to you with the following fundus picture:

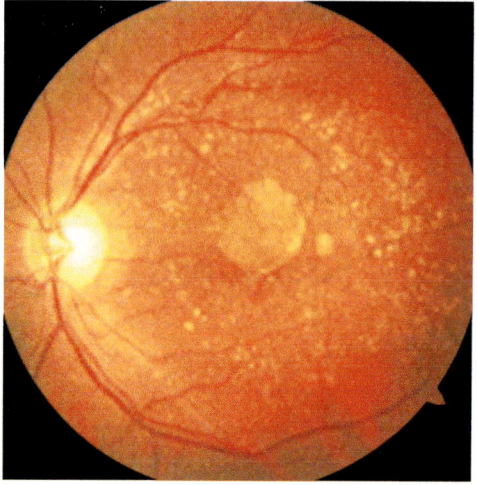

(Image courtesy: Prof. Dipak Kumar Nag, National Institute of Ophthalmology)

A. What are the clinical findings?
B. What could be his chief complaint?
C. Name one appropriate diagnostic tool for this patient and explain why?
D. What treatment you will give to this patient?
E. How you follow-up this patient?

OSPE: 03

A 55-year-old female patient has history of severe diminishing of vision in her right eye. Her fundus picture has following features:

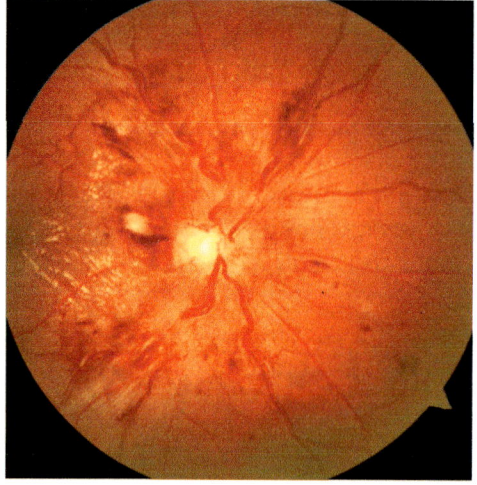

A. Name three clinical findings.
B. What is your clinical diagnosis?
C. Mention one appropriate diagnostic tool in this stage and why?
D. Mention one management option of this case.
E. State reasons for long time follow-up of this patient.

OSPE: 04

A 50-year-old male came to you with sudden severe loss of vision in his left eye.

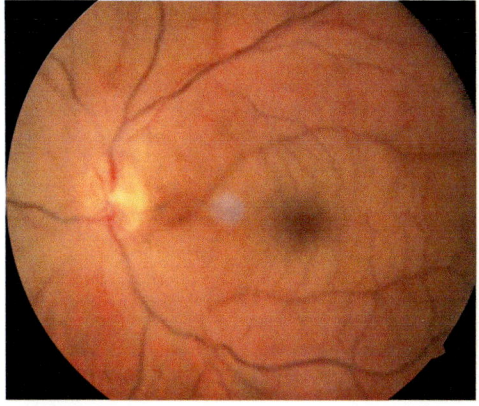

A. What is your clinical finding?
B. What is your clinical diagnosis?
C. Name two differential diagnoses?
D. What you expect in fundus fluorescein angiography (FFA) in such case?
E. What is your immediate plan of management?

OSPE: 05

Look at the fundus picture:

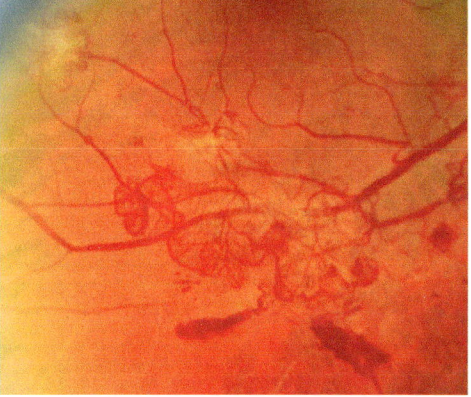

A. Write two clinical findings.
B. Name two common conditions where it may occur.
C. What is the management plan?

D. Write two complications if not treated properly.
E. What investigation is essential for appropriate treatment?

OSPE: 06

A 25-year-old man, nondiabetic and nonhypertensive, came to you with the following fundus picture:

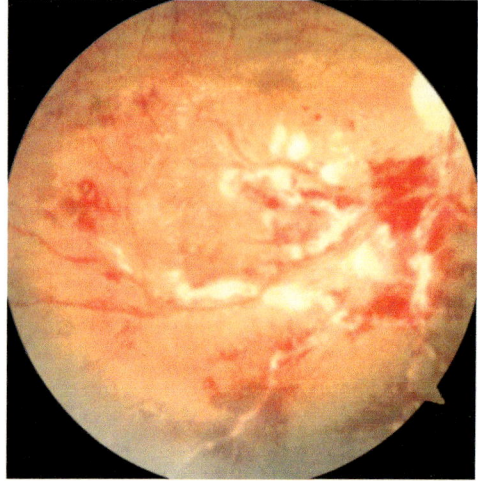

(Image courtesy: Prof. Dipak Kumar Nag, National Institute of Ophthalmology)

A. Write two clinical findings?
B. What is your clinical diagnosis?
C. What could be the most like cause of such condition?
D. What is basic investigations protocol?
E. What could be the treatment options at this stage?

OSPE: 07

A patient having hypertension came to you with marked diminution of vision in his left eye since yesterday.

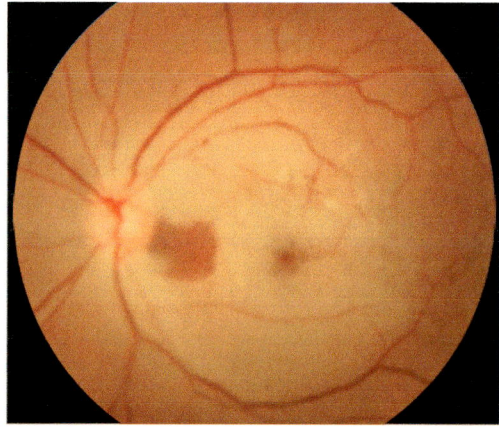

(Image courtesy: Prof. Dipak Kumar Nag, National Institute of Ophthalmology)

A. Name two clinical findings?
B. What is your clinical diagnosis?
C. What are differential diagnoses? Mention two.
D. What would be the most appropriate diagnostic test? And what would be the positive finding?
E. Name two immediate managements?

OSPE: 08

The fundus pictures of a man are given below:

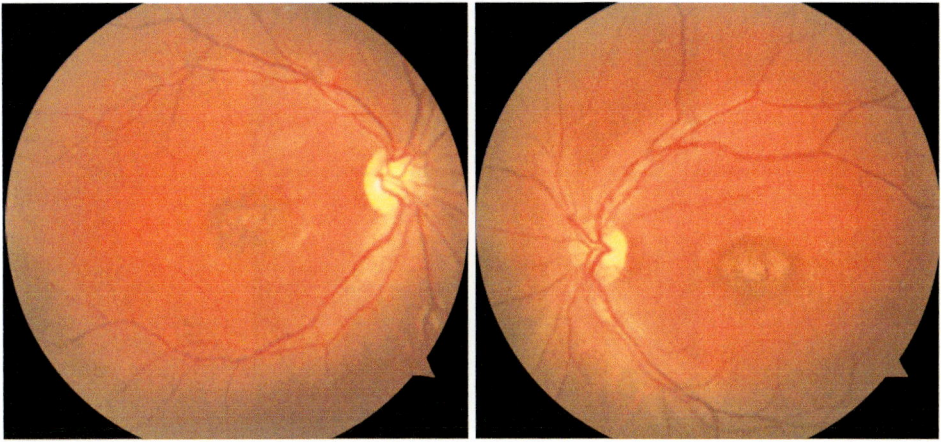

A. How will you describe the macula?
B. What is your clinical diagnosis? Mention two.
C. Mention two differential diagnoses.
D. What may the chief complaint of the patient?
E. What could be the plan of management in such case?

OSPE: 09

A 20-year-old male came to you with the following fundus picture in right eye:

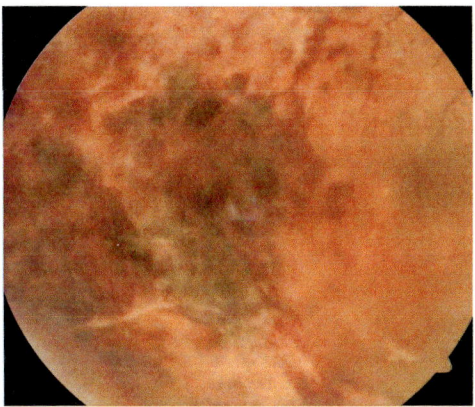

A. Name two clinical findings?
B. What is your clinical diagnosis?
C. Name two differential diagnoses?
D. What may be the common cause of such disease in Bangladesh?
E. What investigation will you prefer for such a patient?

OSPE: 10

A 15-year-old nondiabetic and non-hypertensive patient has the following fundus picture:

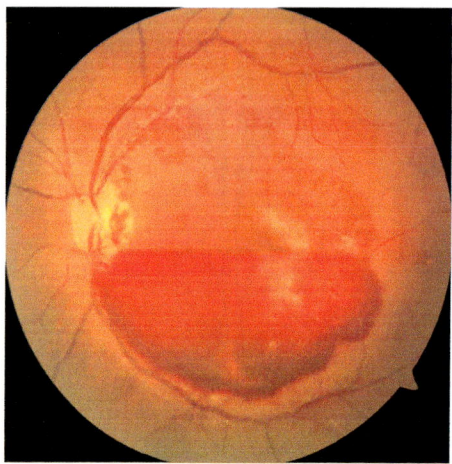

A. Describe the picture.
B. Where could be the site of hemorrhage?
C. What could be the chief complaint?
D. Write two common causes of such case.
E. Name two management options.

OSPE: 11

A 40-year-old male patient came to you with following fundus picture.

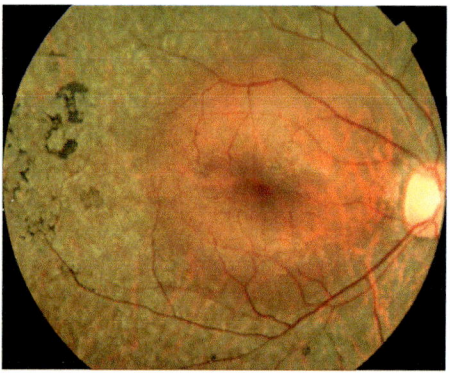

A. Describe two features of the fundus.
B. Mention two symptoms of such case.
C. Name two ocular associations?
D. Name two differential diagnoses.
E. What type of visual field defect is at there?

OSPE: 12

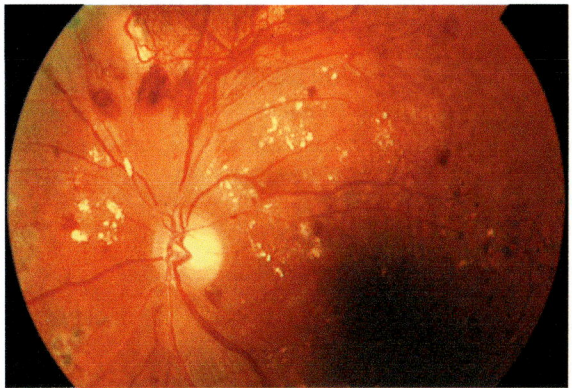

(Image courtesy: Elsevier Inc. 2006. Kanski: Clinical Diagnosis in Ophthalmology)

This is a fundus photograph of a 60-year-old male with blurring of vision. Please observe the photograph and answer the following questions:
A. Write three important positive findings in this photograph.
B. Mention three differential diagnoses.
C. Write two systemic and two ocular investigations to confirm the diagnosis.
D. Name two treatment options.

OSPE: 13

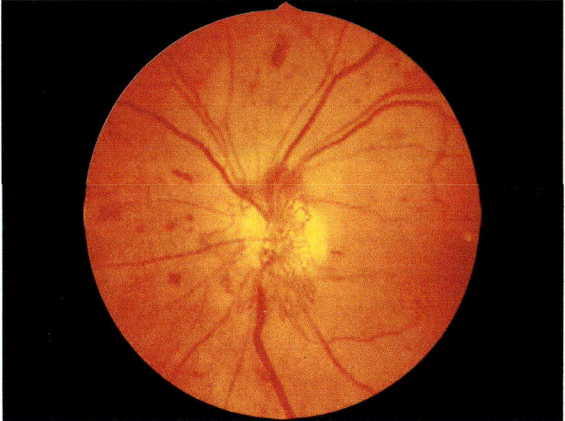

(Image courtesy: Prof. Dipak Kumar Nag, National Institute of Ophthalmology)

A. What are the positive findings in this picture? Mention two.
B. How many areas will be nonperfuse before developing this feature?
C. What is your diagnosis?
D. What other features you may get in this stage? Mention two.
E. What other two general and two ocular investigations will you perform?
F. If you do fundus fluorescein angiography, what positive finding will you get in late phase?

OSPE: 14

Four color fundus pictures are here.
A. What are the positive findings? Mention two in each.
B. What may be the probable diagnosis in each?
C. What clinical examination and laboratory investigation you need to do?

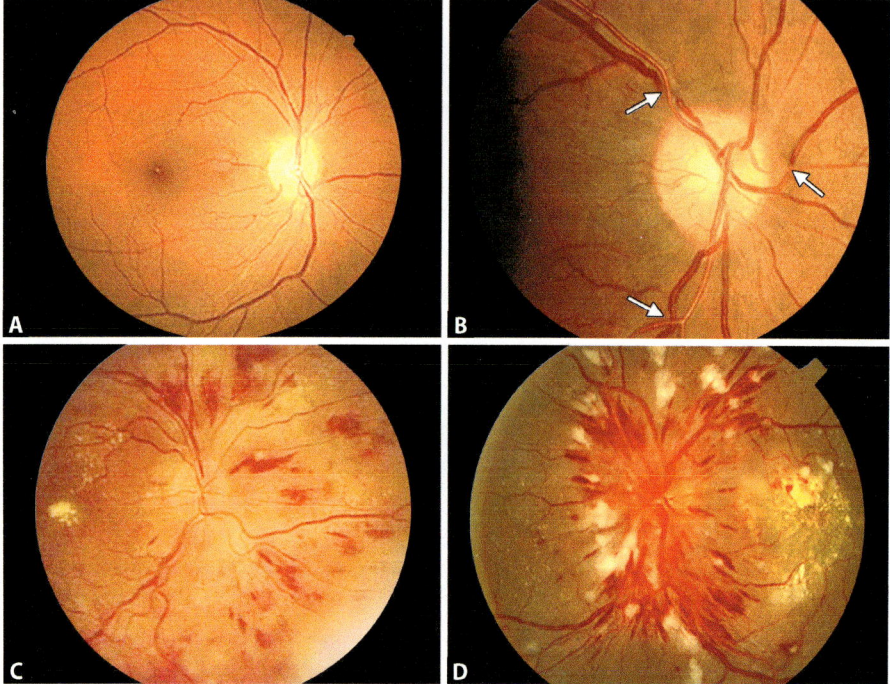

OSPE: 15

A man who is 50-year-old came to you for changing his presbyopic glass. With best corrected glass you see his visual acuity is 6/9 p (OU) and near vision is N8. His pupillary reaction is normal. After dilatation of the pupil you have done the funduscopy and found following features in both eyes. After that you have done blood test.
- Blood sugar is 15 mmol/L
- HbA1c: 8
- Complete blood count (CBC): All the count within normal range except Hb% which is 8 mg/dL.

Retina and Uveal Tissue

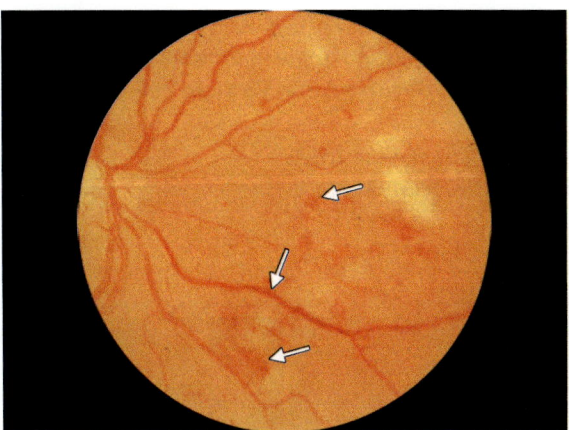

(Image courtesy: Prof. Dipak Kumar Nag, National Institute of Ophthalmology)

A. Write two positive findings from fundus picture.
B. What is your diagnosis?
C. You have done three blood test. What will be the 4th blood test?
D. From the blood picture can you assume, which organ is affected? And to whom should you refer him?

OSPE: 16

This is the fundus photograph of a 70-year-old lady, who was MD of a corporate company and came to you with the complains of reduced vision for both distance and near. She also notices that objects look distorted from the involved eye.

A. What is the diagnosis?
B. The lady wants to know what the problem is going on in her eye. Explain the disease process.
C. If you have one option to ask question her, which one you should to ask?
D. She wants to know who gets this sort of disease.

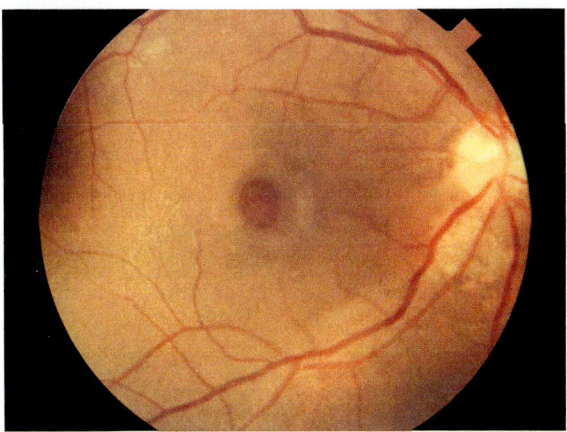

OSPE: 17

A 60-year-old man is suffering from open angle glaucoma for last 20 years. He noticed loss of vision in right eye on waking up this morning; VA right eye 2/60. The fundus picture shows as images below:

A. Mention two positive findings of Figure A.
B. Mention two positive findings of Figure B.
C. What is your diagnosis?
D. Write one grave complication.
E. How long it takes to resolute?

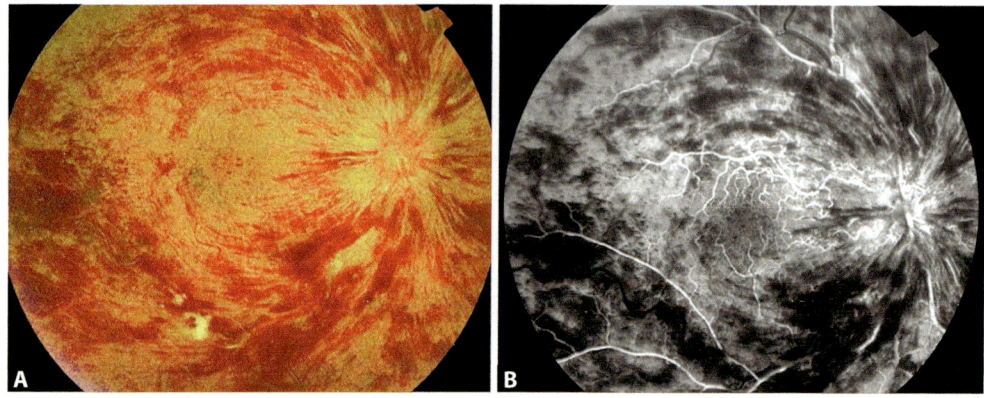

OSPE: 18

This is the fundus photo of a lady of 23-year-old who is suffering from headache for last 2 months which is worse on waking up. Visual acuity is 6/9 both eyes.

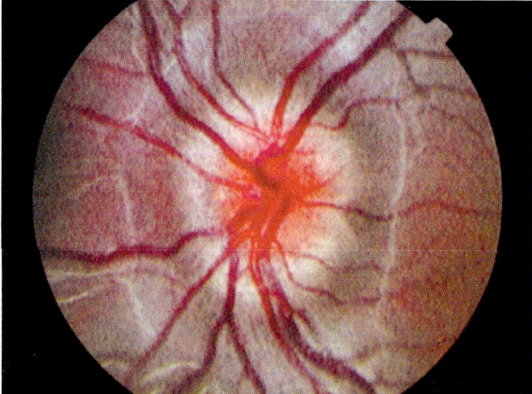

A. What is the most likely diagnosis?
B. Mention one positive finding from the CFP.
C. What are D/Ds? Mention three.

OSPE: 19

In this picture, the patient is 50-year-old suffering from diabetes mellitus and hypertension.

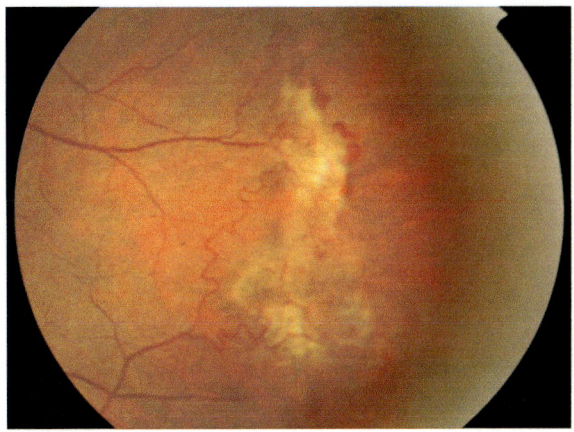

A. What are the positive findings? Mention three.
B. What may be the differential diagnosis? Mention two.
C. Mention three systemic and two ocular investigations.
D. If the patient is 10-year-old, what may be the diagnosis? Mention two.

OSPE: 20

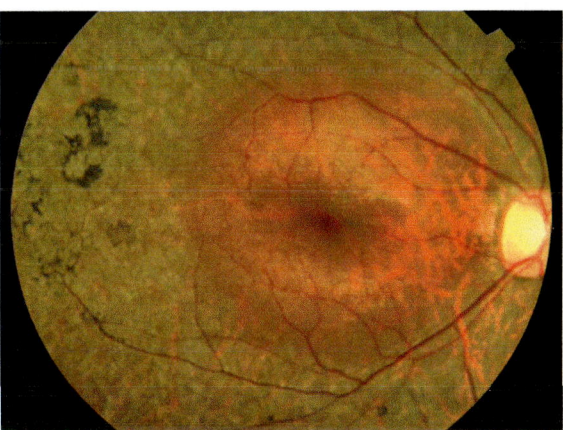

A. Mention three positive findings.
B. What is your diagnosis?
C. What visual field you may expect in this patient?
D. Write two family positive histories you may ask.
E. What is its pathogenesis?
F. Mention two ocular complications.

OSPE: 21

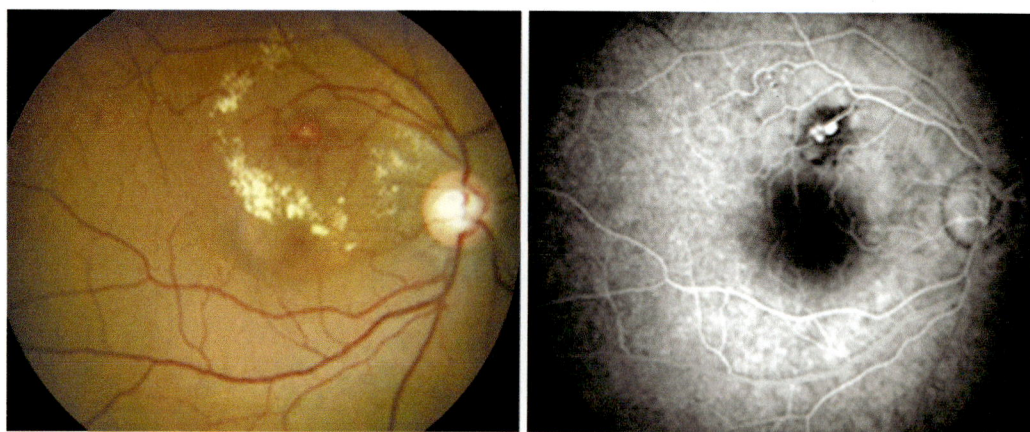

(Image courtesy: Prof. Dipak Kumar Nag, National Institute of Ophthalmology)

The CFP and fluorescein angiography are taken from a patient complaining of distorted right vision.
A. What phase is the fluorescein angiography?
B. What is the diagnosis?
C. What underlying medical condition may be present in this patient?
D. What are the options of treatment in such case? Mention two.
E. Name one differential diagnosis.

OSPE: 22

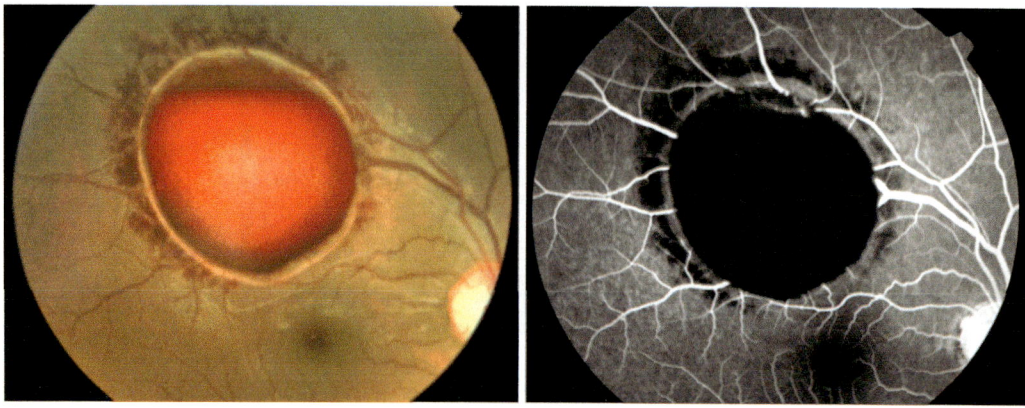

A. These two pictures are from the same patient; mention the name of the investigations.
B. What is your probable diagnosis?
C. What may be the cause? Mention two.
D. What is about visual acuity?
E. Is optical coherence tomography necessary? What investigation would you suggest?
F. What is your treatment?

OSPE: 23

A 45-year-old male diabetic, hypertensive, smoker with visual acuity 6/9 in LE came to you with the following FFA photograph:

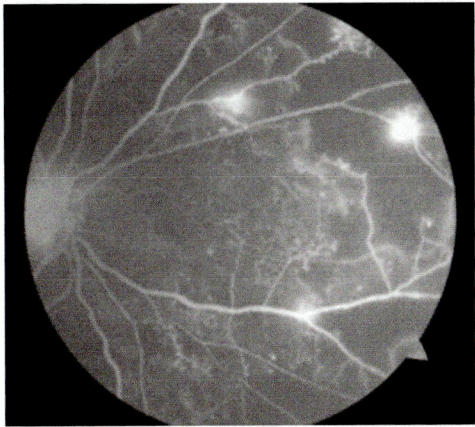

A. Name two angiographic findings of this patient.
B. What is your diagnosis?
C. What are the treatment options for this patient?
D. What would be the most appropriate treatment option for him and why?
E. What advice will you give him to prevent further progression?

OSPE: 24

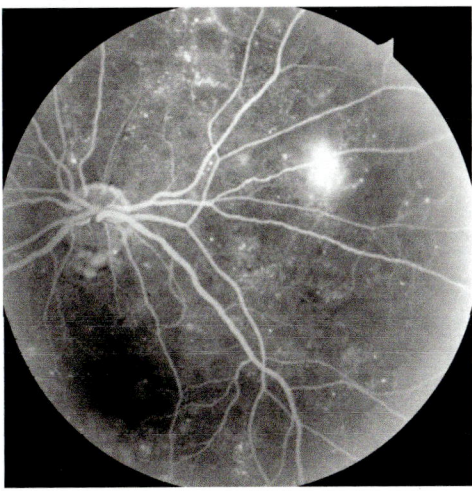

A. Mention three FFA findings.
B. Write down your diagnosis.
C. What treatment will you advice for such case?
D. What advice will you give to prevent further progression? Mention three.

OSPE: 25

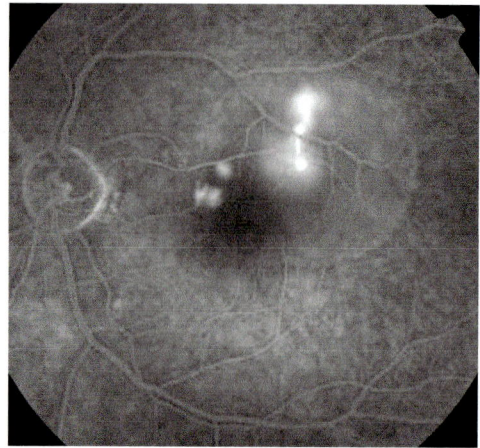

This is an FFA of a 65-year-old man who came to you with blurred and distorted vision.
A. What phase is this frame of fluorescein angiograph?
B. What is the name of this appearance of FFA?
C. What is the diagnosis?
D. What is the treatment?
E. Who suffers more?

OSPE: 26

A 45-year-old male, having history of cataract surgery 2 days back, came to you with severe diminishing of vision and pain in his left eye. On B-scan, he has got the following feature:

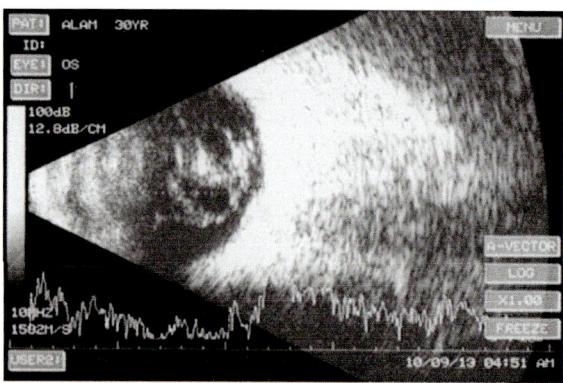

(Image courtesy: Prof. Dipak Kumar Nag, National Institute of Ophthalmology)

A. What has been shown in the B-scan?
B. Name two probable differential diagnoses?
C. Why it is not a retinal detachment?
D. What are the initial steps of management?
E. What is the indication of vitrectomy?

OSPE: 27

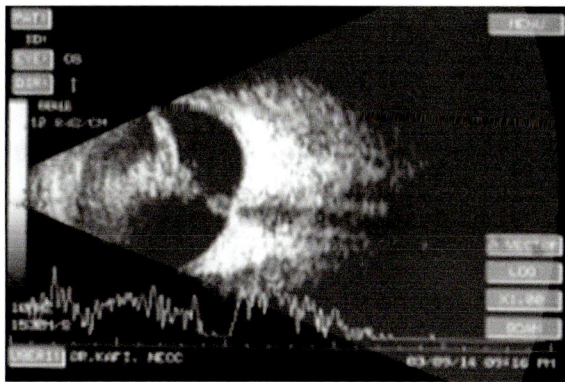

(Image courtesy: Prof. Dipak Kumar Nag, National Institute of Ophthalmology)

A. Write down your diagnosis from the above B-scan findings.
B. Name two differential diagnoses of such condition.
C. Mention four causes for such condition.
D. What management you will try for this particular case?

OSPE: 28

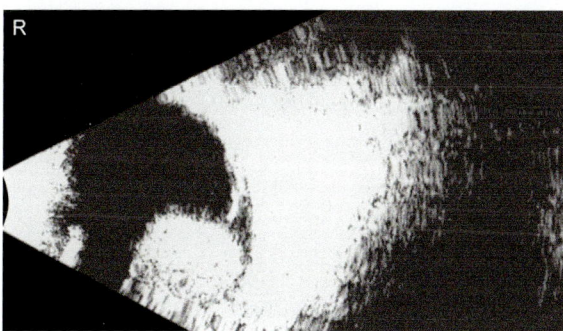

(Image courtesy: Prof. Dipak Kumar Nag, National Institute of Ophthalmology)

A. Name the typical echogenic character of the B-scan.
B. What is the most possible diagnosis?
C. What laboratory tests you need to do in such case?
D. Name three management options for such condition.

OSPE: 29

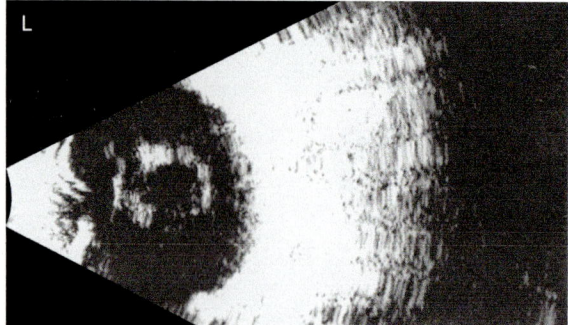

(Image courtesy: Prof. Dipak Kumar Nag, National Institute of Ophthalmology)

A. Mention the findings of B-scan.
B. What is probable diagnosis?
C. Name two conditions where it happened?
D. What is its ideal management?
E. Name two complications that may occur in such case.

OSPE: 30

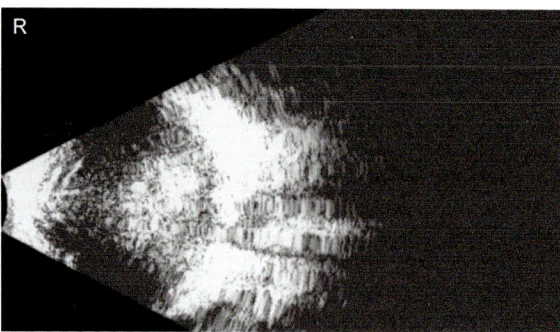

(Image courtesy: Prof. Dipak Kumar Nag, National Institute of Ophthalmology)

A. What the B-scan shows?
B. What is your probable diagnosis?
C. Mention four presenting signs of such case.
D. What is the importance of family history in this case?
E. Name four drugs that can be used for such case.

OSPE: 31

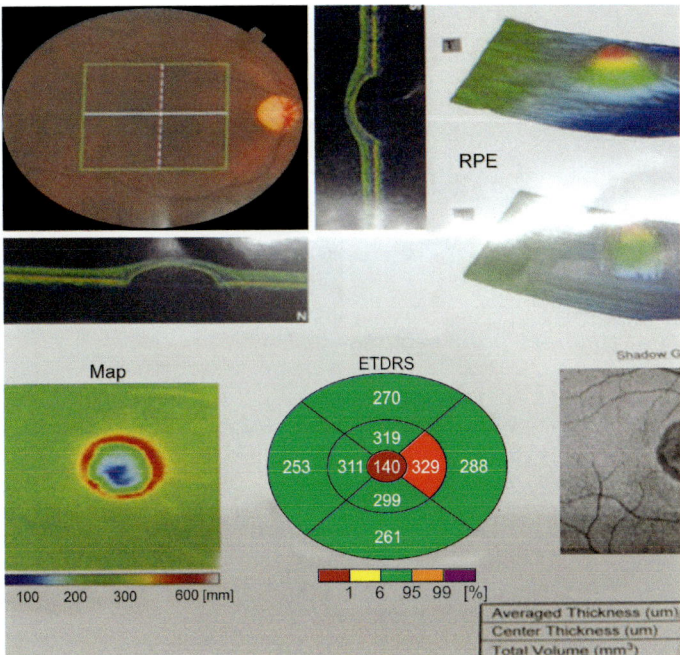

This is OCT macular protocol of a 30-year-old man who came with the complaint of blurred vision for 2 weeks.

A. What is the positive finding here?
B. Mention two other positive findings.
C. What is its basic mechanism?
D. Write two treatment options.
E. Write two natural courses.

OSPE: 32

A. Mention three OCT findings.
B. Mention two common symptoms in such case.
C. Write down three common causes for such condition.
D. Mention two management options.

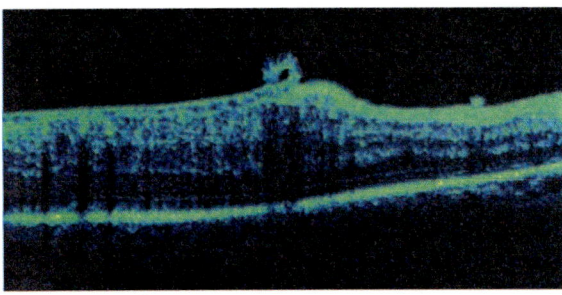

(Image courtesy: Prof. Dipak Kumar Nag, National Institute of Ophthalmology)

OSPE: 33

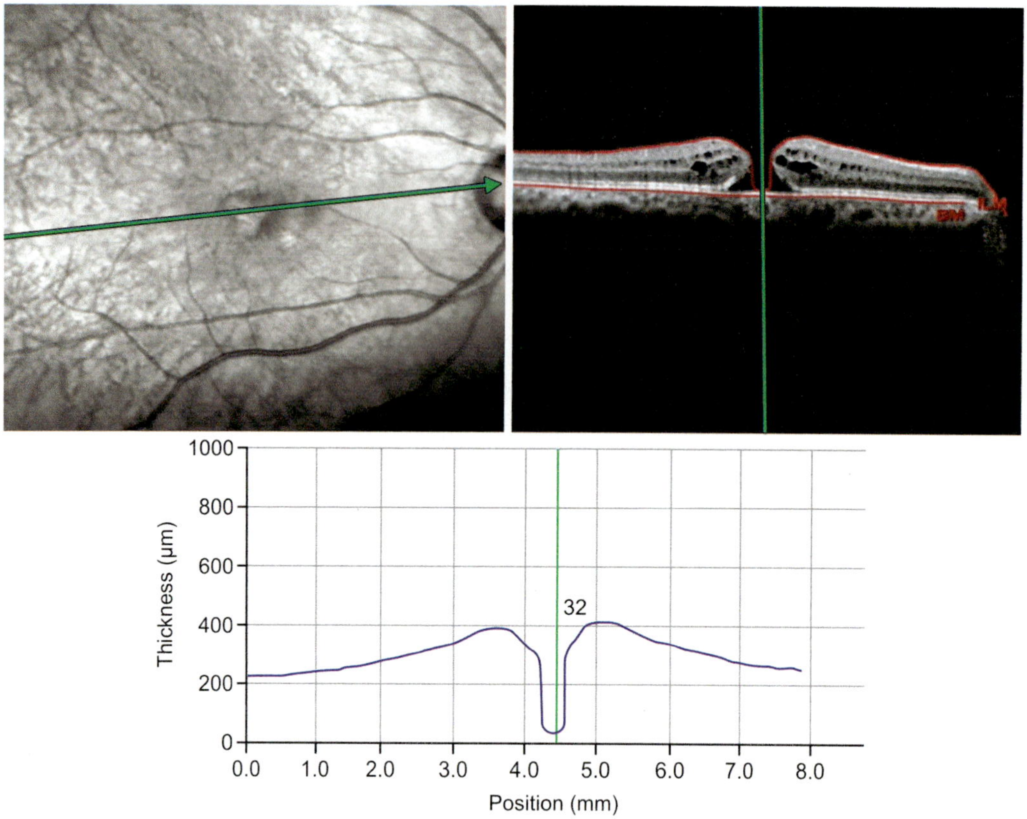

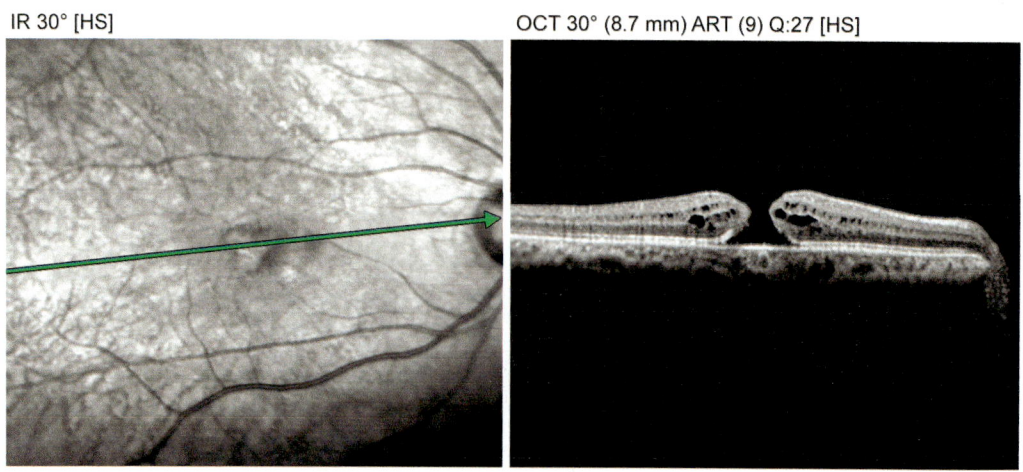

IR 30° [HS]   OCT 30° (8.7 mm) ART (9) Q:27 [HS]

(Image courtesy: Prof. Dipak Kumar Nag, National Institute of Ophthalmology)

Retina and Uveal Tissue

A. Write two positive findings of the given OCT.
B. Mention two most useful clinical diagnostic tests for ophthalmologists to distinguish this from other lesions.
C. Mention two possible causes for such condition.
D. Mention two common initial symptoms of such case.
E. What is the standard surgical management option in this case?

OSPE: 34

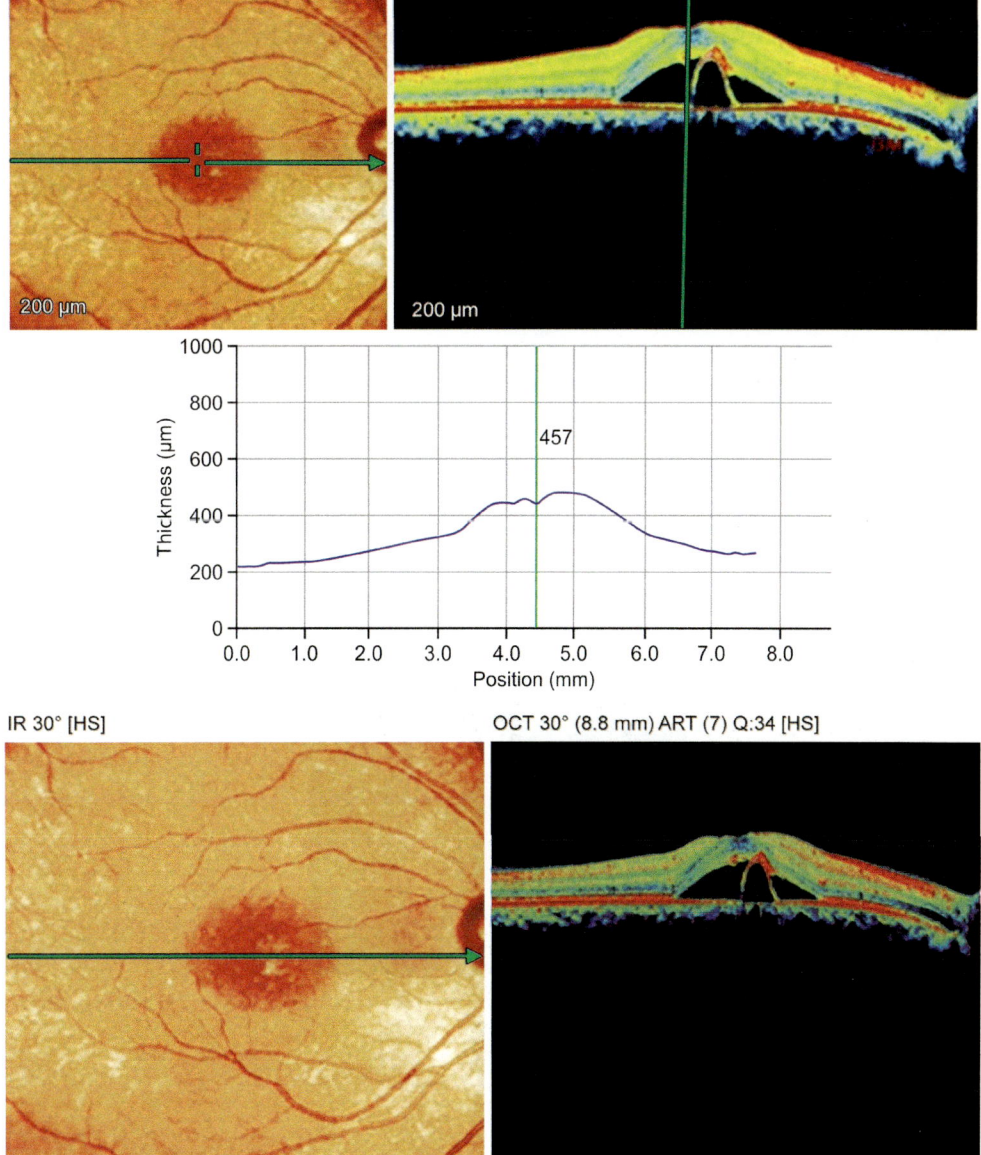

(Image courtesy: Prof. Dipak Kumar Nag, National Institute of Ophthalmology)

A. What are the findings in given OCT?
B. What are the main sites of lesion?
C. Mention two typical presentations that patient may give in the history.
D. What is the type of refractive error in this case?
E. Write three risk factors when such condition may develop.

OSPE: 35

A diabetic patient came to you with NPDR and macular edema in right eye and left eye suspected PDR.
A. Mention four laboratory investigations and two ocular investigations.
B. What findings you deserve to get from these ocular investigations?

OSPE: 36

A 35-year-old man, working as an office executive of a multinational company, normotensive, nonsmoker, and nondiabetic came with the complaints of sudden dimness of vision right eye.
- O/E: VAR = 6/12 improves with +1.00 Dsph. VAL: 6/6 unaided.
- Pupillary reaction normal.
- Slit-lamp examination: NAD.

A. What may be the diagnosis?
B. What finding will you get by ophthalmoscope examination? Mention two.
C. What is the natural course of the disease? Mention three.

OSPE: 37

A. How far should the Amsler's chart be placed in front of the patients?
B. How many degree(s) does each square subtend in the macula when placed in the recommended position?
C. What abnormality is present in above chart? Suggest a possible diagnosis.

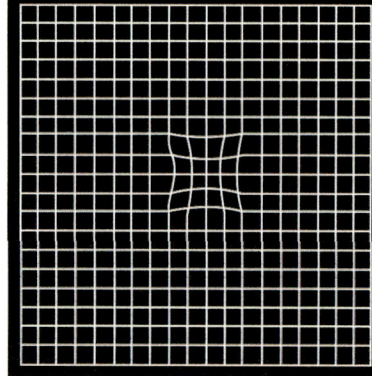

Retina and Uveal Tissue

OSPE: 38

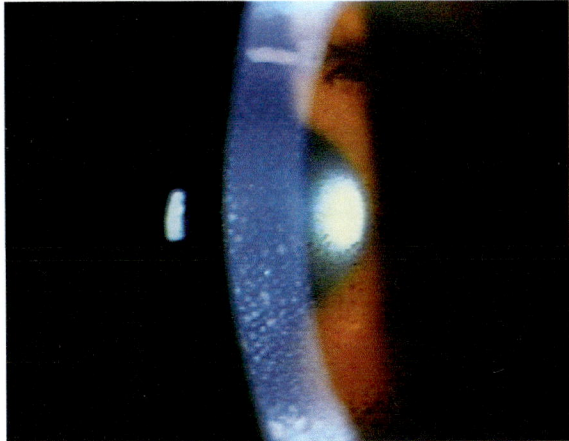

(Image courtesy: Dr. Ishtiaque Anwar, Bangladesh Eye Hospital)

This is a slit-lamp picture of a 25-year-old male patient with irritation, blurred vision, and photophobia on right eye for 3 days. He also gave history of perforating trauma on his left eye 2 months back.

A. What does the picture show?
B. What may be probable diagnosis?
C. Write two fundus findings which support your diagnosis.
D. Write one histopathology findings which you may expect in this condition.
E. Write one preventive and one treatment option.

OSPE: 39

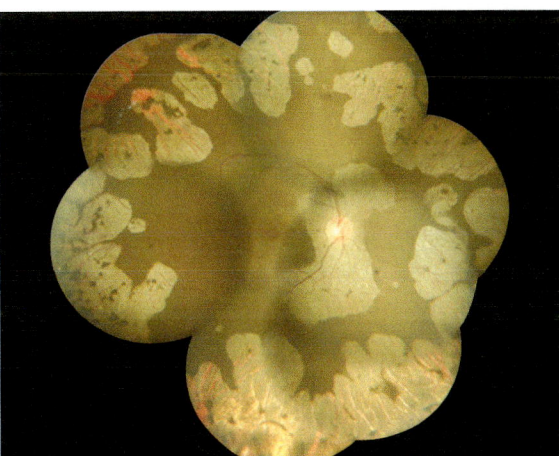

A. What does the picture show?
B. What is your probable diagnosis?
C. Write four other fundal features of this condition.
D. Write two systemic associations.
E. Write two complications.

OSPE: 40

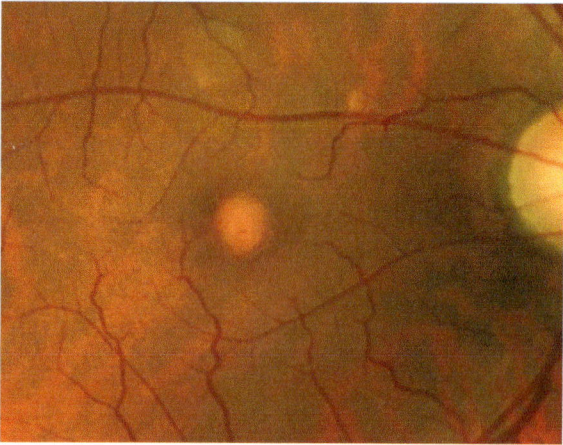

A 42-year-old man presents with decreased vision and not improved with refraction on right eye, no other abnormality found. On funduscopy, you found some changes in macula and you do a CFP.

A. What is your probable diagnosis?
B. What is its fate (mention four)?
C. Mention three investigations.
D. What is it forming in younger age group?

OSPE: 41

A 60-year-old male came to you with sudden profound loss of vision of his right eye. On examination VAR PL+, VAL 6/9, Pupil: Relative afferent pupillary defect (RAPD) (Right). This is the fundus picture of this patient.

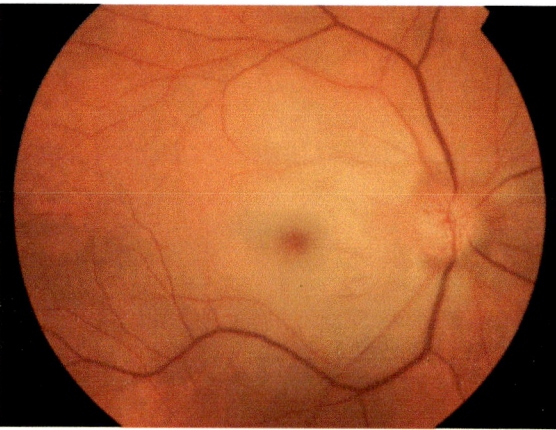

A. Write two findings which help your diagnosis.
B. What is your probable diagnosis?
C. What is the most common etiology?

D. Mention one investigation with interpretation.
E. How will you follow-up the patient?
F. What will you search during follow-up?

OSPE: 42

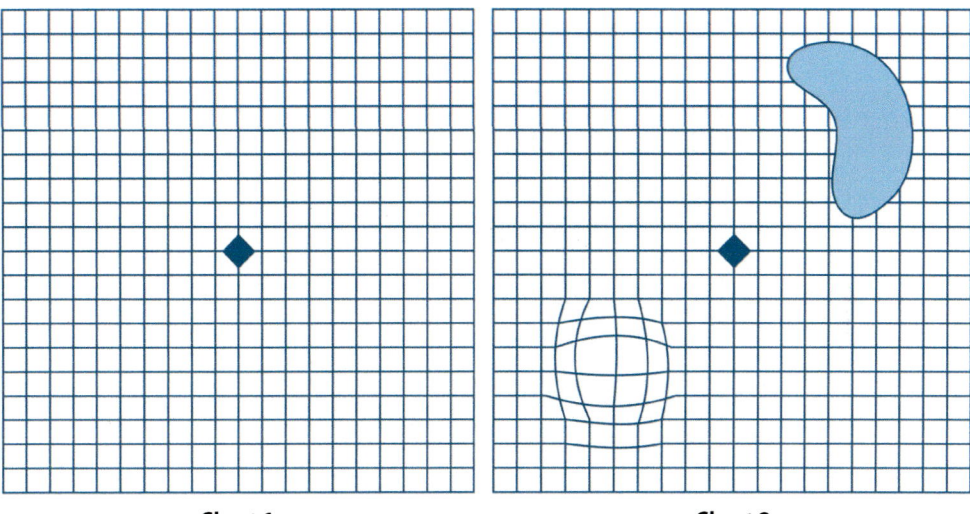

Chart 1 **Chart 2**

These two are Amsler's chart. Chart 1 is normal finding and chart 2 is pathological.
A. How far should the Amsler's chart be placed in front of the patient?
B. How much degree(s) does each square subtend in the macula when placed in the recommended distance?
C. What are the pathological findings in chart 2?
D. What may be the causes?

OSPE: 43

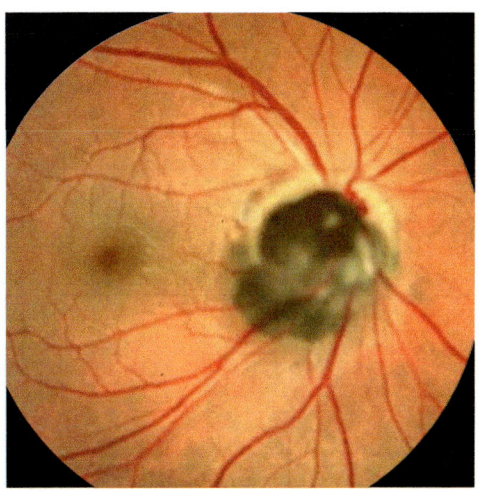

A. What is your probable diagnosis?
B. What type of disease is this?
C. Which gender and race is most commonly affected?
D. What is the mean age?
E. What will be the feature in FFA?
F. What is the fate and complication of it? Mention two of each.

OSPE: 44

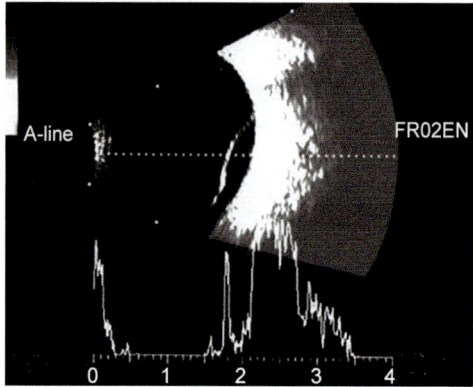

A 16-year-old patient gave history of blunt trauma on his left eye while playing cricket, since then, he complains dimness of vision on his left eye. This is the B-scan of his left eye.
A. Write the positive findings.
B. What is your probable diagnosis?
C. How "gain adjust" support your diagnosis.
D. Mention position of marker on of probe when vertical scan done.
E. Mention marker on probe when horizontal scan done.
F. What frequency wave is used in B-scan?

OSPE: 45

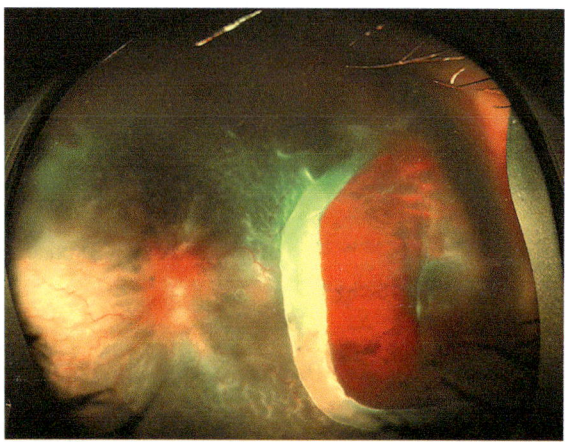

Picture 1

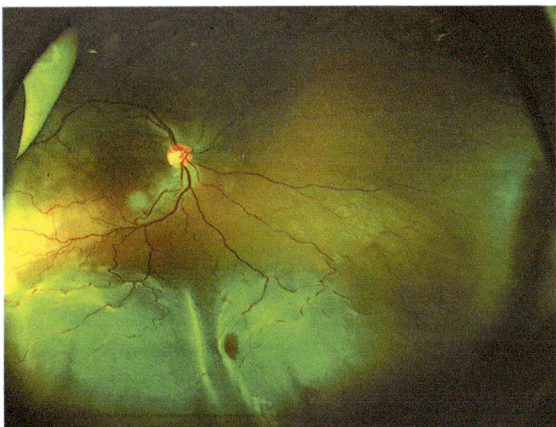

Picture 2

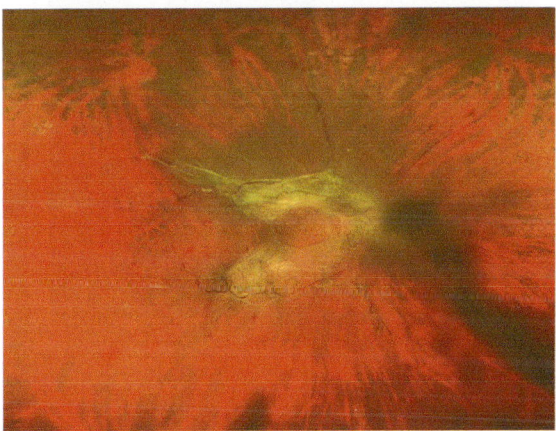

Picture 3

What are the positive findings in pictures 1, 2, and 3?

OSPE: 46

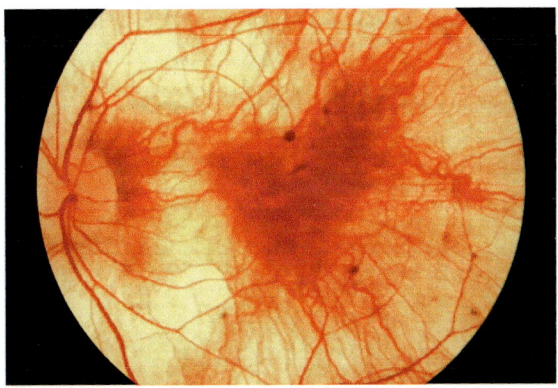

A. What are the positive findings in this picture?
B. What is your diagnosis?
C. What is the other name of the disease?
D. What type of disease is this?
E. What is the prognosis?
F. Who is affected more?

OSPE: 47

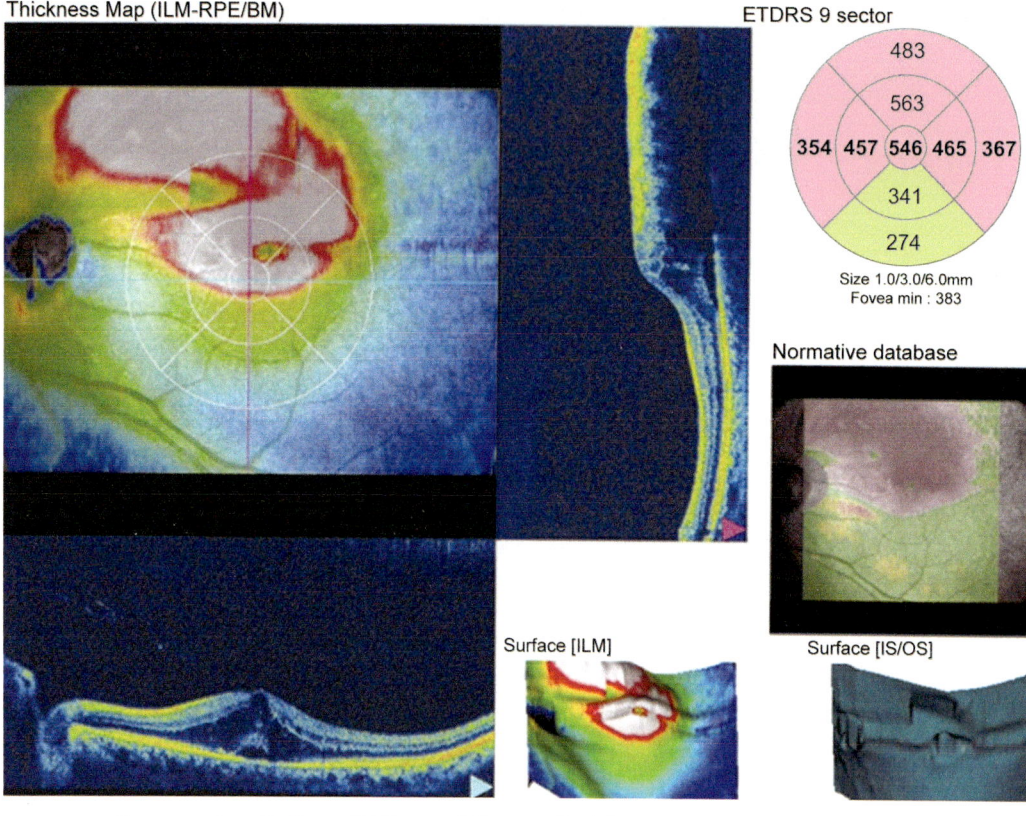

(Image courtesy: Dr. Shams Md. Noman, Chittagong Eye Infirmary & Training Complex of BNSB)

A. What is name of the tracing?
B. What is about vitreomacular interface?
C. What is about neurosensory retina?
D. What is your diagnosis?

Retina and Uveal Tissue

OSPE: 48

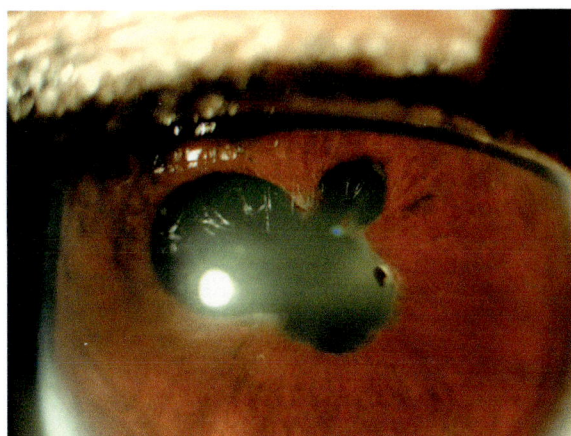

(Image courtesy: Dr. Ishtiaque Anwar, Bangladesh Eye Hospital)

A. What is the appearance of pupil?
B. What it indicates?
C. Why it occurs?
D. What findings you may get in slit-lamp biomicroscope?
E. What is the consequence of this eye?

OSPE: 49

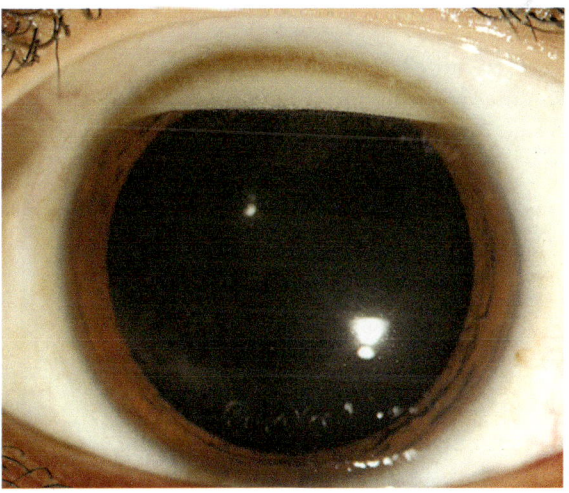

(Image courtesy: Dr. Ishtiaque Anwar, Bangladesh Eye Hospital)

A 38-year-old man presented with painless decrease of vision in his left eye, secondary to a giant retinal tear with surrounding retinal detachment. He underwent surgery, but he did not present for following ocular examinations. After two years, he presented with hand movement.

A. What is the name of the upper whitish area?
B. What is the other name of the condition?
C. What is the material of it?
D. Why it occurs?
E. What complications may occur?

OSPE: 50

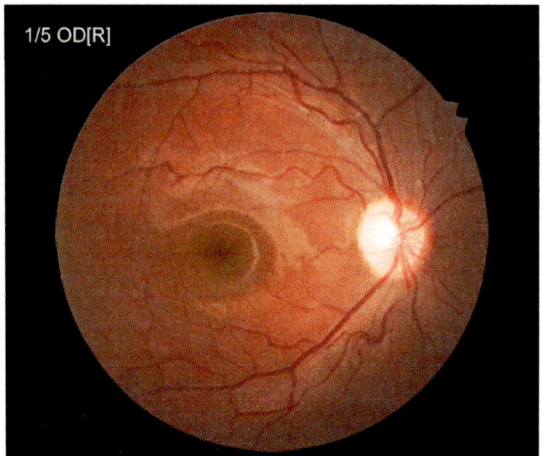

(Image courtesy: Green Eye Hospital, Dhaka)

A. What is the name of the supplied sample?
B. What is your diagnosis?
C. Which gender is affected more?
D. What are the risk factors? Mention four.
E. What are the treatment options? Mention three.

OSPE: 51

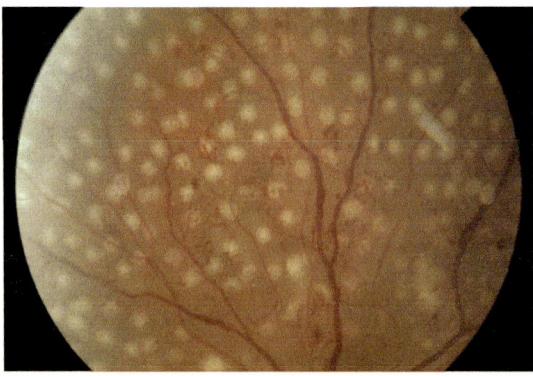

A. What are the positive findings in this picture?
B. What causes these white scars?

C. What are indications of its uses?
D. What are the adverse effects? Mention three.
E. What are the indicators of regression? Mention three.

OSPE: 52

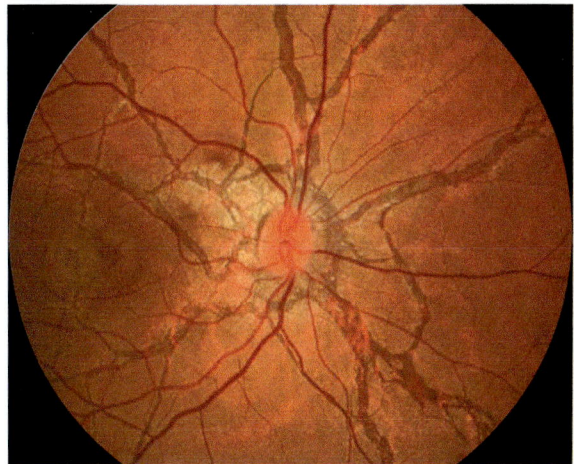

A. Identify the supplied sample and mention two positive findings.
B. What is your diagnosis?
C. What are the common causes of vision loss? Mention two.
D. What are the associations? Mention three.

OSPE: 53

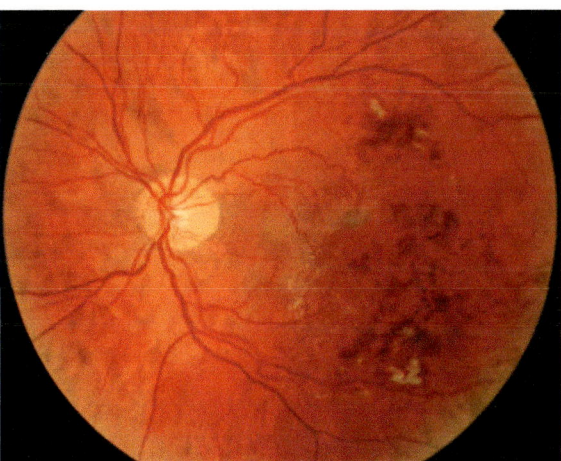

A. Identify the supplied sample. Mention two important positive findings.
B. What is your diagnosis?
C. What are the D/Ds? Mention two.
D. What are the risk factors? Mention four.

OSPE: 54

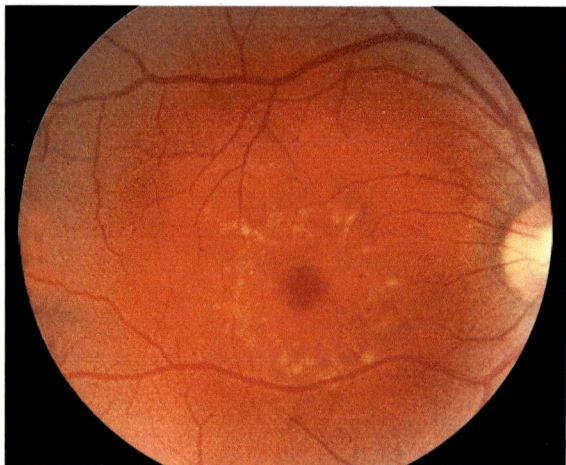

A. What is the name of the specimen?
B. What are the positive findings? Mention two.
C. What is your diagnosis?
D. What is the main pathogenesis?
E. What are the symptoms?

OSPE: 55

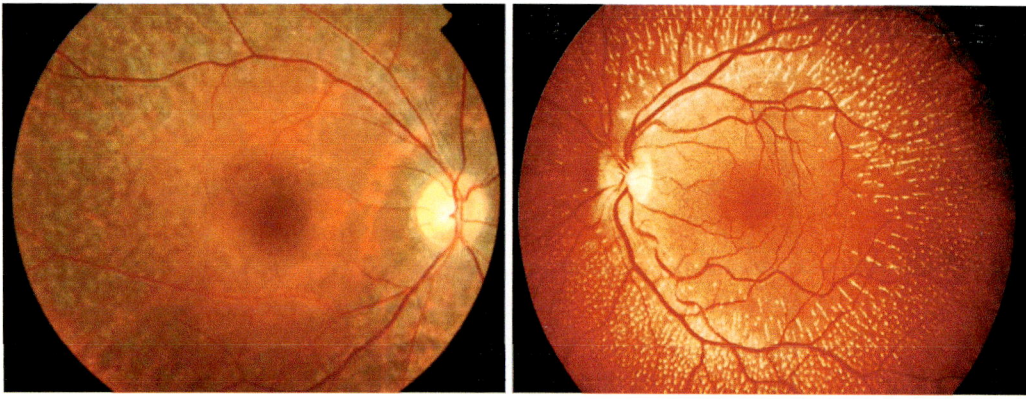

A. What is the similarity between two pictures?
B. What are the differences between two pictures?
C. What are the diagnoses in both cases?

Retina and Uveal Tissue

OSPE: 56

This is the fundus picture of a lady who is suffering from lupus erythematosus and under treatment for last 5 years, now she goes to an ophthalmologist for reduced vision and her fundus picture is shown below:

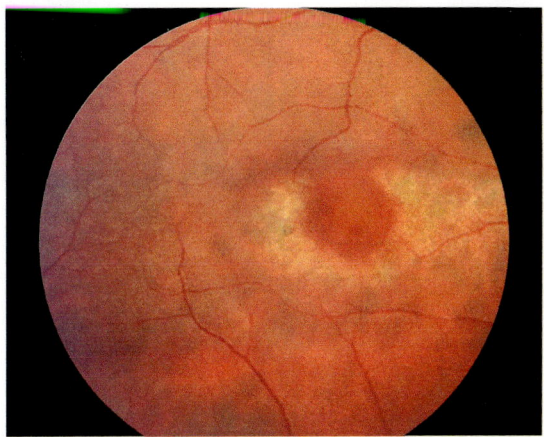

A. What medicine is she using?
B. What is the most common indication of this medicine?
C. Is it reversible or not?
D. What the fundus appearance is called?
E. What is the earliest change of her visual field?

OSPE: 57

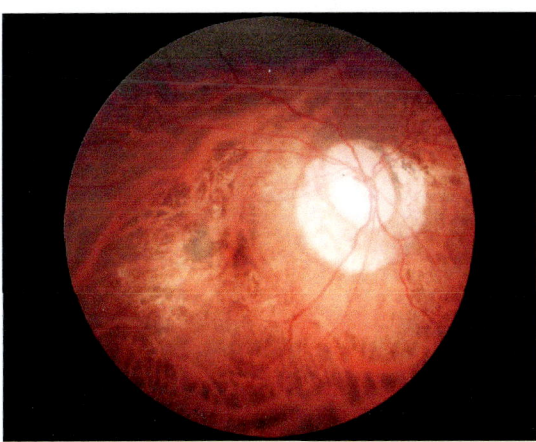

(Image courtesy: Green Eye Hospital, Dhaka)

A. What is the name of the supplied specimen?
B. What are the positive findings? Mention three.
C. What is your diagnosis?
D. What are the systemic associations?

OSPE: 58

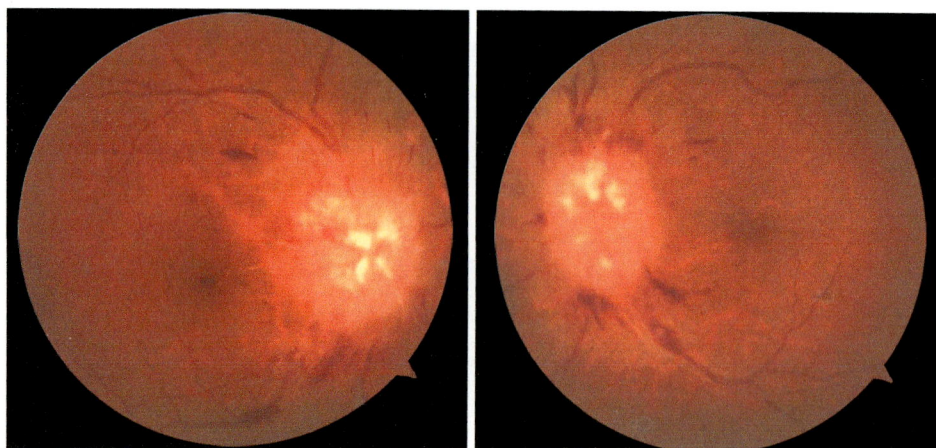

(Image courtesy: Green Eye Hospital, Dhaka)

This is the fundus picture of a 26-year-old man who came to you with the complaints of dimness of vision of both eyes associated with headache and neck ache. Before that, he went to a resident ophthalmologist but the ophthalmologist referred him to neurosurgeon and the neurosurgeon did the MRI of brain, but there was no positive finding in MRI. Then the patient was referred to you by neurosurgeon.

A. What are the positive findings in CFP?
B. Why the resident referred him to neurosurgeon?
C. Why the neurosurgeon referred him to you?
D. What is your diagnosis?
E. What clinical test will diagnose the case?
F. What blood test will you perform? Mention three.
G. To whom you referred him?

OSPE: 59

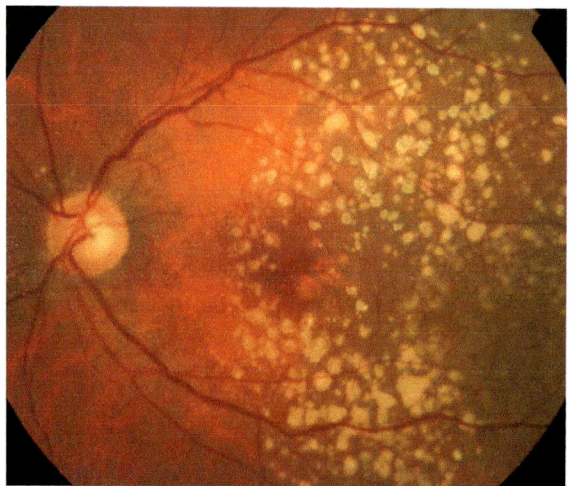

Retina and Uveal Tissue 95

This is the fundus picture of a 76-year-old man who came to you for dimness of vision particularly during reading.
A. What shows the fundus picture?
B. What is your diagnosis?
C. How many types of this disease are there? Name them.
D. What is their alternate name?
E. Which one has the worst prognosis?

OSPE: 60

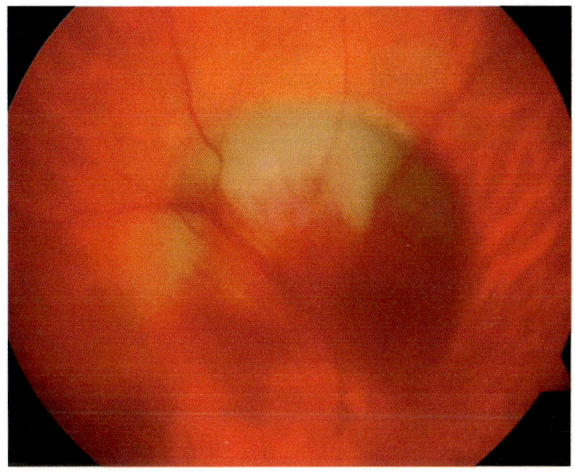

See the above photo and answer the following questions:
A. What is the name of above tracing paper?
B. What are the positive findings?
C. What is your probable diagnosis?
D. What are the D/Ds?

ANSWERS

OSPE: 01. Proliferative diabetic retinopathy
OSPE: 02. Drusen + retinal pigment epithelium (RPE) atrophy
OSPE: 03. Disc swelling
OSPE: 04. Cherry red spot [central retinal artery occlusion (CRAO)]
OSPE: 05. New vessels elsewhere and hemorrhage
OSPE: 06. Vasculitis retinae
OSPE: 07. CRAO with persistent CRA
OSPE: 08. Macular dystrophy
OSPE: 09. Vasculitis retinae
OSPE: 10. Boat-shaped hemorrhage at the macula
OSPE: 11. RP
OSPE: 12. Proliferative diabetic retinopathy (PDR)/Preproliferative diabetic retinopathy (PPDR)
OSPE: 13. PDR
OSPE: 14. Hypertensive retinopathy
OSPE: 15. NPDR
OSPE: 16. Macular hole
OSPE: 17. CRVO
OSPE: 18. Papilledema
OSPE: 19. Fan-shaped neovascularization, intraretinal microvascular abnormalities (IRMA), and hard exudates
OSPE: 20. RP
OSPE: 21. Macroaneurysm
OSPE: 22. Noncentral subhyaloids hemorrhage
OSPE: 23. PDR
OSPE: 24. Microaneurysm (MA), capillary drop outs, and neovascularization elsewhere (NVE)
OSPE: 25. CMO
OSPE: 26. Postoperative endophthalmitis
OSPE: 27. Funnel retinal detachment (RD)
OSPE: 28. Choroidal melanoma
OSPE: 29. Dropped crystalline lens
OSPE: 30. Retinoblastoma
OSPE: 31. Separation of RPE from Bruch's membrane
OSPE: 32. (a) ERM (b) VMT (c) CME
OSPE: 33. Full thickness macular hole
OSPE: 34. Subretinal fluid (central sensory detachment)
OSPE: 35. Right eye NPDR with macular edema and left eye suspected PDR
OSPE: 36. CSCR
OSPE: 37. Amsler's chart
OSPE: 38. Granulomatous KP
OSPE: 39. Focal chorioretinal atrophy
OSPE: 40. Vitelliform macular dystrophy

Retina and Uveal Tissue

OSPE: 41. CRAO
OSPE: 42. CSC or CNVM
OSPE: 43. Optic disc melanocytoma
OSPE: 44. Retinal detachment
OSPE: 45. Giant retinal tear (GRT) with PVR-B (rolled tear margin). Looks total RD.
OSPE: 46. Degeneration of the choroid, RPE, and photoreceptors
OSPE: 47. CMO
OSPE: 48. Festooned pupil
OSPE: 49. Silicon oil
OSPE: 50. CSCR
OSPE: 51. PRP
OSPE: 52. Angioid streak
OSPE: 53. Branch retinal vein occlusion
OSPE: 54. Fundus flavimaculatus/Stargardt diseases
OSPE: 55. Retinitis punctata albescens and fundus albipunctatus
OSPE: 56. Chloroquine toxicity
OSPE: 57. Degenerative myopia
OSPE: 58. Hypertensive retinopathy
OSPE: 59. Age-related macular degeneration (ARMD)
OSPE: 60. Melanoma

ANS: 01

A. Positive findings are:
- NVD and NVE 1.0
- Hard exudates. 1.0

B. Proliferative diabetic retinopathy 2.0
C. Macular edema 1.5
D. Any 3 .... (0.5 × 3) 1.5
- Blood sugar
- HbA1C
- Lipid profile
- Serum creatinine

E.
- FFA for neovessels and capillary dropouts 1.0
- OCT for quantification of macular edema 1.0

F. Antivascular endothelial growth factor (VEGF) + Panretinal photocoagulation .... 1+1
   .... 2.0

TOTAL ***10***

ANS: 02

A. Drusen + RPE atrophy .... 1+1 .... 2.0
B. Loss of central vision 2.0
C. FFA. To see any development of CNVM .... 1+1 .... 2.0
D. Antioxidant vitamin, ARED formula (Age-related eye diseases) 2.0
E. Home Amsler grid chart 2.0

TOTAL ***10***

ANS: 03

A. ....1 × 3..3
   i. Disc swelling
   ii. Dilated tortuous veins and
   iii. Hard exudates in macula
B. CRVO 2
C. OCT macula to quantify macular edema .... 1+1..2
D. Anti-VEGF injection..1
E. To see proliferative retinopathy + NVI................... 1+1..2
TOTAL **10**

ANS: 04

A. Cherry red spot 2
B. Central retinal artery occlusion (CRAO) 2
C. (1) Macular hole. (2) Hemorrhage over macula...... 1+1..2
D. Delayed arterial filling. 2
E. (1) Lowering IOP. (2) Vasodilator-Carbogen .... 1+1..2
TOTAL **10**

ANS: 05

A. New vessels elsewhere and hemorrhage .... 1+1..2
B. (i) Diabetic retinopathy; (ii) CEVO; (iii) Vasculitis retinae (any two)............1+1 2
C. Panretinal photocoagulation..2
D. Vitreous hemorrhage and tractional RD .... 1+1..2
E. FFA and OCT (Macular protocol) .... 1+1..2
TOTAL **10**

ANS: 06

A. (a) Retinal hemorrhage; (b) Vascular sheathing..... 1+1..2
B. Vasculitis retinae 2
C. Tuberculosis..2
D. (a) X-ray chest; (b) Mantoux test .... 1+1..2
E. (a) Anti-TB drug (if X-ray and Monteux positive); (b) Steroid...................1+1..................2
TOTAL **10**

ANS: 07

A. ....(Any two) .... 1+1..2
   i. Redness temporal to disc
   ii. Whitish appearance of the macular area
   iii. Cherry red spot.
B. CRAO with persistent CRA 2
C. ....(Any two) .... 1+1..2
   i. Macular hole
   ii. Hemorrhage over fovea
   iii. Drug toxicity

D. FFA, delay arterial filling... 1+1... 2
E. Message over the globe and IOP lowering agents... 1+1.. 2
TOTAL **10**

ANS: 08
A. Central hypopigmentation surrounded by hyper- and hypopigmentation 2
B. Bull's eye maculopathy, macular dystrophy............. 1+1... 2
C. Stargardt's disease, cone dystrophy, ARMD, drug toxicity.......(Any two)..........1+1.......... 2
D. Loss of central vision 2
E. Counseling, LVA... 1+1... 2
TOTAL **10**

ANS: 09
A. Retinal hemorrhage, vascular occlusion, venous sheathing..............(Any two) 2
B. Vasculitis retinae.. 2
C. BRVO, CRVO, diabetic retinopathy.................... (Any 2)... 2
D. Ocular TB... 2
E. CBE, X-ray chest, MT .... (Any 2)... 2
TOTAL **10**

ANS: 10
A. Boat-shaped hemorrhage at the macula 2
B. Subhyloid, premacular space................................... 1+1... 2
C. Sudden marked loss of vision.. 2
D. ....Any two.. 2
   (a) Valsalva maneuver
   (b) Terson syndrome
   (c) Purtscher's retinopathy
   (d) Retinal artery macroaneurysm
   (e) Blood dyscrasias
E. ....Any two.. 2
   (a) Nd: YAG hyaloidotomy
   (b) Intravitreal tPA
   (c) C_3F_8 injection and positioning pars plana vitrectomy
TOTAL **10**

ANS: 11
A. Pale disc, arterial attenuation, bone spicules...........................(Any two) 2
B. Night blindness, loss of peripheral vision 2
C. PSC, OAG, macular edema, myopia...(Any two) 2
D. Chloroquine toxicity, chorioretinitis, Post RD surgery, PRP......(Any two) 2
E. Tubular field... 2
TOTAL **10**

ANS: 12

A. i. New vessels at elsewhere (NVE) 1.0
    ii. Multiple dot-blot hemorrhage 1.0
    iii. Multiple hard exudates 1.0
B. Any three .... (1 × 3) 3.0
    i. Proliferative diabetic retinopathy (PDR)
    ii. Preproliferative diabetic retinopathy (PPDR)
    iii. Central vein occlusion (CRVO)
    iv. Hypertensive retinopathy
C. i. Blood sugar fasting and 2 hrs after breakfast/GTT 0.5
    ii. HbA_1C 0.5
    Two ocular investigations:
    i. FFA 1.0
    ii. OCT (Macular protocol) 1.0
D. i. PRP 0.5
    ii. Intravitreal anti-VEGF 0.5
TOTAL ***10***

ANS: 13

A. i. NVD 1
    ii. Dot and blot hemorrhage 1
B. More than one quarter of the retina to be non-perfuse to develop this feature 1
C. PDR 2
D. (a) NVE; (b) New vessels in the iris 2
E. RBS. Glycosylated Hb OCT (macular protocol). FFA 2
F. Hyperfluorescence during the later stages 1
TOTAL ***10***

ANS: 14

A. 4
    Picture A: Arterial attenuation, pale disc margin is not well-defined, decrease in number of small blood vessel of disc
    Picture B: Arteriovenous nipping, copper wiring of the arteriole
    Picture C: Flame-shaped hemorrhage all over four quadrants, hard exudates
    Picture D: Disc swelling hyperemic margin not defined, numerous flame-shaped hemorrhage around disc and all over four quadrants, hard exudates, and cotton wool spot.
B. 4
    Picture A: Secondary optic atrophy
    Picture B: Hypertensive retinopathy (Grade 2)
    Picture C. Hypertensive retinopathy (Grade 3)
    Picture D. Hypertensive retinopathy (Grade 4)
C. *Investigation*: Ocular 1
    i. V/A
    ii. Color vision
    iii. RAPD

Investigation: Systemic	1

    i.   Blood pressure
    ii. Serum creatinine
    iii. MRI of brain and orbit
    iv. Lumbar puncture

TOTAL *10*

ANS: 15

A. i. Dot and blot hemorrhage 2.0
     ii. Cotton wool spots 2.0
B. NPDR 2.0
C. Serum creatinine 2.0
D. Nephrologists 2.0

TOTAL *10*

ANS: 16

A. Macular hole 3
B. A macular hole is a disruption of the center of the macula. The interior of the eye is filled with a jelly-like substance called vitreous. As humans age, this jelly begins to shrink and travel toward the front of the eye. Deterioration of this jelly causes it to pull on the macula. In most cases, the vitreous separates without any negative side effects. However, in some cases where the vitreous is firmly attached to the central area of the retina, this pulling away may form a small hole, known as a macular hole 3
C. History of trauma 2
D. Macular holes usually occur in middle older people. People who are very nearsighted, or those who have had blunt injuries to their eyes, may also develop a macular hole 2

TOTAL *10*

ANS: 17

A. .... 1.5 × 2 .... 3.0
    (a) Disc swelling
    (b) Hemorrhage
    (c) Tortuous vessels
    (d) Exudates
B. .... 1.5 × 2 .... 3.0
    (a) Hypofluorescence
    (b) Hyperfluorescence
C. Macular edema 2.0
D. NVI/NVG 1.0
E. 6–12 months 1.0

TOTAL *10*

ANS: 18

A. Papilledema 3.0
B. Swollen optic disc 2.0

C. (a) Intracranial space occupying lesions 2.0
    (b) Raised BP 2.0
    (c) Benign intracranial hypertension 1.0
TOTAL 10

ANS: 19
A. Fan-shaped neovascularization, IRMA, and hard exudates 3.0
B. PDR, CRVO, vasculitis retinae, sickle cell retinopathy ....(any two) .... 1+ 0.5 .... 1.5
C. • *Systemic*: BP, RBS, HbA1C, lipid profile ....(any three) .... 0.5 × 3 ...... 1.5
    • *Ocular:* CFP, FFA, OCT ....(any two) .... 0.5 × 2 ...... 1.0
D. ROP. Sickle cell retinopathy, leukemia ....(any two) .... 1 + 1 .... 2.0
TOTAL 10

ANS: 20
A. .... 1 × 3 .... 3.0
    (a) Bony spicule like pigmentation and tessellated fundus
    (b) Arterial attenuation
    (c) Pale disc
B. RP 2.0
C. Tubular vision 1.0
D. .... 1 × 2 .... 2.0
    (a) Positive family history
    (b) Consanguine marriage of parents
E. Retinal degenerative disease firstly affects rods, then cone 1.0
F. .... 0.5 × 2 .... 1.0
    (a) PSC
    (b) POAG
    (c) Keratoconus
TOTAL 10

ANS: 21
A. The late phase 2
B. Smoke steak pattern 2
C. CMO 2
D. Accumulation of fluid in the outer plexiform and inner nuclear layers of the retina 2
E. Diabetes 2
TOTAL 10

ANS: 22
A. CFP and FFA 2
B. Non-central subhyaloid hemorrhage 2
C. .... 1 × 2 2
    i. Rupture macroaneurysm
    ii. Valsalva retinopathy
    iii. Rupture hemangiomas (mostly due to trauma)
    iv. Blood dyscrasias

Retina and Uveal Tissue

D. Vision should be good, as fovea is unaffected, flat, and healthy looking 1.5
E. OCT seems to be not necessary. B-scan might discover any underlying growth ..... 0.5 + 1
   .... 1.5
F. Treatment is observation + treatment for systemic condition if any 1.0
TOTAL **10**

ANS: 23
A. NVE +capillary dropouts .... 1+1 2
B. PDR 2
C. Anti-VEGF and PRP .... 1+1 2
D. .... 1+1 2
   i. PRP
   ii. It will make hypoxic retina to anoxic retina and will regress new vessels.
E. .... (Any four) .... 0.5 × 4 2
   i. Control DM
   ii. Control hypertension
   iii. Stop smoking
   iv. Control high cholesterol (if any)
   v. Serum creatinine (if any)
TOTAL **10**

ANS: 24
A. .... 1 × 3 .... 3.0
   (a) MA
   (b) Capillary dropouts
   (c) NVE
B. PDR 2.0
C. PRP 2.0
D. (a) Control DM; (b) Control HT; (c) Control cholesterol; (d) Control creatinine; (e) Stop smoking 3.0
TOTAL **10**

ANS: 25
A. The late phase 2
B. Smoke steak pattern 2
C. CSCR 2
D. Observation 2
E. Young male and type A personality 2
TOTAL **10**

ANS: 26
A. Echogenic shadow throughout the vitreous cavity 2
B. .... (Any two) .... 1+1 2
   - Post operative endophthalmitis
   - Toxic anterior segment syndrome (TASS)
   - Vitreous hemorrhage

C. No attachment at the disc and mild to moderate echogenic spike .... 1+1 2
D. Intravitreal vancomycin + ceftadazime. Vitreous tap for Gram stain + KOH + C/S 2
E. No improvement after intravitreal injection + Vision equal to or less than LP 2
TOTAL **10**

ANS: 27

A. Funnel RD 2
B. (a) Choroidal detachment (b) PVD 4
C. (a) Old age; (b) Trauma; (c) Myopia; (d) Aphakia/pseudophakia; (e) Coloboma 2
D. 360-degree band + PPV + SOI 2
TOTAL **10**

ANS: 28

A. Collar button (Mushroom) shape echogenic shadow 3
B. Choroidal melanoma 3
C. Liver enzymes level is indicated in any patient with choroidal melanoma. Because the liver is the most common site of choroidal melanoma 1
D. Management options are: .... (any three)
    i. *Observation*: If the tumor is small and diagnosis is not well-established 1
    ii. *Enucleation*: Preferred treatment for larger than 15 mm and complicated tumor 1
    iii. *Plaque brachytherapy*: Alternative to enucleation 1
    iv. External beam irradiation 1
    v. Pars plana vitrectomy endoresection 0.5
    vi. Laser photocoagulation and transpupillary thermotherapy 0.5
    vii. Orbital exenteration 0.5
TOTAL **10**

ANS: 29

A. Ring-shaped echogenic shadow in the mid-vitreous cavity 2
B. Dropped crystalline lens 2
C. Trauma, cataract surgery 2
D. Pars plana vitrectomy and lensectomy 2
E. Any two: .... 1 × 2 2
    i. Raised intraocular pressure
    ii. Vitreous hemorrhage
    iii. Retinal detachment
    iv. Intraocular inflammation
TOTAL **10**

ANS: 30

A. Mass-like vitreous opacity in the posterior vitreous cavity with internal hyperreflective spots 3
B. Retinoblastoma 2
C. Any four .... 0.5 × 4 2
    i. White/Cat's eye reflex/Leukokoria
    ii. Strabismus

Retina and Uveal Tissue 105

    iii. Orbital cellulitis/Proptosis/Red eye
    iv. Hyphema
    v. Unilateral mydriasis
    vi. Nystagmus
    vii. Heterochromia iridis
D. A positive family history is present in 5–10% of children who developed retinoblastoma 1
E. ....Any four .... 0.5 × 4 2
    i. Vincristine
    ii. Carboplatin
    iii. Etoposide
    iv. Melphalan
    v. Topotecan
TOTAL *10*

ANS: 31
A. Separation of RPE from Bruch's membrane 2
B. 2
    i. An optically empty space in between them
    ii. Serous PED
C. Reduction of hydraulic conductivity of a thickened and dysfunctional Bruch's membrane. 2
D. Any two 2
    i. Observation
    ii. Intravitreal anti-VEGF
    iii. Combined anti-VEGF and PDT
E. Any two 2
    i. Persistence with atrophy and decrease vision
    ii. Resolution with geographical atrophy with visual loss
    iii. RPE tear
    iv. Develop CNV in one-third eye
TOTAL *10*

ANS: 32
A. (a) ERM; (b) VMT; (c) CME 3
B. (a) DoV; (b) Metamorphopsia 2
C. (a) Diabetic retinopathy; (b) Ocular inflammatory disease; (c) Retinal vein occlusion ... 3
D. (a) Anti-VEGF; (b) PPV; (c) Ocriplasmin .... (Any 2) 2
TOTAL *10*

ANS: 33
A. i. Full thickness tissue defects at the center of the macula (full thickness macular hole) 2
    ii. Cystic changes of the retina at the margin of the hole 1

B. i. Watzke-Allen test.. 1
    ii. Laser aiming beam test 1
C. .... (Any two) 2
    i. Trauma
    ii. Progressive high myopia
    iii. Vitreoretinal traction theory
D. i. Blurred central vision.. 1
    ii. Metamorphopsia 1
E. Total vitrectomy with internal limiting membrane (ILM) peeling followed by expansible gas injection in the vitreous cavity 1
TOTAL 10

ANS: 34

A. (a) Subretinal fluid (central sensory detachment)... 1.0
    (b) Pigment epithelium detachment (PED) 1.0
B. (a) Retinal pigment epithelium (RPE) 1.0
    (b) Focal choroidal vasculopathy.. 1.0
C. .... (Any two) 2.0
    (a) Black spot in front of the eye (a positive scotoma)
    (b) Metamorphopsia (Especially micropsia)
    (c) Decreased central vision
D. Hypermetropia... 0.5
E. (a) Steroid use 1.0
    (b) Type A personality.. 0.5
    (c) Systemic hypertension.. 0.5
    (d) Obstructive sleep apnea 0.5
    (e) Pregnancy 0.5
    (f) *Helicobacter pylori* infection 0.5
TOTAL 10

ANS: 35

A. Laboratory investigations (Any four):
    i. Blood sugar. Fasting and 2 hrs after breakfast/glucose tolerance test (GTT) 1.5
    ii. HbA_1C 1.5
    iii. Lipid profile 1.0
    iv. Serum creatinine.. 0.5
    v. Hemoglobin estimation 0.5
    Ocular investigations:
    i. FFA 1.5
    ii. OCT (Macular protocol)...1 + 0.5 .... 1.5
B. i. From OCT: Increase macular thickness in R/E..................1.0 + 0.5 .... 1.5
    ii. FFA, B/E to detect capillary nonperfusion, NVD, and NVE..................................... 1.0
TOTAL 10

Retina and Uveal Tissue

ANS: 36
A. CSCR 3
B. Any two .... 2 × 2 4
   i. Detachment of the sensory retina at macula
   ii. One or more abnormal depigmented RPE foci
   iii. Small patches of RPE atrophy and hyperplasia
C. .... 1 × 3 3
   i. Spontaneous resolution
   ii. Become chronic
   iii. Bullous CSCR

TOTAL **10**

ANS: 37
A. This chart is placed 30 cm from the patient 3
B. When placed at 30 cm each square (which measures 5 mm) subtends 1 degree on the retina 3
C. Central distortion with micropsia (the square look smaller) CMO .... 2 + 2 4

TOTAL **10**

ANS: 38
A. Granulomatous KP 2.0
B. Sympathetic ophthalmitis 2.0
C. Any two
   (a) Multifocal choroidal infiltrates 1.0
   (b) Exudative retinal detachment 1.0
   (c) Vasculitis 0.5
   (d) Optic disc swelling 0.5
D Dalen-Fuchs nodule 1.0
E. (a) *Preventing*: Enucleation of severely injured eye 1.0
   (b) *Treatment*: High dose of oral steroid 1.0

TOTAL **10**

ANS: 39
A. Focal chorioretinal atrophy of periphery and around disc 2.0
B. *Diagnosis*: Myopic fundus 2.0
C. .... 4 × 0.5 .... 2.0
   (a) Lattice degeneration
   (b) Subretinal coin hemorrhage
   (c) Fuchs spot
   (d) Staphyloma
D. Any two .... 2 × 1 .... 2.0
   (a) Down syndrome
   (b) Stickler syndrome
   (c) Marfan syndrome

E. Any two .... 2 × 1 .... 2.0
   (a) RD
   (b) CNV
   (c) Macular hole
TOTAL **10**

ANS: 40
A. Adult onset vitelliform macular dystrophy 2.0
B. 4.0
   (a) Persist
   (b) Absorb
   (c) Break-up
   (d) Disperse
C. 3.0
   (a) *OCT*: (Macular protocol) hyper-reflective material associated with RPE
   (b) *FAF*: Intense hyperautofluorescence
   (c) *FA*: Central hypofluorescence
D. Best Vitelliform macular dystrophy 1.0
TOTAL **10**

ANS: 41
A. (a) Whitish edematous retina 1.5
   (b) Cherry red spot at macula 1.5
B. CRAO 2.0
C. Atherosclerosis-related embolism and thrombus 1.0
D. FFA: Arterial filling defect .... 1 + 1 .... 2.0
E. 3–4 weekly at least 2 follow-up 1.0
F. Neovascularization of posterior and anterior segment 1.0
TOTAL **10**

ANS: 42
A. The chart is placed 33 cm from the patient 2.0
B. When placed at 33 cm each square (which measures 5 mm) subtend 1 degree on the retina 2.0
C. The wavy downward lines resemble fluid accumulation which can be from CSC or CNVM 3.0
D. Upward right side has a shadow which can be from preretinal or subretinal hemorrhage casting shadow 3.0
TOTAL **10**

ANS: 43
A. Optic disc melanocytoma 3.0
B. It is congenital hamartoma 2.0
C. Female, black .... 0.5 + 0.5 .... 1.0
D. 50 years 1.0
E. FA shows persistent dense hypofluorescence due to masking 1.0

Retina and Uveal Tissue

F. Fate ....0.5 × 2... 1.0
   (a) It may be stationary
   (b) Malignant transformation
   Complications...................(any two) ....0.5 × 2... 1.0
   (a) Spontaneous tumor necrosis
   (b) Optic nerve compression and
   (c) Retinal vein obstruction
TOTAL *10*

ANS: 44

A. There is a hypoechoic space in between retina and sclera 3.0
B. Retinal detachment 2.0
C. If gain is low and echo shows then it is RD 1.5
D. Superiorly 1.5
E. Probe more opposite of movement of eye 1.0
F. High frequency 1.0
TOTAL *10*

ANS: 45

Picture: 1
Giant retinal tear (GRT) with PVR-B (rolled tear margin) 2.5
Looks total RD 2.5
Picture: 2
Inferior RD and seems macula on 2.0
Picture: 3
Has FVP at the disc with vitreous hemorrhage suggestive of ADED or complication of previous CRVO 3.0
TOTAL *10*

ANS: 46

A. Degeneration of the choroid, RPE, and photoreceptors, in some area the sclera becomes visible 3.5
B. Choroideremia 2.5
C. Tapetochoroidal degeneration 1.0
D. X-linked 1.0
E. Prognosis is very poor with some exception 1.0
F. Males are only effected 1.0
TOTAL *10*

ANS: 47

A. This is a printout paper of OCT macular protocol 2.0
B. Vitreomacular interface: Normal 3.0
C. Foveal contour lost and elevated. Accumulation of fluid and cystoid spaces in neurosensory retina at foveal and parafoveal 3.0
D. CMO 2.0
TOTAL *10*

ANS: 48

A. Festooned appearance 2.0
B. It is a sign of previous or present iritis 1.5
C. Usually it occurs when posterior synechiae is firm and atropine eye drop could not free the posterior synechiae completely 2.0
D. .... 3 × 0.5 .... 1.5
   (a) KP
   (b) Cell
   (c) Flare
E. .... 6 × 0.5 .... 3.0
   (a) Seclusion papillae
   (b) Secondary angle closure glaucoma
   (c) Iris bombe
   (d) Peripheral anterior synechiae (PAS)
   (e) Occlusio pupillae
   (f) Phthisis bulbi

TOTAL *10*

ANS: 49

A. Inverse hypopyon 2.0
B. Hyperleon 2.0
C. Silicon oil 2.0
D. Emulsified silicone oil migrating from the posterior chamber to the anterior chamber. Because silicone oil has a lower density than aqueous, it has been located in the upper portion of A/C 2.0
E. Cataractous lens and posterior synechiae seen in the eye are secondary to silicone oil-induced inflammatory reaction 2.0

TOTAL *10*

(It is a layered whitish collection in the upper portion of the anterior chamber, known as an upside-down or inverse hypopyon; suggestive of emulsified silicone oil globules. A cataractous lens and posterior synechiae seen in the eye are secondary to silicone oil-induced inflammatory reaction)

ANS: 50

A. Color fundus photography 1.0
B. CSCR 2.0
C. Male 1.5
D. Any four:
   (a) Steroid administration (including intravitreal) 1.0
   (b) Cushing syndrome 1.0
   (c) Helicobacter pylori infection 0.5
   (d) Pregnancy, psychological 0.5
   (e) Stress and 0.5
   (f) Sleep apnea syndrome. 0.5

E. Any three:
   (a) Observation 1.0
   (b) Change of lifestyle to overcome the stress 1.0
   (c) Laser.. 0.5
   (d) PDT 0.5
   (e) Anti-VEGF... 0.5
TOTAL *10*

ANS: 51
A. Laser marks, neovascularization, and hemorrhage... 3.0
B. PRP... 1.0
C. PRP is indicated to treat retinal ischemia and retinal neovascularization, from whatever cause. 1.5
D. To some extent loss of color vision, peripheral vision, and night vision 1.5
E. Indicators of regression include:
   (a) Blunting of vessel tips 1.0
   (b) Shrinking and disappearance of NV, often leaving "ghost" vessels......... 1.0
   (c) Regression of IRMA.. 1.0
   (d) Others are:
   • Decreased venous changes
   • Absorption of retinal hemorrhages
   • Disc pallor
   • Contraction of regressing vessels or associated.
TOTAL *10*

ANS: 52
A. Color fundus photography 1.0
   i. Dark red narrow, irregular lines configured in a radiating fashion from the optic disc 1.0
   ii. The radiating lines are intercommunicating around the disc 1.0
B. Angioid streaks.. 2.0
C. i. CNV... 1.5
   ii. Choroidal rupture 1.0
D. Any three:
   • Pseudoxanthoma elasticum (PXE) 1.0
   • Ehlers–Danlos syndrome.. 1.0
   • Paget disease 0.5
   • Hemoglobinopathies 0.5
TOTAL *10*

ANS: 53
A. Color fundus photography 1.0
   Positive findings are: Any two ....(1 × 2)................................... 2.0
   i. Flame-shaped and blot hemorrhages
   ii. Cotton wool spots
   iii. Venous tortuosity

B. BRVO 2.0
C.   i. Pre-proliferative diabetic retinopathy 1.0
     ii. Vasculitis retinae 1.0
D. Any four
     i. Age 1.0
     ii. Hypertension 1.0
     iii. Hyperlipidemia 0.5
     iv. Diabetes mellitus 0.5
     v. Glaucoma 0.5
     vi. Oral contraceptive pill 0.5
     vii. Smoking. 0.5
TOTAL 10

ANS: 54

A. Color fundus photograph 1
B.   i. Numerous yellow–white round, oval or pisciform lesion around the macula 2
     ii. Bull's-eye configuration at the macula 1
C. Fundus flavimaculatus/Stargardt diseases 2
D. Accumulation of lipofuscin within the RPE 1
E.   i. Impairment of central vision 1
     ii. Reduced color vision 1
     iii. Impairment of dark adaptation. 1
TOTAL 10

ANS: 55

A. *Similarity in fundus picture:*
- Scattered whitish-yellow spots, most numerous at the equator, usually sparing the macula, in upper picture 1.5
- Tiny yellow–white spots at the posterior pole sparing the fovea, in the lower picture 1.5

B. Differences:
Retinal blood vessels are attenuated and disc is pale at the upper 1.5
Retinal blood vessels and disc are normal in most cases in lower picture 1.5
C. Retinitis punctata albescens: upper picture. Fundus albipunctatus in lower picture ... 4.0
TOTAL 10

ANS: 56

A. Chloroquine 2
B. Malaria 2
C. It is reversible in early stage and irreversible in late stage 2
D. Bull's eye 2
E. Bilateral paracentral visual field changes 2
TOTAL 10

Retina and Uveal Tissue 113

ANS: 57
A. Color fundus photography 1.0
B.   i. Pale tessellated (tigroid) fundus.. 2.0
    ii. Peripapillary chorioretinal atrophy 1.5
    iii. Fuchs spot.. 1.5
C. Degenerative myopia.. 2.0
D. ....0.5 × 4.................................. 2.0
    i. Down syndrome
    ii. Stickler syndrome
    iii. Marfan syndrome
    iv. Prematurity
TOTAL *10*

ANS: 58
A. Disc swollen and retinal hemorrhage .... 1.5 + 1.0 .... 2.5
B. He thought it is a case of papilledema 1.5
C. In MRI there was no ICSOL 1.0
D. Hypertensive retinopathy 1.5
E. Measurement of blood pressure 1.0
F. ....Any three ....0.5 × 3 .... 1.5
    (a) CBC
    (b) Serum creatinine
    (c) Lipid profile
    (d) Blood sugar
G. Internist. Or nephrologists if serum creatinine is high 1.0
TOTAL *10*

ANS: 59
A. Drusen cover the macula and perimacular region 2
B. ARMD 2
C. Two types. Dry ARMD and wet ARMD 3
D. (a) Dry ARMD also called non-exudative or non-neovascular 1
    (b) Wet ARMD also called exudative, neovascular 1
E. Wet variety 1
TOTAL *10*

ANS: 60
A. Color fundus photograph 1.0
B. (a) Subretinal brownish elevated mass-like lesion 1.5
    (b) Hemorrhage 1.5
C. Melanoma 3.0
D. (a) Hemangioma 1.0
    (b) Nevus 1.0
    (c) Congenital hypertrophy of RPE 1.0
TOTAL *10*

Glaucoma

CHAPTER 4

QUESTIONS

OSPE: 1
- Uveitis-glaucoma-hyphema (UGH) syndrome
- Secondary pigmentary glaucoma
- Pseudophakic pupillary block
A. Above three types of glaucoma may develop after a surgery. Mention the name of surgery.
B. UGH syndrome is what type of glaucoma?
C. What is the condition of A/C in Pseudophakic pupillary block glaucoma?
D. What is the iris configuration in pseudophakic pupillary block glaucoma?
E. Among these 3 types glaucoma, in one group we use a medication which is contraindicated to other. Mention in which glaucoma? And which medication?

OSPE: 2

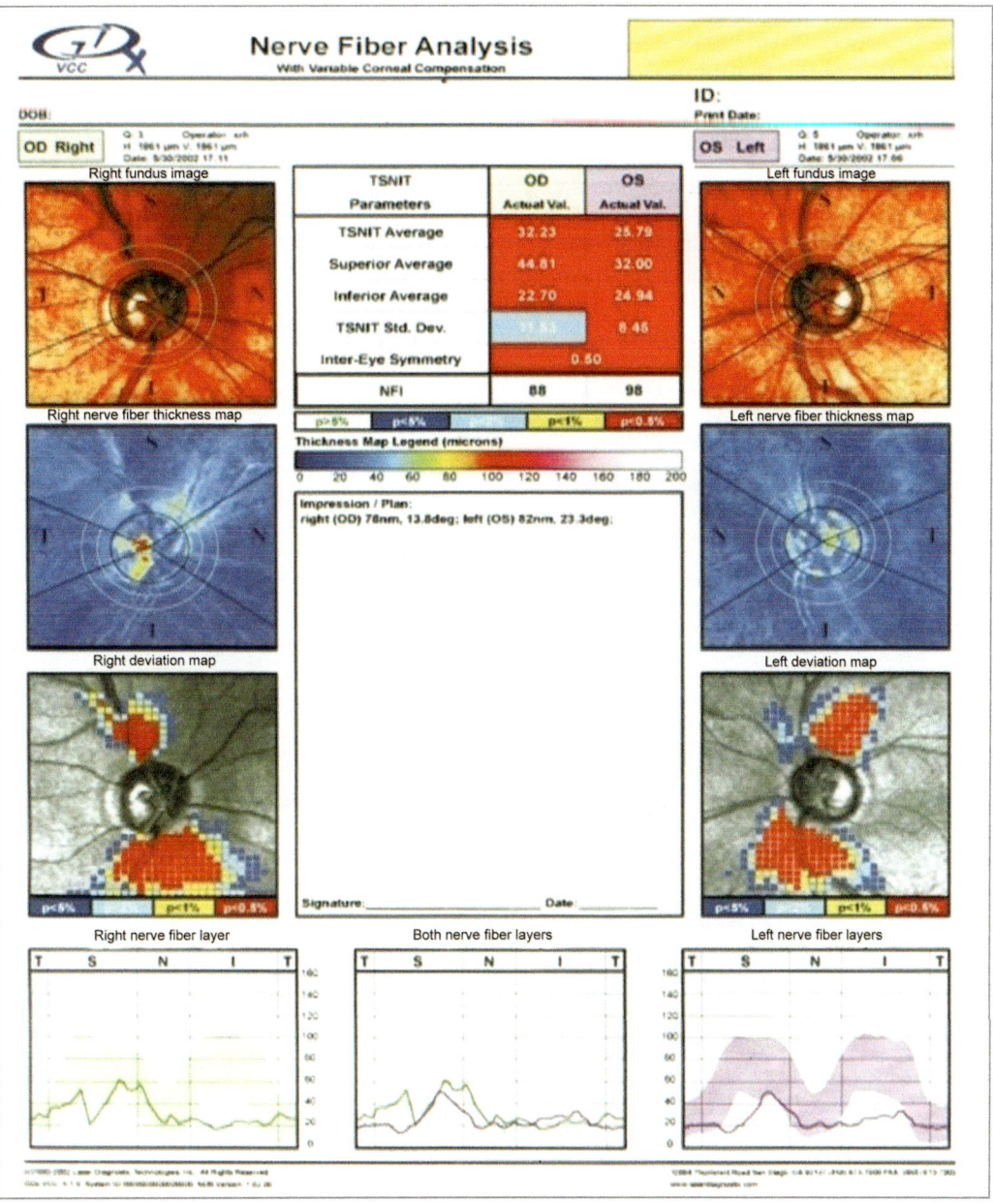

(Image Courtesy: Dr Mosharraf Hossain; NIO)

A. What is the name of the above printout?
B. Describe RNLF thickness map at here?
C. What are the abnormalities in RNFL deviation map?
D. Describe TSNIT (temporal-superior-nasal-inferior-temporal) graphs at here.
E. What is NFI (Nerve fiber indicator) and what does it indicate at here?
F. Mention two additional relevant investigations to confirm your diagnosis.

OSPE: 3

A 42-year-old lady presented with intermittent eye aches. She has shallow anterior chamber in both eyes. Her unaided distant visual acuity is 6/6 in both eyes and her near vision is N5 with +1.25 Dsph lens in both eyes. On slit-lamp examination, anterior segment normal. For proper management:

A. Mention three relevant clinical tests.
B. Mention one important investigation for anterior segment.
C. Name three differential diagnoses.
D. Mention three treatment options.

OSPE: 4

A. Who is more prone to develop glaucoma and who is the least
   Patient (a) has IOP >23.75 to ≤ 25.75 mm Hg and CCT > 555 to ≤ 588 μm.
   Patient (b) has mean IOP 21.0 to 23.75 mm Hg but CCT ≤ 555 μm
   Patient (c) vertical C/D ratio ≥ 0.50 CCT ≤ 555 μm
B. Mention one corneal diseases where IOP is usually below 10 mm Hg

OSPE: 5

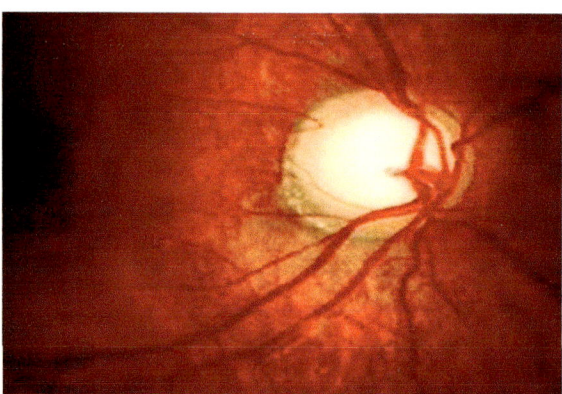

(Image Courtesy: Dr Iftekhar Mohammad Munir, NIO)

A. What are the disc findings present here? Mention 3
B. Write 3 differential diagnosis depend upon findings
C. Write the name of 4 investigations for clinical diagnosis

Glaucoma

OSPE: 6

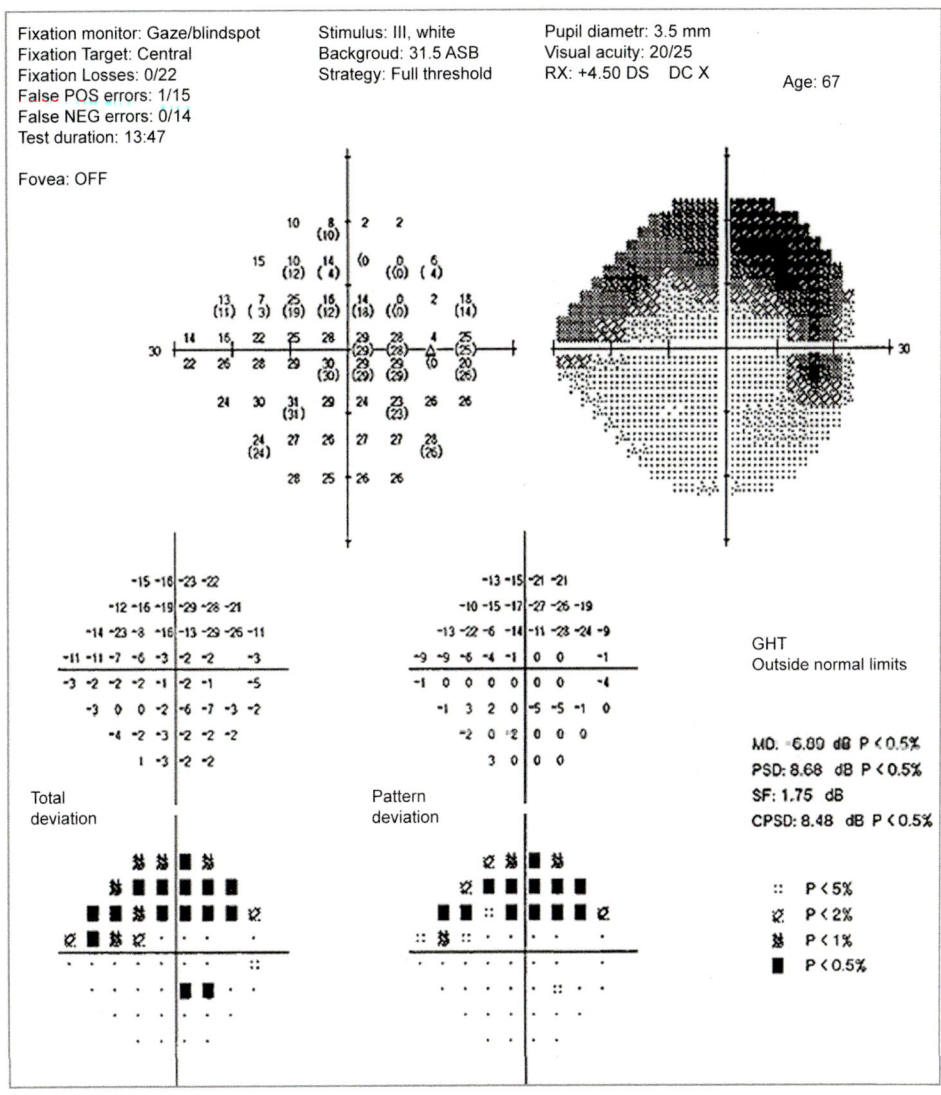

(Image Courtesy: Dr Mosharraf Hossain, NIO)

This is the Humphrey visual field of a 67-year-old woman.
A. What type of perimetry is a Humphrey field analyzer?
B. What does the total deviation measure?
C. What is the pattern deviation?
D. What does the visual field show?
E. List three conditions, which may give this field defect.

OSPE: 7

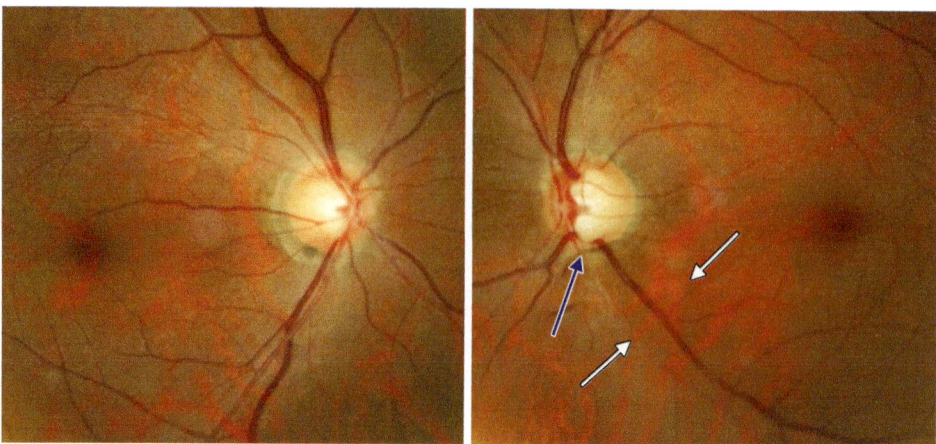

A 69-year-old female presents with intraocular pressure of 15 OD and 14 OS and the fundus appearance is as shown above. He is getting no topical eye drop, or systematic medication.
A. What is your probable diagnosis?
B. Mention two differential diagnoses.
C. What are signs shown by blue and white arrow?

OSPE: 8

A lady of 45-year-old presented with the complaint of sudden loss of vision (one eye) with severe headache, nausea, and vomiting. Slit-lamp examination shows corneal edema, pupil is mid-dilated and vertically oval, there is no light reaction.
A. What is your probable diagnosis?
B. Which systemic condition may mimic with her condition. Mention two.
C. Is it an ocular emergency?
D. What may be the treatment?

OSPE: 9

It is called "silent thief of sight," and is generally bilateral disease of adult onset, it affects both sexes equally. Cell deaths occur predominantly through apoptosis rather than necrosis.
A. What is the name of the disease?
B. What are the risk factors of the disease? Mention 4.
C. What are the routine screening eye examination tests to diagnose the disease?
D. What are end-stage changes in visual field?

OSPE: 10

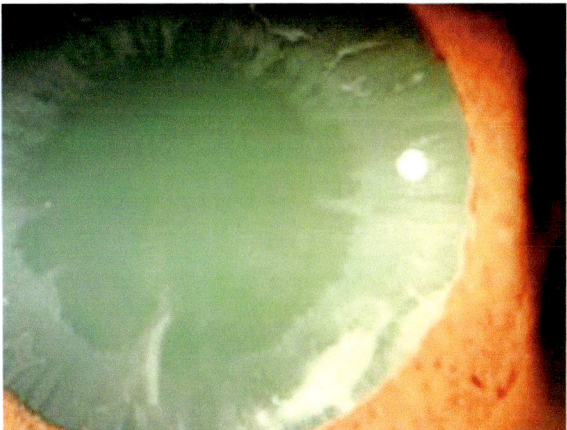

This is the slit-lamp view (pupil is dilated with Atropine 1% eye drop) of right eye of a lady of 70-year-old (housewife), who is also suffering from Alzheimer's disease.
A. What are the slit-lamp findings?
B. What are the compositions of the fibrillin materials?
C. In spite of ocular tissue, mention two other extraocular site where you will get this change.
D. What type of glaucoma it may cause?
E. Why should you face problem during cataract surgery of this lady? Mention 3.

OSPE: 11

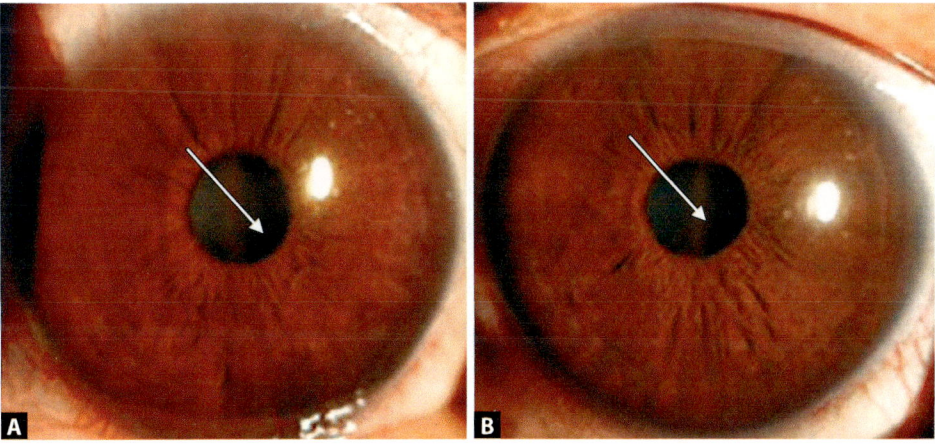

This is the slit-lamp view of both eyes of a patient 43-year-old who came to you for routine follow-up. On slit-lamp examination you got the above appearance of both eyes.
A. What is the specific name of the vertical line? (Arrow given)
B. If this deposition found anterior to the Schwalbe line, what is the name?
C. What other clinical findings should you look for? Mention: 3
D. If your clinical findings are normal should you follow-up this patient and why?

OSPE: 12

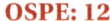

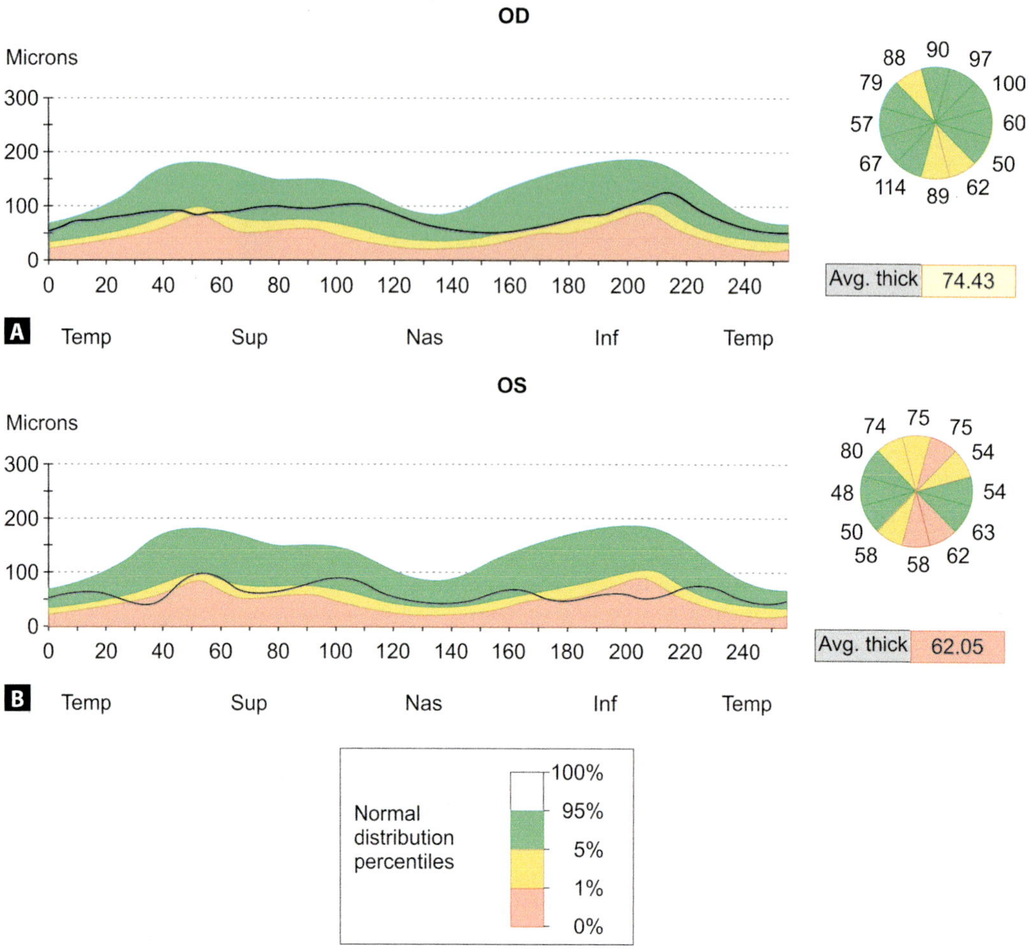

If your clinical findings are within normal limit should you follow up this patient? Explain.
A. What is the name of the above tracing?
B. What are the positive findings at here?
C. What is the average thickness of the nerve layers in right and left eye?
D. What is your diagnosis?
E. What ocular clinical test and investigation you should do for diagnosis?

OSPE: 13

A lady of 60-year-old came to you with the complaints of lengthening, thickening and hyperpigmentation of eyelashes, after using an eye drop for 6 months. Overdose of this drop may causes raised of intraocular pressure.
A. What is the name of the eye drop?
B. In which disease, it is used?

C. What is the mechanism action?
D. What is its dose schedule?
E. Mention name of 4 eye drops of this group.
F. If there is no side effect, you have to stop the medication before cataract surgery
G. Which hyperpigmentation is reversible and which is not?

OSPE: 14

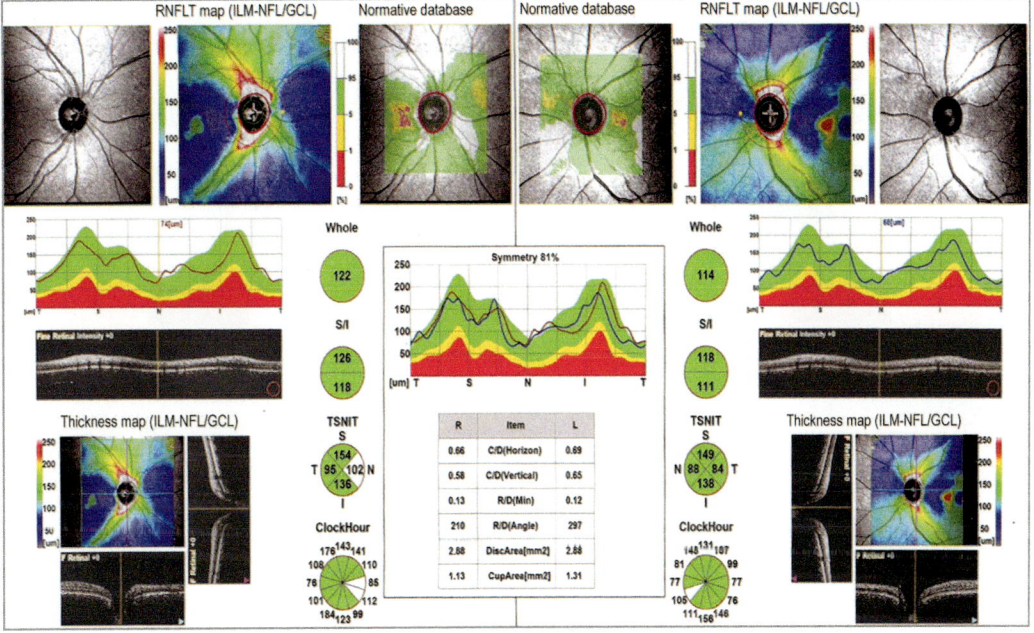

(Image Courtesy: Dr Shams Md Noman, Chittagong Eye Infirmary and Training Complex of BNSB)

A. What is the name of the tracing paper?
B. What is about RNFL thickness map?
C. What is about RNFL deviation map?
D. What is about TSNIT map?
E. What is about color code?
F. What is your conclusion?

OSPE: 15

A. What is the name of the tracing paper?
B. What is about RNFL thickness map in both eyes?
C. What is about RNFL deviation map in both eyes
D. What is about TSNIT curve in both eyes?
E. What is about four quadrants in both eyes
F. What is your diagnosis?

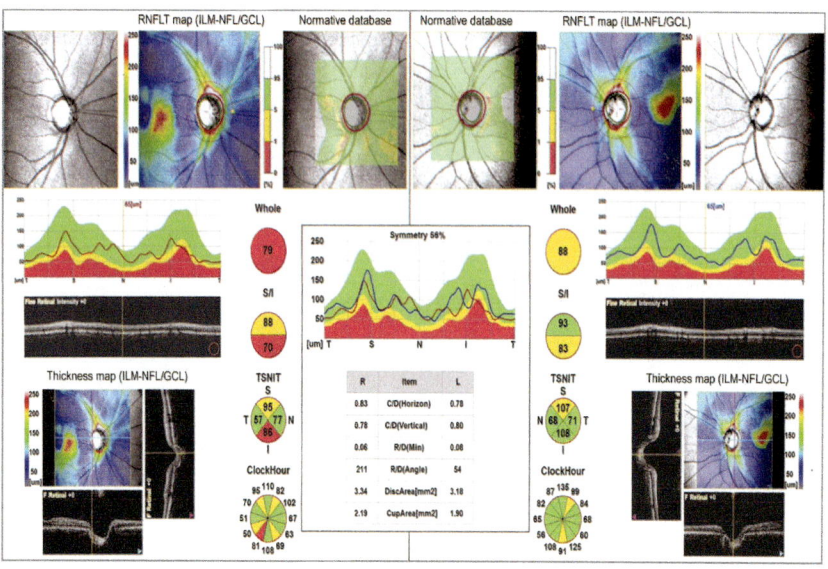

(Image Courtesy: Dr Shams Md Noman, Chittagong Eye Infirmary and Training Complex of BNSB)

OSPE: 16

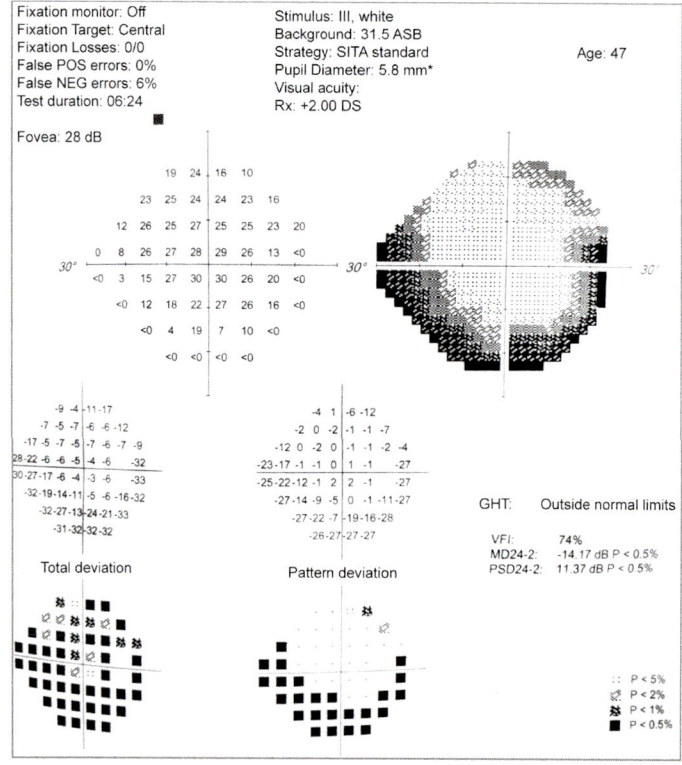

(Image Courtesy: Dr Bipul Kumer De Sarker, Islamia Eye Institute and Hospital)

A. What is the testing pattern at here?
B. What other testing pattern at there?
C. Which pattern we like for glaucoma?
D. What is the field defect at here?
E. What is your diagnosis at there?
F. If the diseases progress, what will be the next finding?

OSPE: 17

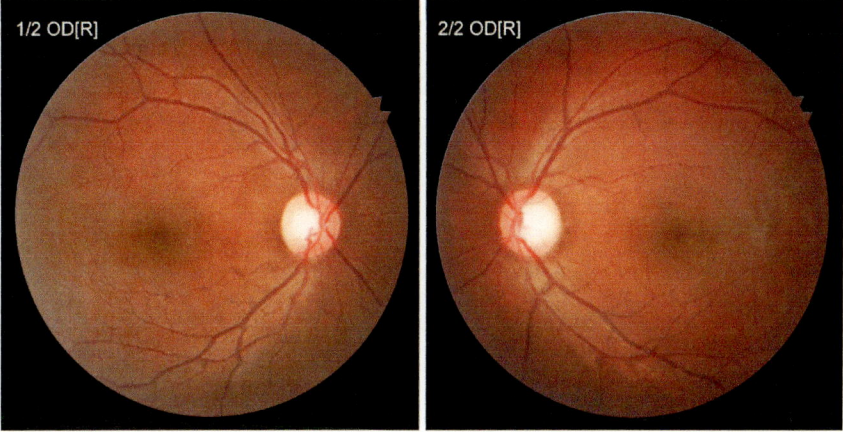

(Image Courtesy: Green Eye Hospital, Dhaka)

This is the investigation report of a patient of 56 year-old, who came to with the complaints of frequent change of presbyopic glass. He is nondiabetics but hypertensive.
A. What is the name of above investigation?
B. What is your probable diagnosis?
C. What are the positive findings in the picture in favor of your diagnosis?
D. What other investigations you have to do for your diagnosis? Mention: 2 clinical and 2 laboratory investigations.

OSPE: 18

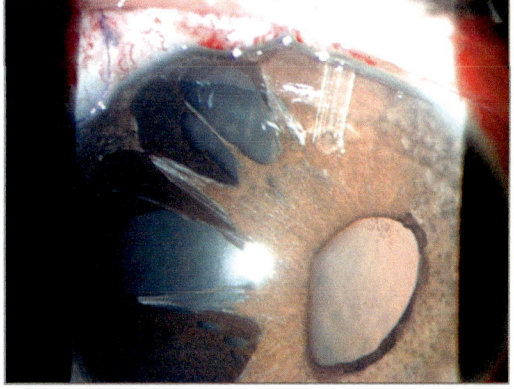

(Image Courtesy: Dr Ishtiaque Anwar, Bangladesh Eye Hospital)

A. What are the positive findings? Mention 2.
B. What is your diagnosis?
C. What is the name of the tube at upper limbus?
D. Why it is at here?
E. What is the indication of the tube?

OSPE: 19

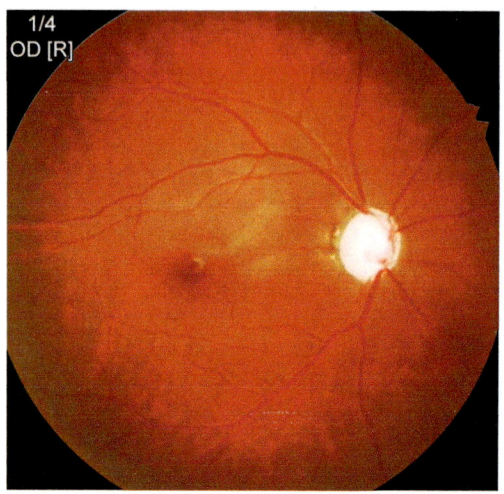

(Image Courtesy: Green Eye Hospital, Dhaka)

This is the fundus photograph of both eyes of a man of 24-year-old. His visual acuity is 6/60 of right eye and 3/60 of left eye. In his teen, he was suffering from vernal keratoconjunctivitis (VKC) and used some eye drop for a long time, but forgot the name of the eye drop.

A. What is your probable diagnosis?
B. Which eye drop he used?
C. What may be cause?
D. How will you treat this case? Mention: 3.
E. What will be the visual field?

OSPE: 20

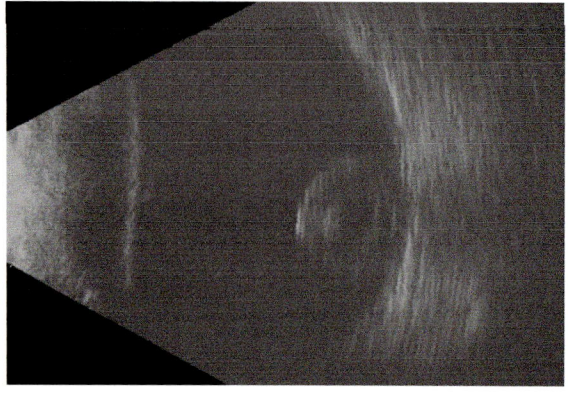

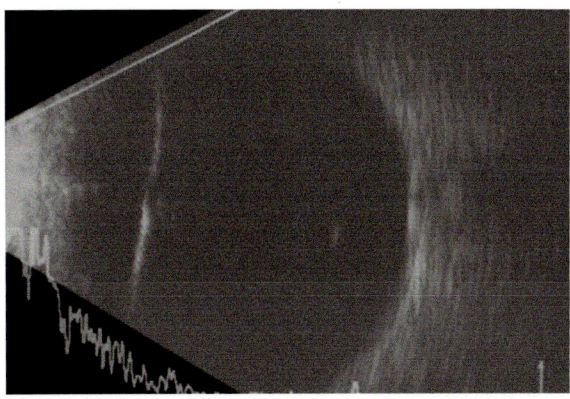

Images 1 and 2. These are ultrasounds from a 56-year-old man with history of congenital glaucoma OU and diabetes since 1999, who presents with VA: OD: PL and OS: NPL. Ocular tension is 13 OU. Anterior segment shows band keratopathy OU and mature cataract OS. Ultrasound was requested to evaluate the posterior pole OD.
A. Mention 2 positive findings in B Scan (Both are horizontal views)
B. What is the most likely diagnosis and the differential diagnosis?
C. Why is important to have kinetic studies in this case?
D. What is the axial length and is it consistent with the patient's ocular history?
E. What other medical history may be important for this diagnosis?

ANSWERS

OSPE: 01. Uveitis-glaucoma-hyphema (UGH) syndrome
OSPE: 02. GDx printout for RNFL analysis
OSPE: 03. Angle closure suspect
OSPE: 04. Who is prone to develop glaucoma and who is the least?
OSPE: 05. Optical disk
OSPE: 06. Humphrey field analyzer
OSPE: 07. Normotensive glaucoma
OSPE: 08. Acute congestive angle-closure glaucoma
OSPE: 09. Silent thief of sight
OSPE: 10. Pseudoexfoliation syndrome (PXF)
OSPE: 11. Krukenberg's spindle
OSPE: 12. OCT (optic nerve fibers) protocol
OSPE: 13. Prostaglandin analogue
OSPE: 14. OCT optic nerve head and RNFL of BE
OSPE: 15. Right eye: Glaucomatous change present. Left eye: Borderline glaucomatous change
OSPE: 16. Inferior arcuate scotoma
OSPE: 17. Open-angle glaucoma
OSPE: 18. Axenfeld–Rieger anomaly
OSPE: 19. Steroid-induced glaucoma
OSPE: 20. Congenital glaucoma

ANS: 01

A.	Cataract surgery	2.0
B.	Secondary, inflammatory .... 1 + 1	2.0
C.	Shallow	2.0
D.	Iris bombe	2.0
E.	Pseudophakic pupillary block...Atropine .... 1 + 1	2.0
	TOTAL	**10**

ANS: 02

A.	GDx printout for RNFL analysis of both eyes	1.0
B.	Absence of warm colors (red and yellow) in both eyes, more in left eye, is indicating thinning/loss of RNFL	2.0
C.	Appearance of square pixels in superior and inferior quadrants of both eyes	2.0
D.	(a) Double hump patterns of TSNIT graphs are absent	1.0
	(b) Graphs are flat	0.5
	(c) Inferior humps are more flat	0.5
E.	Nerve fiber indicator, it is a Global index ranging from 1 to 100	0.5
	(a) 1–30 indicates normal RNFL thickness	0.5
	(b) 31–50 indicates borderline	0.5
	(c) 51–100 indicates thinning of RNFL	0.5
F.	(a) Digital optic disk photography	0.5
	(b) SAP (HVFA/octopus VFA)	0.5
	TOTAL	**10**

ANS: 03

A. .... 1 × 3 3
    (a) Measurement of IOP
    (b) Gonioscopy
    (c) Examination of optic nerve head (ONH) and peripapillary nerve fiber layer
B. UBM/AS-OCT 1
C. .... 1 × 3 3
    (a) Primary angle-closure suspect (PACS)
    (b) Primary angle closure (PAC)
    (c) Primary angle-closure glaucoma (PACG)
D. .... 1 × 3 3
    (a) Anti-glaucoma drugs/Pilocarpine 2%
    (b) Laser peripheral iridotomy (LPI)
    (c) Trabeculectomy
TOTAL ***10***

ANS: 04

A. Patient C is more prone to develop glaucoma and patient A is least prone to develop glaucoma .... 2 × 4 8
B. Keratoconus 2
TOTAL ***10***

ANS: 05

A. ....(Any three) .... 1 × 3 3
    (a) Increased CDR
    (b) Narrow neuroretinal rim (NRR)
    (c) Peripapillary atrophy (PPA)
    (d) Vascular signs
B. .... 1 × 3 3
    (a) Suspicious disk
    (b) Physiological cup
    (c) Glaucomatous cupping
C. ....(Any four) .... 1 × 4 4
    (a) IOP
    (b) CCT
    (c) VFA
    (d) OCT
    (e) HRT
TOTAL ***10***

ANS: 06

A. Humphrey field analyzer is a static automated perimetry 2
B. The total deviation measures the difference (in dB) between the patient's threshold values and that of the age-corrected values 2
C. The pattern deviation adjusts the total deviation for any shift in the patient's overall sensitivity. This allows localized area of field loss to be clearly demonstrated 2

D. Superior arcuate scotoma 1
E.   i. Open angle glaucoma with inferior loss of arcuate nerve fiber layer 1
    ii. Optic disk pit 1
    iii. Inferior branch retinal vein occlusion 1
TOTAL **10**

Explanation:

A. Humphrey field analyzer is a static automated perimetry (In this test, the patient maintains fixation on a central target and the computer randomly presents a brief [about 0.2 seconds] and non-moving, i.e. static light stimulus at different loci throughout the visual field. The intensity of the light stimulus that the patient can see is then recorded).

B. The total deviation measures the difference (in dB) between the patient's threshold values and that of the age-corrected values.

C. The pattern deviation adjusts the total deviation for any shift in the patient's overall sensitivity. This allows localized area of field loss to be clearly demonstrated (Many conditions other than glaucoma can cause poor vision, for example cataract or corneal edema. Therefore, to find out how much of a patient's relative insensitivity to light is due to glaucoma rather than to something else, it is important to "subtract out" these other factors. This can be done because these other conditions tend to produce a similar pattern of diffuse visual field loss, while glaucoma tends to produce localized areas of visual field loss).

D. Superior arcuate scotoma.

E. Open angle glaucoma with inferior loss of arcuate nerve fiber layer. Optic disc pit Inferior branch retinal vein occlusion (Visual field should not be interpreted without reference to ocular examination. An arcuate scotoma can occur in conditions other than open angle glaucoma as mentioned above).

ANS: 07

A. Normotensive glaucoma 3
B.   i. Physiological cupping 1.5
    ii. Normal fundus 1.5
C. The bayoneting and thinning of the inferior optic nerve rim (blue arrow) and the nerve fiber layer defect (white arrows) are .... 1.5+1.5+1 .... 4.0
TOTAL **10**

ANS: 08

A. Acute congestive angle-closure glaucoma 3.0
B. .... 1.5 × 2 .... 3.0
    i. Acute abdomen, and
    ii. Intracranial space-occupying lesion
C. Yes 1.0
D. .... 1 + 1 + 1 .... 3.0
    (a) Treatment is surgical, before that IOP should be control with Tab Acetazolamide and Inj Mannitol.
    (b) And then go for peripheral iridectomy (P,I) or trabeculectomy according to synechiae.
    (c) Fellow eye should have treated with laser PI or Pilocarpine 2% eye drop
TOTAL **10**

Glaucoma

ANS: 09
A. Primary open-angle glaucoma (POAG) 3.0
B. Any three
   (a) IOP 1.0
   (b) Age 1.0
   (c) Race 1.0
   (d) Family history of POAG 1.0
   (e) Diabetes mellitus 0.5
C. For routine screening, following test should be included:
   (a) Visual field examination 1.0
   (b) Tonometry 1.0
   (c) Ophthalmoscopy 0.5
D. Changes are characterized by:
   (a) A small island of central vision 1.0
   (b) Accompanied by a temporal island 0.5
TOTAL 10

ANS: 10
A. Deposits of white material on the anterior lens surface 2.0
B. It is a gray-white fibrillary amyloid-like material 1.5
C. PXF has been found in skin and visceral organs .... 1 + 1 .... 2.0
D. Chronic open-angle glaucoma 1.5
E. There is a higher risk of complications, due to: .... 1 × 3 .... 3.0
   (a) Poor mydriasis
   (b) Increased fragility of the zonule and lens capsule, and
   (c) Endothelial deficiency
TOTAL 10

ANS: 11
A. Krukenberg's spindle 2.0
B. Sampaolesi line 1.5
C. .... 1.5 × 3 .... 4.5
   i. IOP
   ii. C/D ratio
   iii. Gonioscopy
D. Yes, because there is a chance of development of pigmentary glaucoma .... 0.5 + 1.5 .... 2.0
TOTAL 10

ANS: 12
A. This is the OCT (optic nerve fibers) protocol .... 1.5 + 0.5 .... 2.0
B. (a) Both eyes have lost double hump pattern (more in left) 1.0
   (b) The ISNT rule of RNFL distribution is broken. As there is thinning of inferior and superior quadrants of both eyes (more in left eye) 1.0
C. Right eye shows loss of nerve fiber layer with an average thickness of 74.43 microns. Left eye shows more substantial loss of nerve fiber layer with an average thickness of 62.05 microns 2.0

D. The probable diagnosis is POAG...1.0
E. • *Ocular test*................................3 × 0.5 ....1.5
       i. IOP
       ii. C/D ratio
       iii. Gonioscopy
   • Ocular investigation................................3 × 0.5..1.5
       i. Color fundus photo
       ii. VFA
       iii. AC-OCT
TOTAL...*10*

ANS: 13

A. Prostaglandin analogue..2.5
B. Glaucoma 2.0
C. Enhancement of uveoscleral aqueous outflow, although increased trabecular outflow facility 1.5
D. Once in a day
E. 2.0
       i. Latanoprost
       ii. Travoprost
       iii. Bimatoprost
       iv. Tafluprost
F. To prevent cystoid macular edema 1.0
G. Hyperpigmentation of periocular skin is common but reversible. Irreversible iris hyperpigmentation 1.0
TOTAL...*10*

ANS: 14

A. The name of the tracing paper is OCT optic nerve head and RNFL of BE....................2.0
B. RNFL thickness map normal...1.5
C. RNFL deviation map normal..1.5
D. TSNIT curve shows well maintained of double hump pattern 2.0
E. The four quadrants show green color and clock hour map also shows green color...2.0
F. Normal OCT of ONH and RNFL...1.0
TOTAL...*10*

ANS: 15

A. The name of the tracing paper is OCT retinal nerve fiber layer of both eyes 2.0
B. RNFL thickness map: Disappearance of warm colors of both eyes 1.0
C. RNFL deviation map: Appearance of warm colors of both eyes 1.0
D. .... 1 × 2 ....2.0
   • TSNIT curve of RE shows double hump pattern lost and Inferiorly it touches the red color
   • TSNIT curve of RE shows partially lost of double hump pattern and Inferiorly it touches the yellow line

Glaucoma

E. .... 1 × 2 .... 2.0
- Right eye: Four quadrants show inferior red color and clock hours' map shows three clock thinning.
- Left eye: Four quadrants show superior and inferior yellow color and clock hours show yellow color.

F. .... 1 × 2 .... 2.0
- Right eye: Glaucomatous change is present
- Left eye: Borderline glaucomatous change is present

TOTAL 10

ANS: 16

A. 24–2 2
B. (a) 30–2 1
   (b) 10–2 1
C. 24–2 1
D. Inferior arcuate scotoma 2
E. POAG 2
F. Ring scotoma 1

TOTAL 10

ANS: 17

A. CFP 1.0
B. Open-angle glaucoma 2.0
C. i. C/D ratio is more in L/E than that of R/E and difference is more than 2, so it is in favor of glaucoma 2.0
   ii. Blood vessels are nasally shifted in B/E 1.5
   iii. Neuroretinal rim is thin nasally in B/E 1.5
D. .... 0.5 × 4 .... 2.0
   Clinical investigation:
   - Measurement of IOP
   - Gonioscopy to assess angle structure
   Laboratory investigation:
   - Visual field analysis
   - OCT (RNFL protocol)

TOTAL 10

ANS: 18

A. - Corectopia and full-thickness iris defects—pseudopolycoria 3
   - Upper limbus shows a tube is protruding 1
B. Axenfeld–Rieger anomaly 3
C. One end of glaucoma shunt 1
D. To drain aqueous 1
E. Intractable glaucoma 1

TOTAL 10

ANS: 19

A.	Steroid-induced glaucoma	2
B.	Steroid group of eye drops	2
C.	Injudicious use of steroid	2
D.	• Stop steroid eye drop	1
	• Antiglaucoma eye drop	1
	• Trabeculectomy	1
E.	Tubular field of vision	1
TOTAL		**10**

ANS: 20

A. Any two:
  (a) A large globe with normal contour 1.0
  (b) Aphakia 1.0
B. Most likely diagnosis is:
  • An echogenic round mobile structure within the vitreous cavity 1.0
  Differential diagnosis:
  • Choroidal melanoma 1.0
  • Intraocular foreign body 1.0
C. By kinetic studies we can make a difference between a tumor and luxated lens 1.0
D. (a) Axial length is approximately 30 mm 1.0
  (b) Past history of congenital glaucoma and is consistent with the diagnosis of buphthalmos 1.0
E. (a) History of trauma 0.5
  (b) Marfan's syndrome 0.5
  (c) Homocystinuria 0.5
  (d) Weill–Marchesani syndrome 0.5

TOTAL 10

Explanation: The ultrasound shows a large globe with normal contour. There is no obvious lens or posterior capsule within the iris plane. There are low-reflective vitreous echoes. The retinochoroidal layer is attached without presence of mass lesion. There is an echogenic round mobile structure within the vitreous cavity with acoustically irregular internal structure.

This is likely a cataractous lens in the vitreous of a buphthalmic eye. But, this image may be mistaken for a tumor of the retinochoroidal such as a choroidal melanoma; and if there is as history of trauma, it may be mistaken for an intraocular foreign body.

Kinetic studies will be helpful in the differentiation between a tumor and luxated lens. An immobile mass would be more consistent with a tumor; however, immobile adherent lenses can also be seen.

The axial length is approximately 30 mm, which is expected from the past history of congenital glaucoma and is consistent with the diagnosis of buphthalmos.

A dislocated lens can be seen in a variety of conditions such as trauma, Marfan's syndrome, homocystinuria, Weill–Marchesani syndrome, syphilis, and retinitis pigmentosa, so it is important to obtain a thorough medical history.

CHAPTER 5

Neuro-ophthalmology

QUESTIONS

OSPE: 01
A patient came to you with the complaints of binocular horizontal diplopia, worse for distance than near, most pronounced in the direction of paretic muscle.
A. What is your probable diagnosis?
B. What may be the causes?
C. In the same case, child does not suffer from double vision. Why?
D. What may be the cause in case of children?

OSPE: 02
A lady of 30-year-old came to you with the complaints of sudden loss of vision of right eye for 3 days, she also complains colored flushes of light in front of the eye and there is feeling of discomfort during ocular movements associated with frontal headache.
On examination:
- VAR: 6/36, VAL: 6/9 (not improved with pin hole)
- Pupillary light reflex: RAPD is present
- *Fundus:* Normal in right eye, and temporal pallor in left eye

A. What is your probable diagnosis?
B. Which systemic diseases you may think first
C. Why temporal pallor in opposite eye?
D. What positive findings you may get in visual field analysis? Mention 3.

OSPE: 03
A child of 3-year-old developed fever after schedule immunization, after two weeks of immunization the child developed sudden loss of vision both eyes.
A. What may be the cause?
B. What is the usual prognosis?
C. When she/he needs treatment?
D. Mention name of two drugs to treat.

OSPE: 04

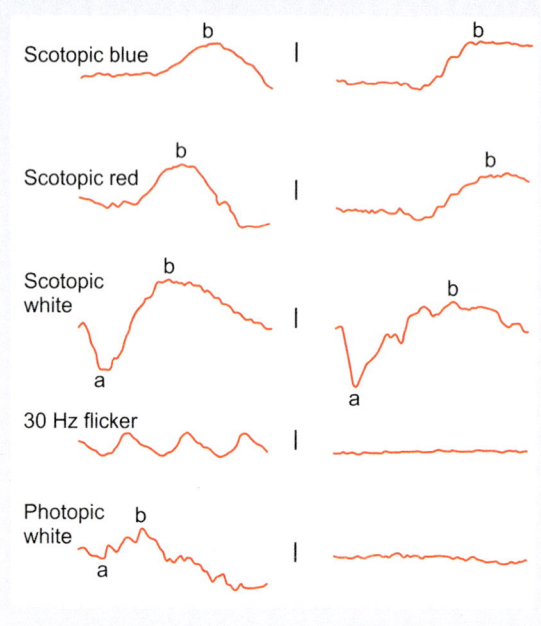

A. What is the name of this tracing?
B. What looks like a normal pattern in this tracing?
C. What it indicates here "a" wave?
D. What it indicates here "b" wave?
E. What is your diagnosis at here?

OSPE: 05

A 40-year-old obese lady complains of transient loss of vision. Examination reveals Best Corrected Visual Acuity (BCVA) 6/6 and disc swelling in both eyes.
A. What is the provisional diagnosis?
B. Name 3 differential diagnoses.
C. Name 4 investigations to confirm the diagnosis.

OSPE: 06

It is an autosomal-dominant disease with irregular penetrance and variable expressivity. It forms a characteristic S-shaped deformity of the upper eyelid. It affects 2.5/10,000 individuals. They develop anywhere along the course of the peripheral and autonomic nerves, but do not occur on purely motor nerve.
A. What is your probable diagnosis?
B. What is the other name of the disease?
C. What is the feeling by hand of the S-shaped deformity of the upper lid?
D. What change will you get in cornea?
E. How many types of this disease are? And what are their names?

Neuro-ophthalmology

OSPE: 07

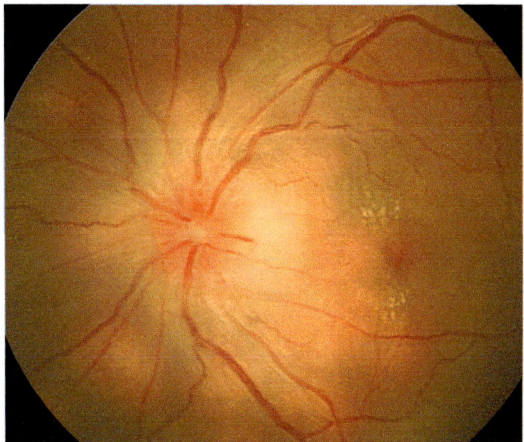

A. Mention two positive findings.
B. What is your provisional diagnosis?
C. Write three causes of this condition.
D. Write two ocular investigations.
E. What is the prognosis of this condition?

OSPE: 08

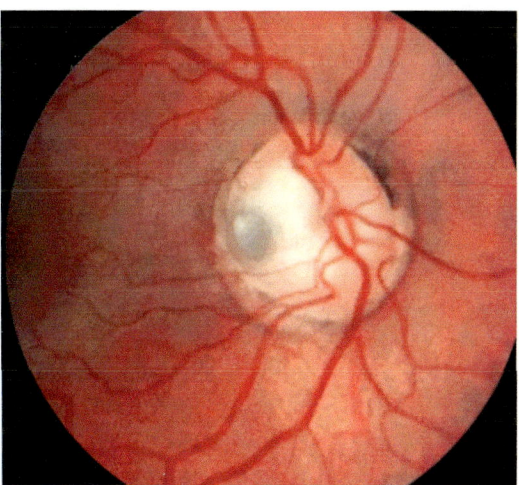

A. What does the picture show?
B. What may be the diagnosis?
C. What is the anomaly in intrauterine life to develop this?
D. What is the significance of this case?

OSPE: 09

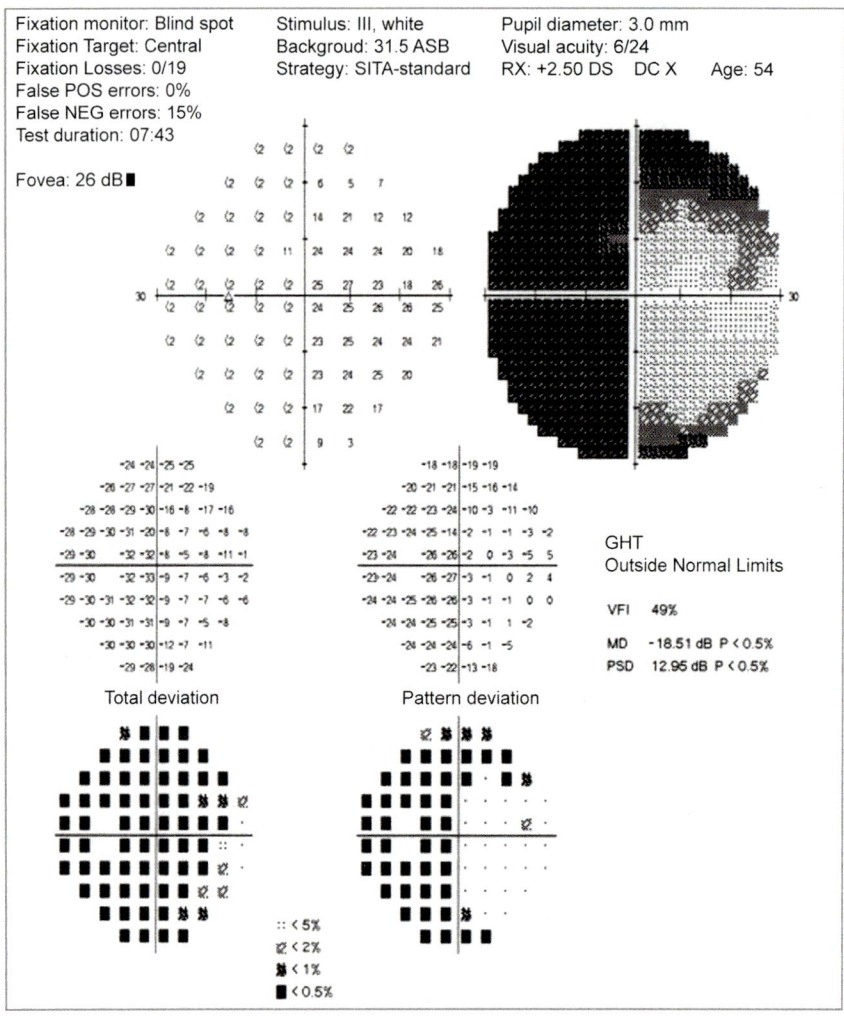

Neuro-ophthalmology

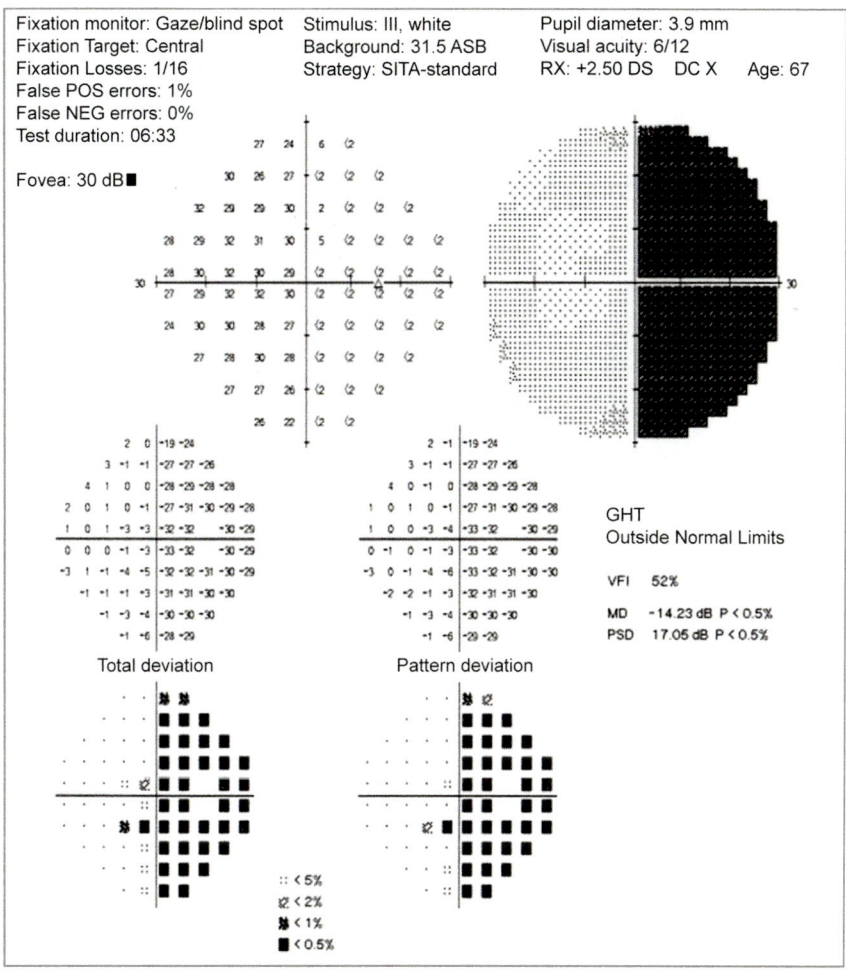

(Image Courtesy: Dr Bipul Kumer De Sarker, Islamia Eye Institute and Hospital)

This is the Humphrey visual analysis of both eyes of a patient 67 years' old who came to you for the treatment of headache with some unexplained visual defect. When you asked him go through the Snellen's chart he missed some letters at the periphery of the row. He also complains frequently bumps into objects like door-frames or people and fear or anxiety in walking through unfamiliar areas.

A. What shows the visual field analysis?
B. What may be the most common probable cause?
C. What are the differential diagnoses?
D. Is this a heteronymous hemianopia?
E. To whom you should refer the patient?
F. What will be the role of an ophthalmologist?

OSPE: 10

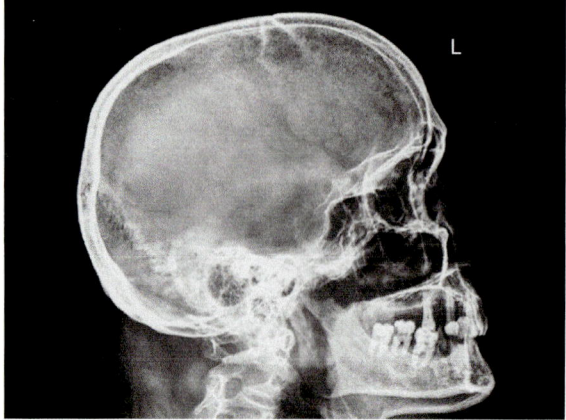

Look at the X-ray film and answer the following questions:
1. What type of X-ray is this?
2. Which view it shows?
3. What are other investigations which you have to do for diagnosis?
4. If the patient complains of double vision, what may be the cause?
5. If there is presence of nystagmus, what type of nystagmus it is?
6. Mention three differential diagnoses.

OSPE: 11

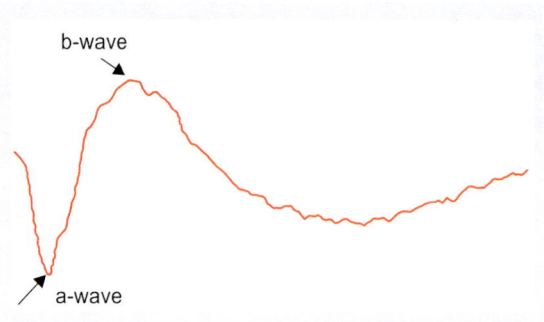

A. What is the name of this tracing?
B. What it measures?
C. What it indicates here "a" wave?
D. What it indicates here "b" wave?

OSPE: 12

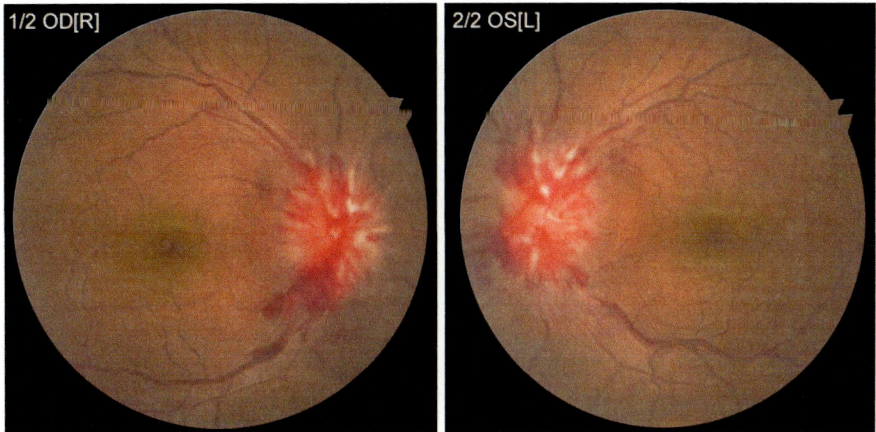

(Image Courtesy: Green Eye Hospital, Dhaka)

A. What are the signs you can get from this picture?
B. What is your diagnosis?
C. What may be the cause?
D. Mention an important differential diagnosis.
E. What is visual field?

ANSWERS

OSPE: 01. 6th cranial nerve palsy
OSPE: 02. Retrobulbar neuritis
OSPE: 03. Postimmunization optic neuritis
OSPE: 04. Electroretinogram (ERG)
OSPE: 05. IIH
OSPE: 06. Neurofibroma
OSPE: 07. Disc swelling
OSPE: 08. Optic disc pit
OSPE: 09. Bitemporal visual field defect
OSPE: 10. Plain X-ray of orbit
OSPE: 11. Ocular electroretinogram
OSPE: 12. Papilloedema

ANS: 01

A.	6th cranial nerve palsy	3.0
B.	Any three	
	(a) Diabetes	1.0
	(b) Hypertension	1.0
	(c) Atherosclerosis	1.0
	(d) Trauma	0.5
	(e) Idiopathic	0.5
C.	Due to suppression	2.0
D.	(a) Traumatic	1.0
	(b) Neoplastic	1.0
TOTAL		**10**

ANS: 02

A.	Retrobulbar neuritis	3.0
B.	MS	2.0
C.	Previous attack of optic neuritis	2.0
D.	(a) Decreased sensitivity in central 30 degree	1.0
	(b) Altitudinal/Arcuate scotoma	1.0
	(c) Central/Centrocecal scotoma	1.0
TOTAL		**10**

ANS: 03

A.	Postimmunization optic neuritis	3.0
B.	It is usually self-limiting	3.0
C.	(a) When visual loss is severe and bilateral	1.0
	(b) When there is involvement of only seeing eye	1.0
D.	(a) Intravenous steroid	1.0
	(b) Systemic antiviral	1.0
TOTAL		**10**

Neuro-ophthalmology

ANS: 04
A. Electroretinogram (ERG) 2.0
B. The normal ERG is predominantly biphasic 2.0
C. The a-wave indicates-negative deflection generated by the photoreceptors 2.0
D. The b-wave is a slower + large amplitude deflection. It is generated from Müller and bipolar cells 2.0
E. Here, left one is normal finding. And right shows cone dystrophy 2.0
TOTAL **10**

ANS: 05
A. IIH 2.0
B. (a) ICSOL 1.5
    (b) Malignant hypertension 1.5
    (c) Diabetic papillopathy 1.0
C. .... 1 × 4 .... 4.0
    (a) CT/MRI of brain
    (b) Blood sugar
    (c) Blood pressure
    (d) CSF study
TOTAL **10**

(*Courtesy:* Dr Md Lutfor Rahman, Assoc Prof. Neuro-ophthalmology)

ANS: 06
A. Neurofibroma 3.0
B. Van Recklinghausen 1.0
C. Bag of worm 1.5
D. Prominent corneal nerve 1.5
E. 2 types 1.0
    (a) Neurofibromatosis type: 1 and 0.5
    (b) Neurofibromatosis type: 2 .... 0.5
TOTAL **10**

ANS: 07
A. (a) Disc swelling 1.0
    (b) Macular star 1.0
B. Neuroretinitis 2.0
C. .... 1 × 3 .... 3.0
    (a) Idiopathic
    (b) Syphilis
    (c) Lyme disease, mumps
D. .... 1 × 2 .... 2.0
    (a) OCT (Optic nerve protocol)
    (b) FFA
E. Normal or near normal VA within 6–12 months 1.0
TOTAL **10**

ANS: 08

A. Focal depression on the temporal aspect of the optic disc 2.5
B. Optic disc pit 2.5
C. The pit is thought to arise from incomplete closure of the superior end of the embryonic fissure 2.5
D. The most important significance is serous retinal detachment 2.5
TOTAL **10**

ANS: 09

A. Bitemporal visual field defect 2.0
B. Pituitary adenoma 2.0
C. (a) Craniopharyngioma 1.0
   (b) Aneurysm in the anterior communicating artery 1.0
D. No 1.0
E. Neurosurgeon 1.0
F. .... 1 × 2 .... 2.0
   (a) Pituitary adenoma can ophthalmologist will do the visual field regularly to check the progression
   (b) The first sign of recurrence may be visual loss; therefore, baseline visual fields and visual acuity testing are recommended 2–3 months after treatment and at intervals of 6–12 months afterwards.
TOTAL **10**

ANS: 10

1. Plain X-ray 1.5
2. Lateral view 1.5
3. CT/MRI of brain 1.5
4. The diplopia is due to bitemporal hemianopia causing hemifield slips 1.5
5. See-saw nystagmus is the classical sign but rarely observed 1.0
6. (Any 3) .... 1 × 3 .... 3.0
   (a) Pituitary macroadenoma
   (b) Craniopharyngioma
   (c) Meningioma
   (d) Glioma
TOTAL **10**

ANS: 11

A. Ocular electroretinogram 2
B. It measures retinal electrical activity 2
C. The a-wave is an initial first corneal-negative deflection generated by the photoreceptors 3
D. The b-wave is a subsequent slower positive large amplitude deflection. It is generated from Müller and bipolar cells, it is directly dependent on functional photoreceptors 3
TOTAL **10**

ANS: 12

A. Any 3
    (a) Venous engorgement 1.5
    (b) Hemorrhages over and/or adjacent to the optic disc 1.5
    (c) Blurring of optic margins 1.5
    (d) Elevation of the optic disc 1.0
B. Papilloedema 1.5
C. ICSOL 1.5
D. Optic disc Drusen 1.5
E. Enlargement of the blind spot 1.0
TOTAL 10

Lens and Cataract

CHAPTER 6

QUESTIONS

OSPE: 01

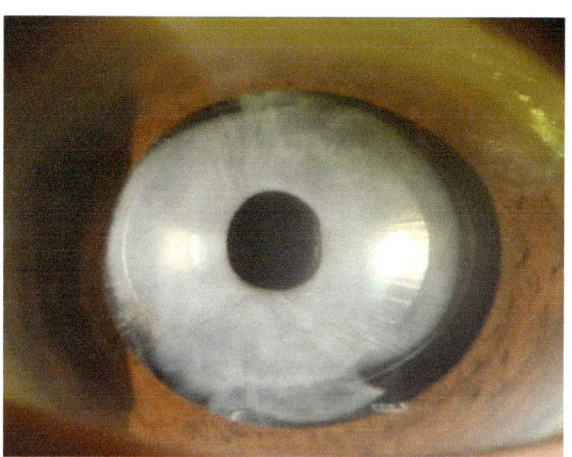

(Image courtesy: Dr Ishtiaque Anwar, Bangladesh Eye Hospital)

This is the slit-lamp view of a 67-year-old patient. Phacoemulsification with posterior chamber intraocular lens (PC IOL) implantation was done 6 months before and the surgery was uneventful. Now he came to you with gradual dimness of vision. B-scan shows no posterior segment abnormality (slit-lamp view has been taken after full dilatation).

A. What is your diagnosis?
B. What complications may arise? Mention there.
C. What is the main factor to develop this problem?
D. How can we overcome it during surgery?

OSPE: 02

In phaco surgery, a proverb can be used by the trainee surgeon "Tiger on the land and crocodile in water".

A. Can you write which structure is "land" and which one is "water"?
B. If you injured "water", what consequence may happen?
C. If you injured "land", what consequence may happen?

OSPE: 03

A 56-year-old woman complains of increasing difficulty reading the newspaper in the morning, especially in bright sunlight.
A. What may be the cause?
B. What will be the treatment of choice?
C. Before doing the treatment proper, what investigation you should do? Mention one general and three ocular investigations.

OSPE: 04

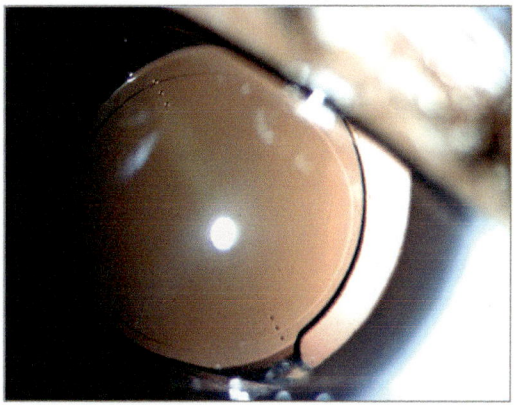

(Image courtesy: Dr Ishtiaque Anwar, Bangladesh Eye Hospital)

This is the postoperative image of a cataract patient, where pupil is fully dilated, optical portion of the lens is clearly visible. From the image, answer the following questions:
A. What operation has been carried out?
B. Optic of the lens is 6 mm; can you predict what will be the size of the capsulorhexis?
C. At 5'O clock and 11'O clock position, there are dotted marking, what indicate for?
D. When the lens uses?
E. What is the difficult part to introduce this lens?

OSPE: 05

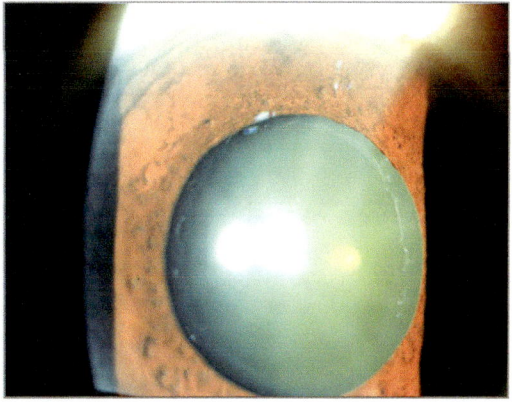

(Image courtesy: Dr Ishtiaque Anwar, Bangladesh Eye Hospital)

The picture has been taken before cataract surgery and patient was tried to maximum dilation, but it was mid-dilated:
A. Which type of cataract is this?
B. What is associated with the scenario?
C. How will you manage small pupil? Mention two.
D. What problems you may face during the surgery? Mention three important points.
E. What may be the postoperative complications? Mention four.

OSPE: 06

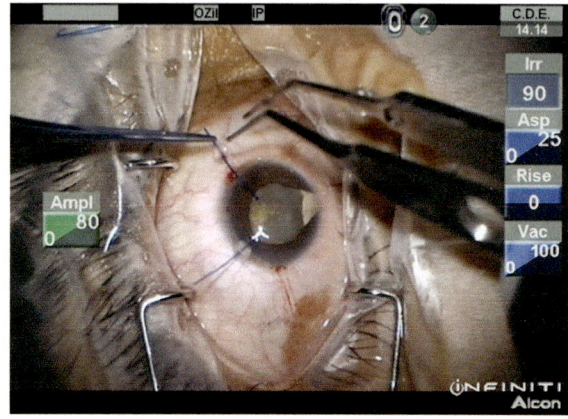

(Image courtesy: Dr Ishtiaque Anwar, Bangladesh Eye Hospital)

This is the image of cataract surgery. Answer the following questions regarding this picture:
A. Why there is more white at 3'O clock position?
B. What material is pushed inside the eye by surgeon?
C. Why he is doing this?
D. At the end of the surgery, what will be done with this material?

OSPE: 07

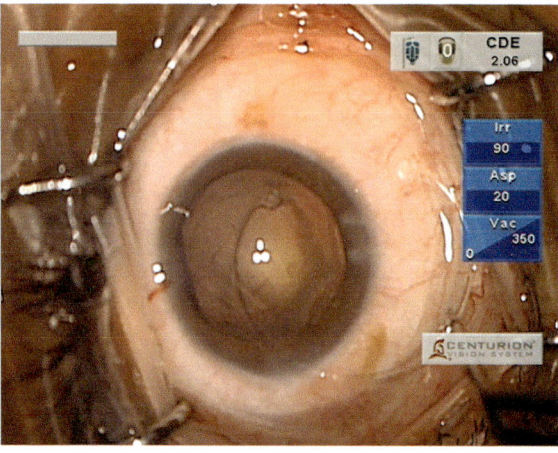

(Image courtesy: Dr Ishtiaque Anwar, Bangladesh Eye Hospital)

This image has been taken during cataract surgery.
A. What is the name of this white circular ring?
B. Why it is introducing inside the eye?
C. What are the indications of this device?
D. What benefit will you get?

OSPE: 08
In the preassessment clinic, you came across patient with following biometry. Give the reasons why the patient is not suitable for the inexperienced surgeon to carry out cataract extraction.

	Right eye	Left eye
K1	= 42.75	42.25
K2	= 42.50	42.50
Axial length	= 21.75 mm	22.0 mm
Refraction	= −8.25 D	−7.50
VA	= 6/24	6/36

OSPE: 09

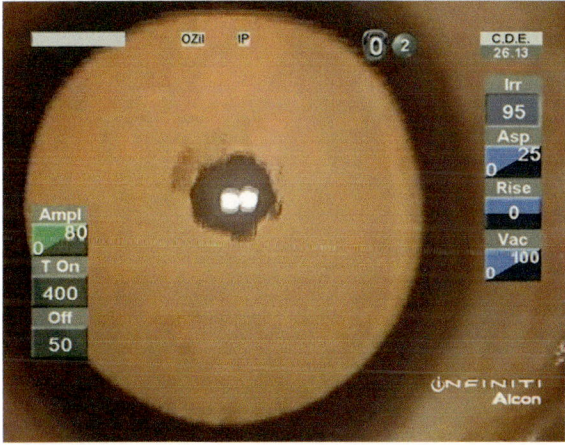

(Image courtesy: Dr Ishtiaque Anwar, Bangladesh Eye Hospital)

This is the preoperative view of the pupil under operating microscope which was dilated with Tropicamide and Phenylephrine eye drops?
A. What is the type of cataract?
B. What may be the complaints of patient?
C. What major complication may arise during surgery?
D. What precaution measures he will take to avoid complication?
E. What changes of phacodynamics will help you to avoid complication?

OSPE: 10

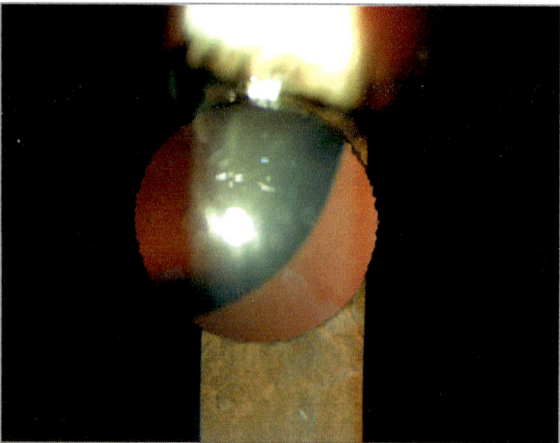

(Image courtesy: Dr Ishtiaque Anwar, Bangladesh Eye Hospital)

This is the slit-lamp view of left eye. Answer the following:
A. What is your diagnosis?
B. What is the most common systemic cause?
C. What are the D/Ds?
D. What other ocular complications may be associated with it?

OSPE: 11

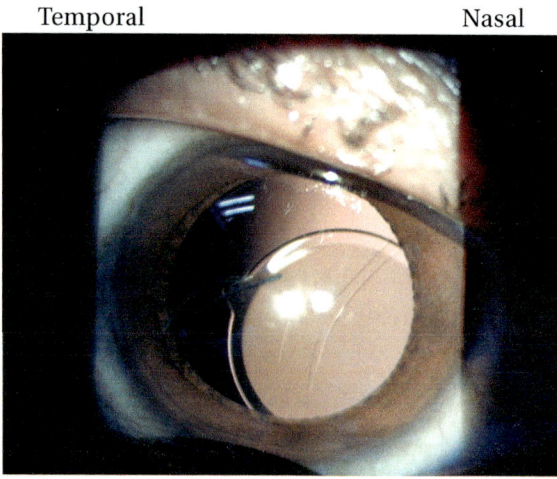

(Image courtesy: Dr Ishtiaque Anwar, Bangladesh Eye Hospital)

This is the postoperative image of phacoemulsification.
A. What is the condition of the IOL?
B. Why it occurs?
C. Behind the lens there is a crescent-shaped white line, what does it indicate?
D. How will you manage the condition? Mention two.

OSPE: 12

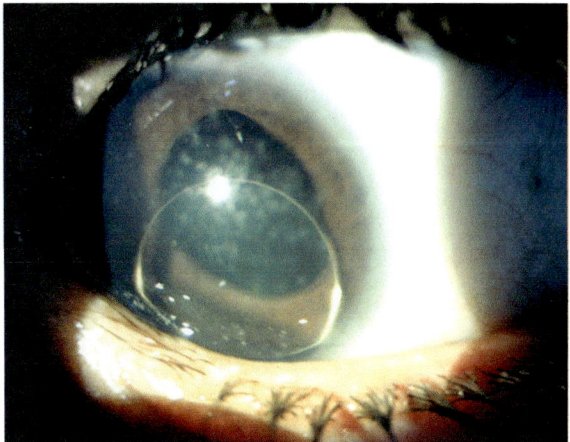

Image courtesy: Dr. Ishtiaque Anwar. Bangladesh Eye Hospital

A. What is your diagnosis?
B. What indicates corneal opacity?
C. What are the systemic associations? Mention three.
D. Is the patient myopic, hypermetropic, or emmetropic and why?
E. Sometimes it may be found in isolation with a systemic association. What is name of the systemic association?

OSPE: 13

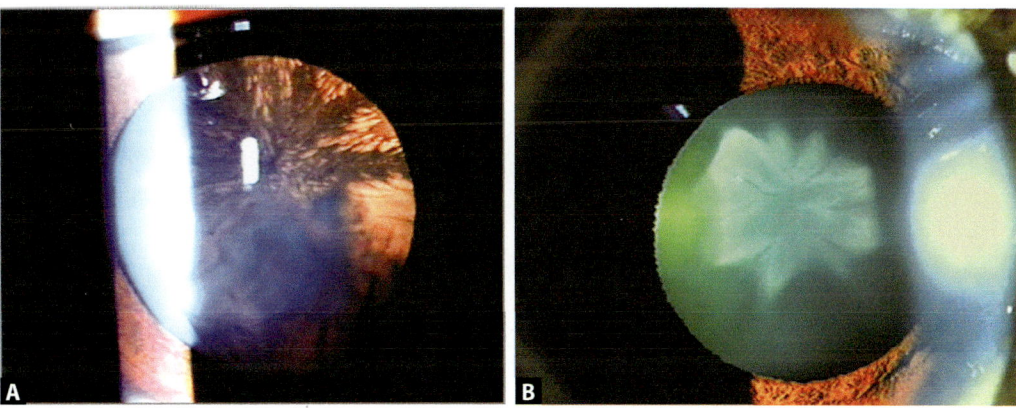

(Image courtesy: Dr Ishtiaque Anwar, Bangladesh Eye Hospital)

A 28-year-old man complained of a gradual decreased vision of left eye. 2 year earlier, he sustained a left traumatic hyphema after being hit with a cricket ball.

A. What does the picture show?
B. What is the name of the appearance?
C. What other lens abnormalities may occur with blunt trauma?
D. Is this patient can develop glaucoma due to trauma? What is the name of the glaucoma?

OSPE: 14

A 1-month-old baby is diagnosed with unilateral anterior polar cataract that is approximately 1.5 mm in diameter.
A. What is the most appropriate initial management?
B. What is the other name of this cataract?
C. How many bigger are they?
D. Do they usually require surgery?
E. Why the vision is usually affected?
F. What should you do to preserve the vision?

Lens and Cataract

ANSWERS

OSPE: 01. Anterior capsular phimosis syndrome
OSPE: 02. "Tiger on the land and crocodile in water"
OSPE: 03. Posterior subcapsular cataracts
OSPE: 04. Phaco with PCIOL Implantation
OSPE: 05. Pseudoexfoliative cataract
OSPE: 06. Coloboma
OSPE: 07. Capsular Tension Ring (CTR)
OSPE: 08. Biometry
OSPE: 09. Posterior Polar cataracts (PPC)
OSPE: 10. Subluxation of the lens (upper temporal region)
OSPE: 11. The IOL is dropped inferior nasal quadrant
OSPE: 12. Microspherophakia and lens is at A/C
OSPE: 13. Traumatic cataract
OSPE: 14. Pyramidal cataract

ANS: 01

A. Anterior capsular phimosis syndrome 3
B. There may be: .... 1 × 3 3
    (a) Pseudophacodonesis and IOL tilt
    (b) Decent ration, or
    (c) Dislocation
C. Small capsulorhexis 2
D. Bigger capsulorhexis 2
TOTAL **10**

ANS: 02

A. i. Cornea 2
    ii. Posterior capsule 2
B. i. Vitreous prolapsed 2
    ii. Drop nucleus 2
C. Endothelium decomposition 2
TOTAL **10**

ANS: 03

A. Posterior subcapsular cataracts 3
- *(Posterior subcapsular cataracts create more difficulty with glare and near vision. Nuclear and cortical cataracts affect distance vision more than near vision. Progressive loss of vision from oil droplet or anterior polar cataracts is not often seen in this age group)*
B. Phacoemulsification with posterior chamber intraocular lens implantation 2
C. General:
    - Blood sugar 2
    Ocular:
    - Biometry 2
    - IOP 1
    - SPT 1
TOTAL **10**

ANS: 04
A. Phaco with PCIOL implantation 1.5
B. 5.5 mm 1.5
C. Marking of the axis of the toric lens 1.5
D. When astigmatism is corneal, and regular .... 2 + 2 .... 4.0
E. Rotation inside the bag 1.5
TOTAL 10

ANS: 05
A. Pseudoexfoliative cataract 2.0
B. Pseudoexfoliation glaucoma 1.0
C. Management of small pupil:
    (a) By iris hook 1.0
    (b) Visco dilation 1.0
D. There is a higher risk of complications, due to .... 1 × 3 .... 3.0
    i. Poor mydriasis,
    ii. Increased fragility of the zonule and lens capsule, and
    iii. Endothelial deficiency
E. Postoperative problems comprise (Any 4) .... 0.5 × 4 .... 2.0
    (a) IOP spikes   (b) Corneal edema
    (c) IOL deposits   (d) Cystoid macular edema
    (e) IOL subluxation/dislocation
TOTAL 10

ANS: 06
A. Coloboma 2.5
B. Iris hook 2.5
C. To enlarge the pupil 2.5
D. Remove 2.5
TOTAL 10

ANS: 07
A. Capsular tension ring (CTR) 2.0
B. To stabilize the capsule in eyes with zonule weakness or dehiscence 2.0
C. .... 4 × 1 .... 4.0
    (a) Advanced or mature cataract
    (b) Post-traumatic cataract
    (c) Pseudoexfoliation syndrome
    (d) Subluxated lens
D. (a) Circular expansion of the capsule and stabilization of the bag 1.0
    (b) Centration of IOL 0.5
    (c) Minimize the risk of capsular fibrosis 0.5
TOTAL 10

ANS: 08
The patient's biometry shows average keratometric readings and axial length but high minus refraction. These changes are seen in patient with significant nuclear sclerosis.

The lenses are likely to be large and hard. A large lens will give a shallow A/C, making capsulorrhexis difficult for the inexperienced surgeon. A hard nucleus increases the phaco time and in the hand of inexperienced surgeon complication such as corneal edema increased.

ANS: 09

A. Posterior polar cataracts (PPC) 3.0
B. (a) Despite normal visual acuity patient may complaints glare and haloes 1.0
    (b) Vision will have reduced in bright light even day light but will be better in dusk .. 1.0
    (c) There will be complaints during reading because of miosis 0.5
C. Posterior capsular tear and vitreous prolapsed 2.0
D. .... 0.5 × 2 .... 1.0
    (a) Try to avoid hydrodissection
    (b) Minimal rotation of lens material is advised to avoid extraneous capsule manipulation and stress
E. .... 0.5 × 3 .... 1.5
    (a) Lower energy parameters
    (b) Torsional cutting as available with newer generation platforms
    (c) Lower than typical aspiration flow rates may be advised.
TOTAL *10*

ANS: 10

A. Subluxation of the lens (upper temporal region) 2.0
B. Marfan's syndrome 2.0
C. (a) Traumatic 1.0
    (b) Weill–Marchesani syndrome 1.0
    (c) Pseudoexfoliation 1.0
D. .... any 6 .... 0.5 × 6 .... 3.0
    (a) Flattened cornea (causing astigmatism)
    (b) Keratoconus
    (c) Increased globe length (causing myopia)
    (d) Iris coloboma
    (e) Cataracts, glaucoma
    (f) Strabismus
    (g) Amblyopia
TOTAL *10*

ANS: 11

A. The IOL is dropped inferior nasal quadrant 3.0
B. Due to PC rent at this region 2.0
C. It indicates rent margin of posterior capsular 2.0
D. Explanation of the IOL followed by 1.0
    (a) A/C lens or 1.0
    (b) Sclera fixation lens 1.0
TOTAL *10*

ANS: 12

A. Microspherophakia and lens is at A/C.
B. It indicates, it is at A/C for a long time.
C.
- Marfan syndrome
- Weill–Marchesani syndromes,
- Hyperlysinemia and
- Congenital rubella.

D. Myopic. The spherical shape of the lens results in increased refractive power, which causes the eye to be highly myopic.
E. Lowe syndrome

ANS: 13

A. Traumatic cataract 2.0
B. Stellate or rosette-shaped opacity 2.0
C. Apart from cataract, the following changes may occur: .... 1.5 × 3 .... 4.5
   i. Subluxation
   ii. Dislocation
   iii. Vossius ring
D. Yes, angle recession glaucoma .... 0.5 + 1.0 .... 1.5
TOTAL 10

ANS: 14

A. Close observation 2.0
B. Pyramidal cataract 2.0
C. They are less than 3 mm. 1.0
D. No 1.0
E. There is an increased incidence of anisometropia in patients with anterior polar cataracts 3.0
F. Refraction. 1.0
TOTAL 10

Explanation: Anterior polar cataracts are typically small (3 mm) white opacities located centrally in the anterior lens capsule. They are not progressive and are not large enough to interfere with vision. However, there is an increased incidence of anisometropia in patients with anterior polar cataracts; refractions should therefore be monitored in these patients.

Anterior polar cataract may be flat or project as a conical opacity into the anterior chamber (pyramidal cataract) flat anterior polar opacities are central, less than 3 mm in diameter, bilateral in one-third of cases and visually insignificant. Pyramidal opacities are frequently surrounded by an area of cortical opacity and may affect vision. Occasional associations of anterior polar cataracts include persistent pupillary membrane, Aniridia, Peters anomaly, and anterior lenticonus.

Oculoplasty

CHAPTER 7

QUESTIONS

OSPE: 01

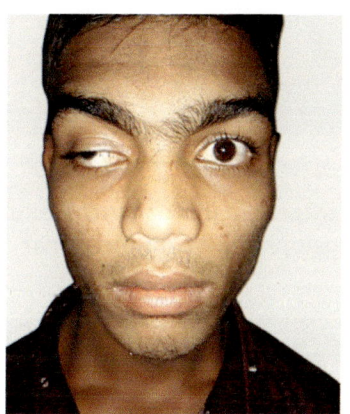

(Image courtesy: Dr Mukti Rani Mitra)

See the photograph and answer the following questions:
A. What are the presenting features in this patient? Mention three.
B. Give two differential diagnoses.
C. What other clinical findings you want to know to reach the diagnosis?

OSPE: 02

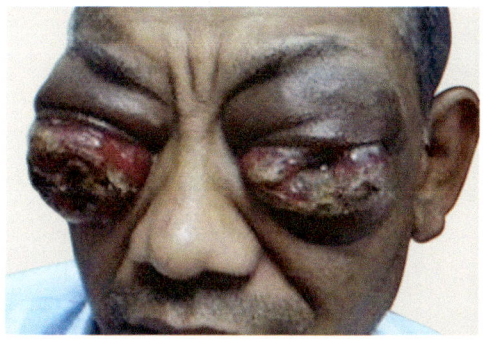

Fig. 1

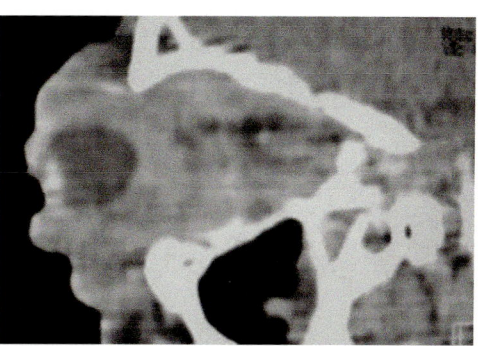

Fig. 2

Figure 1 is the ocular findings of a 50-year-old patient and Figure 2 is the computed tomography (CT) scan of this patient.

What are the findings in Figure 1? Mention five. And what are the CT findings? Mention five.

OSPE: 03

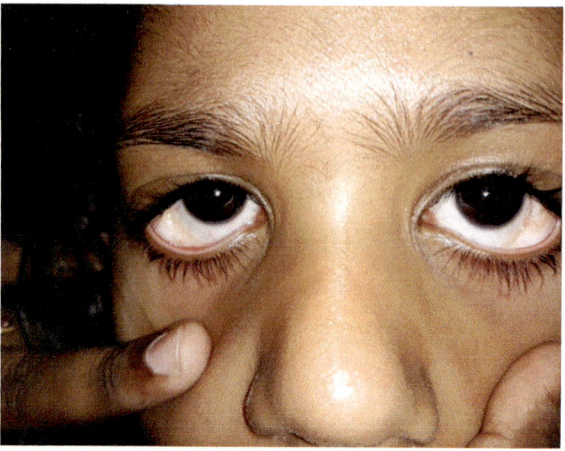

(Image courtesy: Dr Mukti Rani Mitra)

A. What are the indications of surgery in this patient? Mention two.
B. What may be the possible postoperative complications?

OSPE: 04

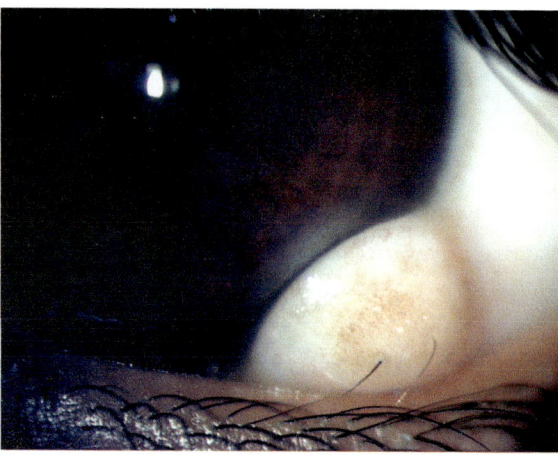

(Image courtesy: Dr Mukti Rani Mitra)

A. What is your diagnosis?
B. What are the differential diagnoses?
C. What are the indications of surgery?

Oculoplasty 157

OSPE: 05

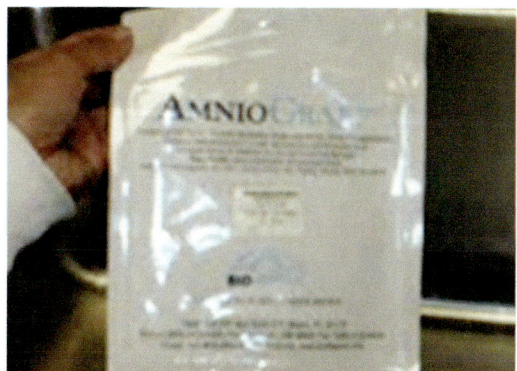

Supplied sample is oven-dried amniotic membrane.
Answer the following questions:
A. From where it was collected?
B. How it was collected?
C. How it was sterilized?
D. In which temperature it is preserved?
E. Mention four important properties.
F. Enumerate two important ophthalmic uses.

OSPE: 06

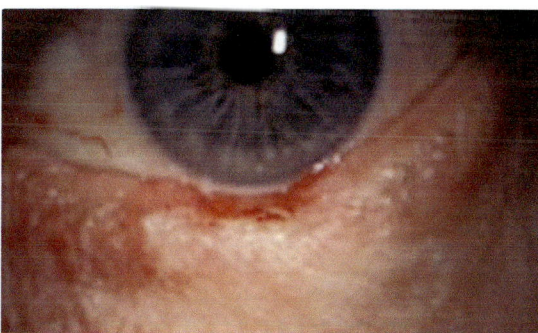

Usually, basal cell carcinoma (BCC) forms a nodule in the eyelid but here in the picture, it does not make a nodule and grow within the eyelid; it induces pulling of the eyelid.
A. What is the name of this variant?
B. Why this is more difficult to treat?
C. Write one differential diagnosis.
D. Which is the most common site in the eye?
E. In which location of the eye it has the worst prognosis?
F. Which will you prefer? Excisional biopsy or incisional biopsy and why?

OSPE: 07

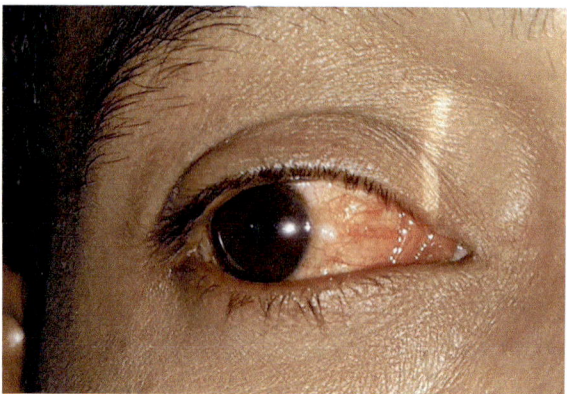

A 12-year-old girl came to you with the complaints of chronic irritation and redness at the medial bulbar conjunctiva. On examination, you observed an elevated area near to nasal limbus.

A. What is your diagnosis?
B. What is the most common causative organism?
C. What type of disease is this?
D. What is the treatment?

OSPE: 08

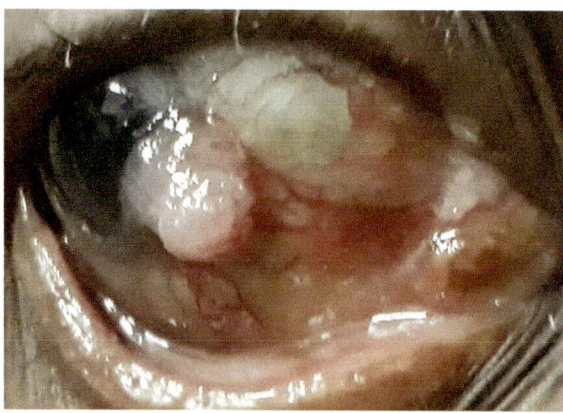

A 70-year-old man came to you with the complaints of visible mass in one eye, accompanied by conjunctivitis-type symptoms. The growth starts from the limbal area and encroaching the cornea with 4 months.

A. Describe two points about the growth.
B. What is your probable diagnosis?
C. How will you estimate the depth of invasion? Mention two investigations.

OSPE: 09

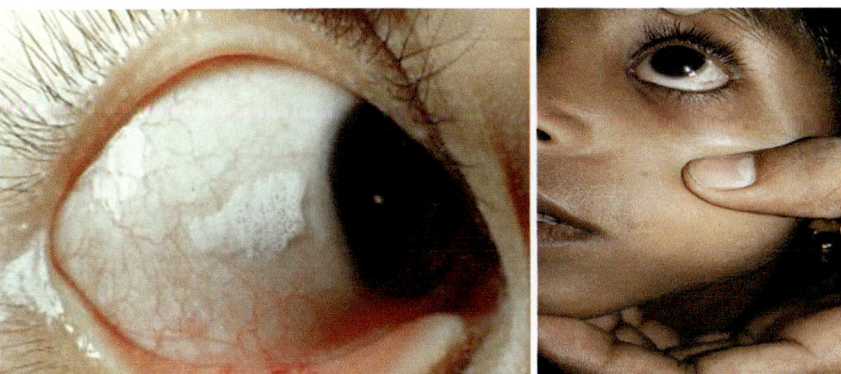

(Image courtesy: Dr Mukti Rani Mitra)

- These two pictures are taken from the same girl who is 10 years old. She came to you after recovery from severe diarrhea, she develops whitish lesion consisting of a dry, scaly patch with a foamy appearance on the temporal conjunctiva of both eyes. Corrected visual acuity was 6/6 in both eyes; the remainder of the ocular examination was normal.

A. What may be the diagnosis?
B. What is the cause?
C. What other finding you may get?
D. What is the most common site?
E. What is the composition of this lesion?

OSPE: 10

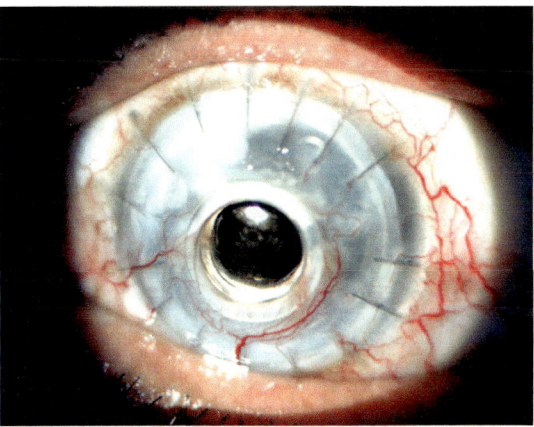

(Image courtesy: Dr Ishtiaque Anwar, Bangladesh Eye Hospital)

A. What is the name of this implantation?
B. What are the indications?
C. What are the parts of it?

OSPE: 11

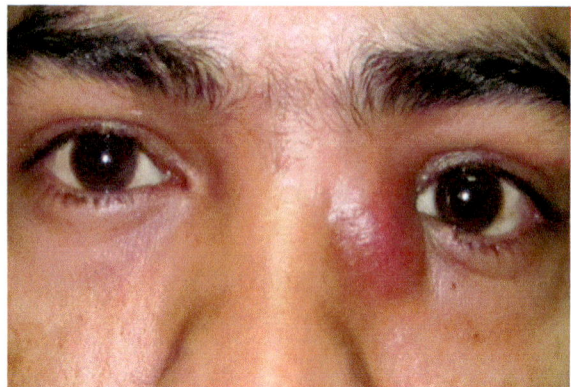

(Image courtesy: Dr Murtuza Nuruddin, Chittagong Eye Infirmary and Training Complex of BNSB)

This is the picture of a 25 years old male farmer, living in a village and usually takes bath in stagnant pond water. He came to you with the complaints of
- Bloody discharge through nose
- Epiphora
- Blocked lacrimal passage

On palpation of the swelling, you feel it is a doughy swelling over lacrimal sac region:
A. What is your probable diagnosis?
B. What is the importance of bathing in stagnant pond water?
C. What is the specific treatment?
D. What drug you can use if recurrence is there?

OSPE: 12

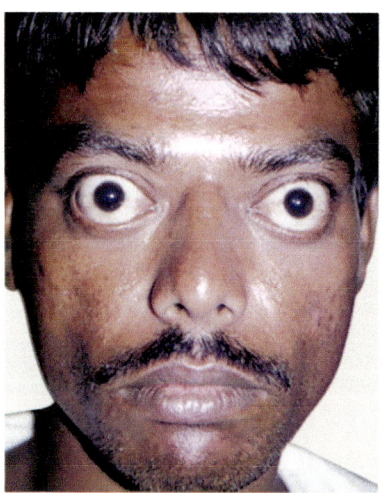

(Image courtesy: Dr Murtuza Nuruddin, Chittagong Eye Infirmary and Training Complex of BNSB)

This is the photography of a 40-year-old man. It is diagnosed with a case of thyroid ophthalmopathy. Mention three positive findings from the photo.

OSPE: 13

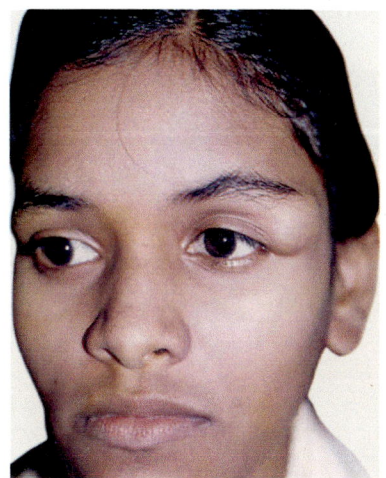

(Image courtesy: Dr Murtuza Nuruddin, Chittagong Eye Infirmary and Training Complex of BNSB)

The 15-year-old girl came to you with the complaints of a mass in the upper and outer quadrant of the orbit since childhood, and last two years it gradually increases in size and came to this shape.
A. What is your diagnosis?
B. Mention two differential diagnoses.
C. What is the most common site for this growth?
D. What is the preferred radiological investigation for this growth?
E. What may be the sequel if left untreated? Any 2.

OSPE: 14

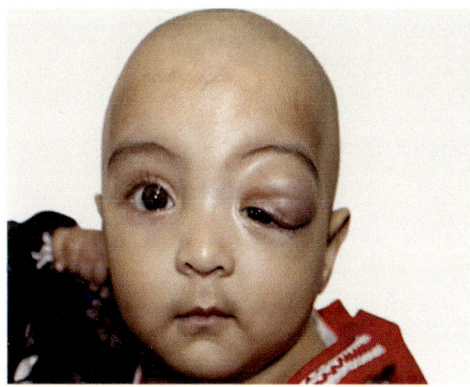
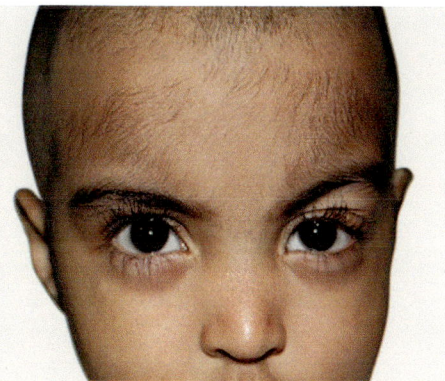

(Image courtesy: Dr Murtuza Nuruddin, Chittagong Eye Infirmary and Training Complex of BNSB)

Here are pictures of two babies aged 2 years and 3 years, respectively. Both are suffering from same disease but different grades.
A. What is your probable diagnosis?
B. Who suffers more, boys or girls?

C. What is the natural course of the disease?
D. Who needs urgent treatment? And why?

OSPE: 15

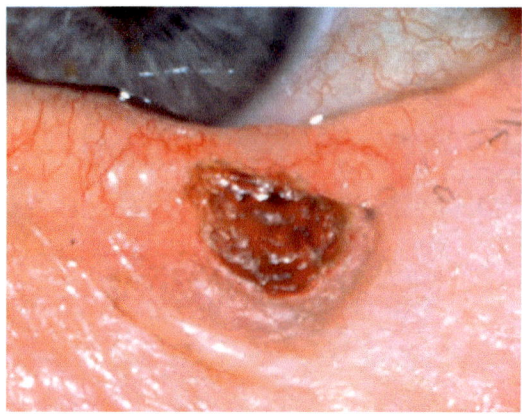

A. Mention three positive findings of the ulcerated area.
B. What is your diagnosis?
C. What are the D/Ds?
D. How many varieties are there? Name them.

ANSWERS

OSPE: 01. Right exotropia
OSPE: 02. Bilateral severe proptosis
OSPE: 03. Dermoid
OSPE: 04. Limbal dermoid
OSPE: 05. Amniotic membrane
OSPE: 06. Sclerosing BCC
OSPE: 07. Phlyctenular keratoconjunctivitis
OSPE: 08. Ocular surface squamous neoplasia (OSSN)
OSPE: 09. Bitot's spot
OSPE: 10. Boston keratoprosthesis
OSPE: 11. Lacrimal sac rhinosporidiosis
OSPE: 12. Axial proptosis
OSPE: 13. Superficial dermoid
OSPE: 14. Capillary hemangiomas
OSPE: 15. BCC

ANS: 01

A. i. Right exotropia 2.0
    ii. Brow elevation 2.0
    iii. Moderate ptosis 2.0
B. Right third nerve palsy and congenital ptosis with exotropia due to amblyopia. 2.0
C. Extraocular motility. 2.0
TOTAL *10*

ANS: 02

Any 5 5
  A. Bilateral severe proptosis 1
  B. Bilateral severe chemosis 1
  C. Right eye sloughed out cornea 1
  D. Left keratopathy 1
  E. Deposition of crust and keratinization of bilateral bulbar conjunctiva 1
  F. Fullness of superior and inferior sulcus with engorged dilated vessels 1
CT scan findings .... **Any 5** 5
  A. Sagittal view 1
  B. Noncontrast 1
  C. Severe proptosis 1
  D. No bony lesion 1
  E. Diffuse heterogeneous lesion occupying whole of the retrobulbar region up to the orbital apex 1
  F. Extraocular muscles and optic nerve are not visualized 1
  G. Intraocular lens is opacified with no corneal contour or anterior chamber is seen ... 1
  H. Diffuse vitreous haze present 1
TOTAL *10*

ANS: 03

A. (a) Increasing in size causing irritation 2
 (b) Cosmetic 2
B. (a) Injury to the lateral rectus muscle causing strabismus 2
 (b) Injury to the ducts of the lacrimal gland causing dry eye 2
 (c) Injury to the levator muscle (lateral horn) causing ptosis 2

TOTAL 10

ANS: 04

A. Limbal dermoid 3.0
B. Conjunctival growth—ocular surface squamous neoplasia) 2.0
C. Indication of surgery
 (a) Cosmetics 2.0
 (b) Astigmatism 2.0
 (c) Dellen formation 1.0

TOTAL 10

ANS: 05

A. From human placenta 2
B. Elective cesarean section 2
C. Gamma radiation 1
D. 4°–8° centigrade temperature 1
E. 0.5 × 4 2
 (a) Anti-inflammatory
 (b) Antifibroblastic
 (c) Antiangiogenesis
 (d) Acts as a scalped for epithelization
F. ...... (Any 2) 2
 (a) Chemical injury of the cornea
 (b) Persistent epithelial defect
 (c) Symblepharon release and fornix reconstruction
 (d) Excision of pterygium with amniotic membrane transplantation (AMT)

TOTAL 10

ANS: 06

A. Sclerosing BCC or morpheaform variant 2
B. Much more difficult to treat because its edges are harder to define 2
C. Chronic blepharitis 1
D. Lower eyelid 1
E. Medial canthus 1
F. Excision biopsy ...... (1 + 2) 3

TOTAL 10

(Because tumors that recur following incomplete treatment tend to be more aggressive)

Oculoplasty

ANS: 07
A.	Phlyctenular conjunctivitis	3.0
B.	*Staphylococcus aureus*	2.0
C.	Hypersensitivity type 4	2.0
D.	Treatment	
	(a) Steroid eye drop	1.5
	(b) Artificial tear	1.5
TOTAL		**10**

ANS: 08
A.	(a) A fleshy, gelatinous, and leukoplakic lesion at the medial palpebral fissure, encroaching the cornea	2
	(b) Feeder vessels are seen	2
B.	Ocular surface squamous neoplasia	2
C.	(a) Ultrasonic biomicroscope (UBM)	2
	(b) Anterior segment optical coherence tomography (OCT)	2
TOTAL		**10**

ANS: 09
A.	Bitot's spot	2
B.	Vitamin A deficiency	2
C.	Conjunctival xerosis	2
D.	Lesion is usually seen on the bulbar conjunctiva near the limbus, at the 3 O'clock or 9 O'clock positions	2
E.	The white deposit consists of keratinization	2
TOTAL		**10**

ANS: 10
A.	Boston keratoprosthesis	2
B.	i. Multiple failed penetrating keratoplasties	1
	ii. Stevens–Johnson syndrome	1
	iii. ocular cicatricial pemphigoid	1
	iv. Aniridia	1
	v. Chemical injury	1
C.	It consists of three components:	
	i. Front plate with optical stem	1
	ii. Back plate	1
	iii. Titanium locking C-ring	1
TOTAL		**10**

ANS: 11
A.	Lacrimal sac rhinosporidiosis	4
B.	It is a water-borne disease	2
C.	DCT	2
D.	Dapsone (diaminodiphenyl sulfone)	2
TOTAL		**10**

ANS: 12

A. Axial proptosis 4
B. Lid retraction both upper and lower lids 2
C. Staring and frightened appearance (Kocher sign) present 4
TOTAL **10**

ANS: 13

A. Superficial dermoid 3.0
B. (a) Lacrimal gland tumor 1.0
    (b) Upper lid plexiform neurofibroma 1.0
C. Along the embryonic lines of closure 2.0
D. CT scan of orbit 1.0
E. Any 2 .... 2.0
    (a) Chronic granulomatous inflammation
    (b) May remain as it is
    (c) Infection followed by abscess formation
TOTAL **10**

ANS: 14

A. Capillary hemangiomas 3
B. Girls 2
C. • Rapid growth 3–6 months after diagnosis 1
    • Followed by a slower phase of natural resolution in which 30% of lesions resolve by the age of 3 years 1
    • About 75% by the age of 7 1
D. The first baby needs early treatment because there is chance of amblyopia 2
TOTAL **10**

ANS: 15

A. i. Centrally ulcerated 2.0
   ii. Pearly raised rolled edges and 1.5
   iii. Dilated and irregular blood vessels 1.0
B. BCC 2.0
C. (a) Squamous cell carcinoma. (b) Skin ulcer 2.0
D. Three types. (a) Nodular; (b) Rodent; (c) Sclerosing .... 0.5 × 3 .... 1.5
TOTAL **10**

Cornea

CHAPTER 8

QUESTIONS

OSPE: 01

Suppose you are working in a primary eye care hospital at upazila level. A boy of 7 year-old boy came to you with penetrating corneal injury and iris prolapse.
A. Before referring the boy at tertiary eye care center, give him two treatments.
B. Mention name of three essential instruments required to repair in tertiary center.
C. What will be your instruction to anesthetist?
D. How will you decide for reposition of the iris?

OSPE: 02

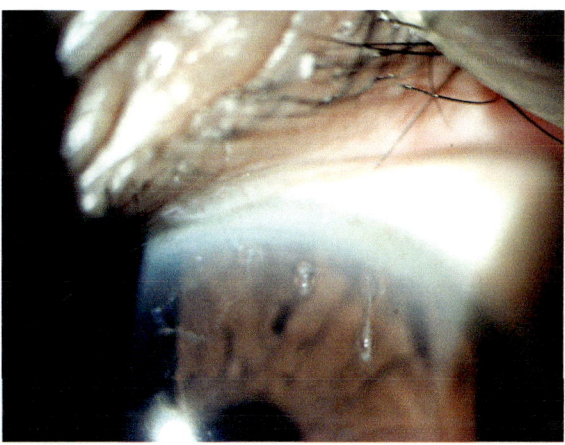

(Image courtesy: Dr Ishtiaque Anwar, Bangladesh Eye Hospital)

This is the enlarge view of cornea with slit-lamp biomicroscope:
A. What is the illumination?
B. Mention one positive finding.
C. What are the compositions of it?
D. What is the diagnosis?
E. What are the causes? Mention: 3.

OSPE: 03

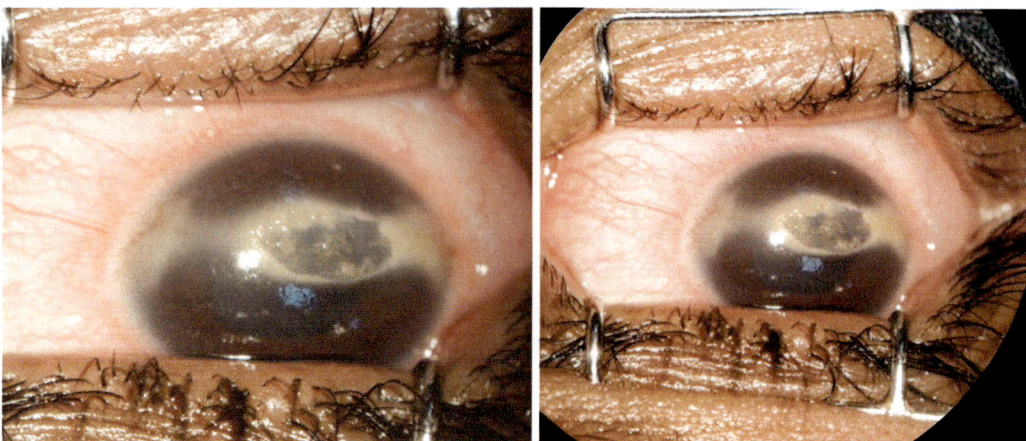

These two pictures have been taken from the left eye of a farmer. Answer the following questions
A. Write three positive findings from the pictures.
B. What is the probable diagnosis?
C. What may be other name?
D. What may be the cause?
E. What is the difference between primary and secondary condition in this case?
F. Is this primary or secondary?
G. What treatment is needed?

OSPE: 04

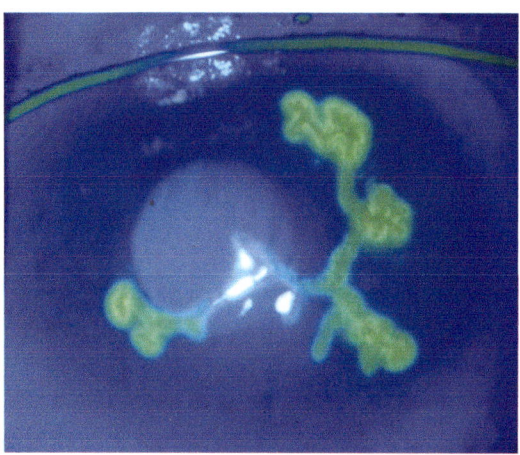

(Image courtesy: Dr Ishtiaque Anwar, Bangladesh Eye Hospital)

A. What is the name of the ulcer?
B. What may be the cause? Mention 3.
C. In which layer it involves?

D. What is the name of the stain?
E. Mention other stain that can be used.
F. What is the difference between these two?

OSPE: 05

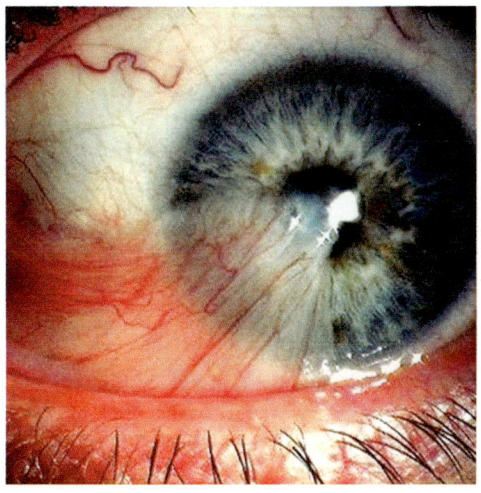

A. What is your diagnosis?
B. What type of disease is this?
C. What are the predisposition factors? Mention two.
D. What are the differential diagnoses? Mention two.

OSPE: 06

This is the feature of a patient's right eye, 15 days after pterygium surgery (surgery was done by bare sclera technique followed by mitomycin (MMC)-C eye drop).

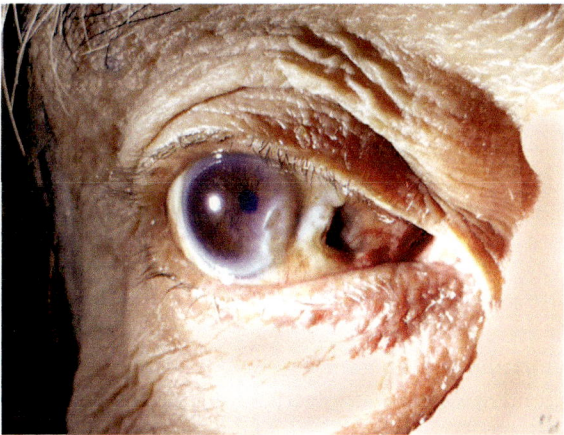

A. What is the feature now?
B. What is the most probable cause?

C. Mention two symptoms.
D. What grievous complication impending to occur?
E. How can you manage it?

OSPE: 07

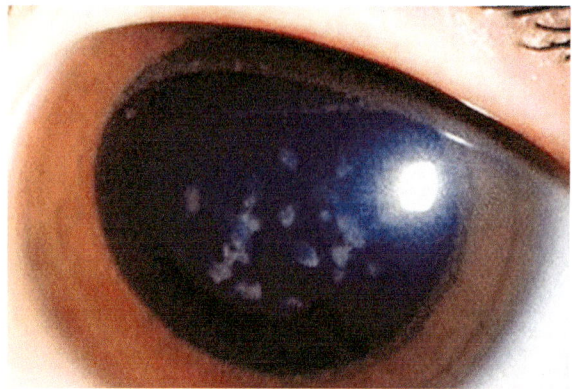

A. What does the picture show?
B. What is the type of illumination?
C. Describe the lesion.
D. Do you think 2nd eye have to be examined? If yes, or no explain the reason.

OSPE: 08

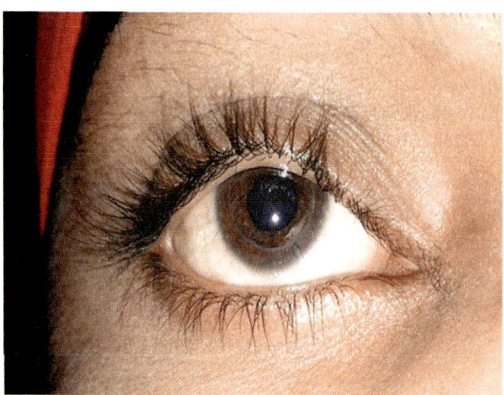
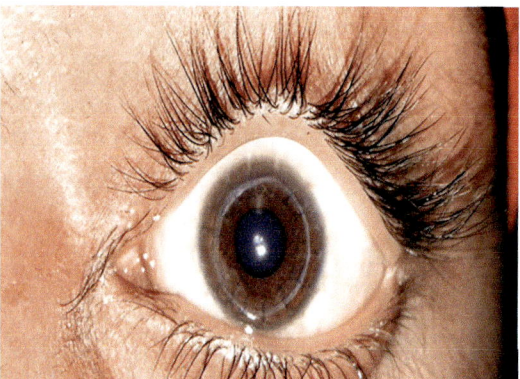

This is the picture of a patient of 35-year-old man. His both eyes were operated (penetrating keratoplasty). One eye was operated one year before and the other was two years before.

A. Can you say which eye was operated earlier?
B. How can you confirm about your comment?
C. What is deep anterior lamellar keratoplasty (DALK)
D. Which one is better? Why?

OSPE: 09

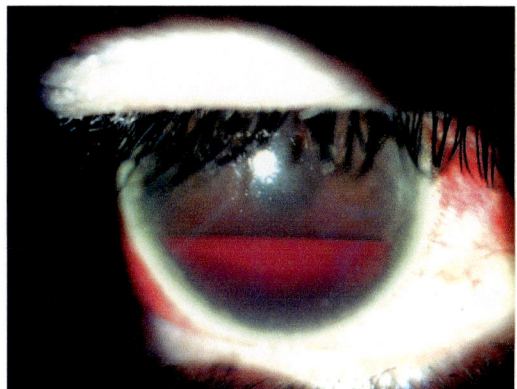

(Image courtesy: Dr Ishtiaque Anwar, Bangladesh Eye Hospital)

A 10-year-old boy came to you with above feature, he is also suffering from sickle-cell hemoglobinopathies.
A. He has more chance to develop increased intraocular pressure (IOP). What is the reason?
B. What sort of rest you have to advise him?
C. What will be his sleeping posture?
D. Should you prescribe miotic? Give one explanation.
E. What advices should you give after discharge?

OSPE: 10

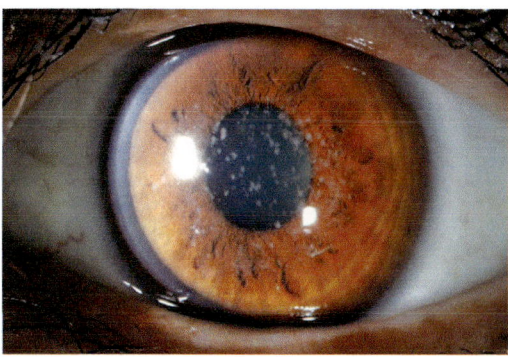

A 20-year-old man was seen in the eye clinic because his father had a corneal graft. His vision was 6/9 in both eyes.
A. What is the diagnosis?
B. Mention two points from this photo in favor of your diagnosis.
C. What is responsible for the corneal appearance?
D. What is the natural history of this condition?

OSPE: 11

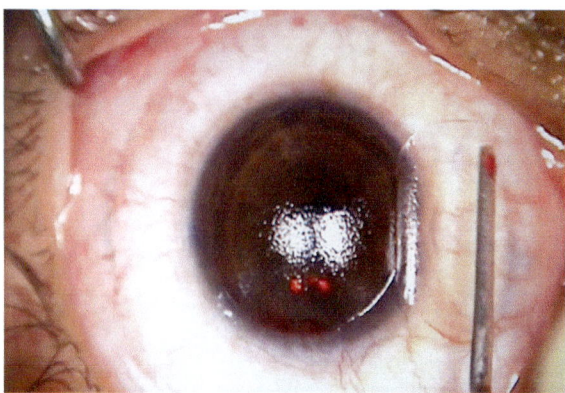

A. What is the name of the surgery?
B. Which step is going on at here?
C. Which instrument we used during this step?
D. What complications may arise during this step? Mention 2.
E. What is the next step?

Cornea 173

ANSWERS

OSPE: 01. Penetrating corneal injury and iris prolapsed.
OSPE: 02. Corneal filaments
OSPE: 03. Spheroidal degeneration
OSPE: 04. Dendritic ulcer
OSPE: 05. Pterygium
OSPE: 06. Thinning of sclera
OSPE: 07. Multiple discrete stromal opacity
OSPE: 08. DALK
OSPE: 09. Sickle-cell hemoglobinopathies
OSPE: 10. Granular dystrophy
OSPE: 11. Lasik

ANS: 01

A. Light pad and bandage of the eye (no drop or ointment inside the eye).......1 + 0.5...... 1.5
   Systemic analgesic and antibiotics .... 0.75 + 0.75.. 1.5
B. Any three .... 1 × 3.. 3.0
   - Eye speculum
   - Barraquer needle holder
   - Corneal forceps/St Martin
   - Two tying forceps
C. Please caring about raised IOP (avoid suxamethonium) 2.0
D. If iris is viable, it will be reposed 2.0
TOTAL *10*

ANS: 02

A. Diffuse illumination.. 2.0
B. Filaments... 1.5
C. Degenerated epithelial cells and mucus .... 1 + 1... 2.0
D. Filamentary keratopathy or filamentous keratitis 1.5
E. (a) Aqueous deficiency (keratoconjunctivitis sicca) 1.0
   (b) Excessive contact lens wear 1.0
   (c) Corneal epithelial instability.. 1.0
   (d) Bullous keratopathy 0.5
   (e) Neurotrophic keratopathy 0.5
TOTAL *10*

ANS: 03

A. (a) Amber-colored granules in the superficial stroma of the peripheral interpalpebral
       cornea 1
   (b) Slough out of the epithelium and Bowman's layer 1
   (c) Surrounding stroma is often hazy 1
B. Spheroidal degeneration 2
C. Labrador keratopathy/climatic droplet keratopathy 1
D. Ultraviolet exposure is likely to be an etiological factor1

E. The primary form is an aging process which affects only the peripheral cornea. The secondary form is constantly associated with other ocular pathology such as absolute glaucoma, phthisis bulbi, post-traumatic scars, and lattice corneal dystrophy. 1
F. This is secondary 1
G. Protection against ultraviolet damage with sunglasses, and superficial keratectomy or lamellar keratoplasty 1
TOTAL **10**

ANS: 04

A. Dendritic ulcer 2
B. i. Varicella zoster virus 1
    ii. Recurrent corneal erosion 1
    iii. Acanthamoeba keratitis 1
C. Epithelial layer 1
D. Fluorescein 1
E. Rose Bengal 1
F. Terminal buds and its bed stains well with fluorescein. The virus-laden cells at the margin of the ulcer stain with rose Bengal 2
TOTAL **10**

ANS: 05

A. Pterygium 2
B. Degenerative 2
C. (a) Ultraviolet exposure 2
    (b) Chronic surface dryness 2
D. (a) Pinguecula 1
    (b) Pseudopterygium 1
TOTAL **10**

ANS: 06

A. Thinning of sclera 2
B. Mitomycin-C 2
C. Severe pain and photophobia 2
D. Perforation of sclera 2
E. Patch scleral graft 2
TOTAL **10**

ANS: 07

A. Multiple discrete stromal opacity 3.0
B. Sclerotic scatter 2.0
C. Discrete central ant stromal opacity like sugar granule or bread crumb, margin is free and area in between opacity is clear 2.0
D. Yes, because corneal dystrophy affects both eyes .... 1 + 2 .... 3.0
TOTAL **10**

ANS: 08

A. Above eye (R/E) was operated earlier 3.0
B. There is no stitch in the R/E, but stitch is in L/E 3.0
C. Deep anterior lamellar keratoplasty 2.0
D. Deep anterior lamellar keratoplasty. Chance of rejection is less than penetrating keratoplasty (PKP) 2.0
TOTAL 10

ANS: 09

A. Due to trabecular meshwork obstruction by deformed red cells 3
B. Strict bed rest is probably unnecessary, but substantially limiting activity is prudent 1
C. Semiupright posture, including during sleep 2
D. Miotics should be avoided as they may increase pupillary block and disrupt the blood–aqueous barrier 2
E. Avoid any activity with a risk of even minor eye trauma for several weeks 2
TOTAL 10

ANS: 10

A. Granular dystrophy 3
B. (a) The lesions appear as well-demarcated granular opacities 1
   (b) Cornea between the lesions is clear 1
C. Hyaline deposits 2
D. The lesions appear early in life but usually remains asymptomatic years. The dystrophy is slowly progressive and tends to enlarge and involve the deeper layer. The vision seldom drops below 6/60 3
TOTAL 10

ANS: 11

A. Lasik 2
B. Corneal flap creation 2
C. Laser or microkeratome 2
D. Any two .... 1 × 2 2
   - Buttonholing' (penetration) of the flap
   - Flap amputation
   - Incomplete or irregular flap creation
E. Ablation of the stroma by laser 2
TOTAL 10

CHAPTER 9

Drug Preparation

QUESTIONS

OSPE: 01. Prepare injection mydricaine.
OSPE: 02. Make fortified gentamicin.
OSPE: 03. Prepare 2.5% phenylephrine and 0.75% tropicamide.
OSPE: 04. Prepare intravitreal injection of ceftazidime for endophthalmitis.
OSPE: 05. Prepare intravitreal injection of vancomycin for endophthalmitis.
OSPE: 06. Prepare pilocarpine 0.125% drop.
OSPE: 07. Preparation of methylprednisolone.
OSPE: 08. Preparation of mitomycin C (MMC) for trabeculectomy.
OSPE: 09. Fitting of bandage contact lens (BCL) into the dummy's right eye.
OSPE: 10. Prepare amphotericin B for fungal corneal ulcer.
OSPE: 11. Prepare botulinum toxin A for the treatment of essential blepharospasm.
OSPE: 12. Prepare topical voriconazole eye drops 1% and voriconazole for intrastromal injection 50 μg/0.1 mL separately.

ANSWERS

ANS: 01
Prepare injection of mydricaine for subconjunctval administration with the supplied drugs and disposables for an adult.

Checklist
A. Wearing gloves 0.5
B. Taking 3 cc syringe 0.5
C. Drawing drugs
    (a) Atropine—1 mL (0.6 mg) 2.0
    (b) Adrenaline—0.12 mL (1 in 1,000 dilution) or 0.1 mL 2.0
    (c) 2% lignocaine—0.3 mL or 0.4 mL 2.0
    Total = 1.42–1.5 mL
D. Fixing of 26 G needle.. 1.0
E. 0.3–0.5 mL is ready for use (given in divided doses in four quadrants)......................... 1.0
F. Waste disposal... 1.0
TOTAL *10*

Explanation: The preparation of injection mydricaine is quoted from Stallard's Eye Surgery, 7th edition (the dose is 0.3 mL for each quadrant with atropine 1 mg and procaine 3 mg which is not available in our country). That is why, the dose is modified here for practical purpose what we usually use in our clinical practice with the available drugs and available dosage.

ANS: 02
Make fortified gentamicin eye drop for bacterial corneal ulcer with the supplied materials (gentamicin eye drop, 10 cc syringe, Injection Gentamicin, signature pen, and micropore).

Checklist
A. Wearing gloves 2.0
B. Draw 5 mL Gentamycin drop and discard.. 3.0
C. Mix the whole injection Gentamicin into the vial.. 3.0
D. Leveling of the vial 2.0
TOTAL *10*

ANS: 03
For the detection of retinopathy of prematurity (ROP), you have to dilate the pupil of premature infant with 2.5% phenylephrine and 0.75% tropicamide, but which is commercially not available.
    Prepare above concentration with the supplied materials.

Checklist

		Done
1.	Discard 2 mL from the tropicamide	2.5
2.	Take 1 mL from phenylephrine	2.5
3.	Mix the phenylephrine with tropicamide	2.5
4.	Discard disposals	2.5
TOTAL		*10*

ANS: 04

Prepare intravitreal injection of ceftazidime for endophthalmitis.

Checklist
1. Wearing of the gloves 2.0
2. Add 10 mL water for injection (WFI) 1.5
3. Draw up 1 mL of the solution, containing 50 mg of antibiotic 1.5
4. Add 1.5 mL WFI or saline giving 50 mg in 2.5 mL 1.5
5. Draw up about 0.2 mL 1.5
6. Fit the fresh needle 1.0
7. Discard all but 0.1 mL 0.5
8. Discard disposable 0.5
TOTAL 10

ANS: 05

Prepare intravitreal injection of vancomycin for endophthalmitis with the following supplied materials:
1. Injection Vancomycin (500 mg)
2. Gloves
3. 10 mL syringe
4. 3 mL syringe
5. 1 mL syringe
6. 26 G needle
7. Water for injection.

Checklist
Only saline, not WFI, should be used with vancomycin. As 1–8 above, again preferably starting with a 500 mg ampoule.

ANS: 06

Prepare pilocarpine 0.125% drop. With 2% pilocarpine drop, 10 mL bottle of artificial tear, 5 cc syringe, and hexisol for hand wash.

Checklist
A. Wash hand with hexisol hand washes 1.0
B. Take 2.5 mL of artificial tear in a 5-cc syringe and discard it 3.5
C. Take 0.5 mL of 2% of pilocarpine drops in a 5-cc syringe and pour it in a 7.5 mL containing artificial tear bottle 3.5
D. Mix and shake well 1.0
E. And label it with 0.125% pilocarpine drops 1.0
TOTAL 10

(Courtesy: Dr Md Lutfor Rahman, Associate Professor, Neuro-ophthalmology, NIO).

ANS: 07

Preparation of methylprednisolone from 1 gm vial with this supplied materials for the patient of RBN.
1. 1 g methylprednisolone

2. 10 mL distilled water
3. 500 mg normal saline
4. Syringe
5. Butterfly needle.

Checklist

A.	Wearing of the gloves	2.5
B.	Mix 10 mL distilled water in the vial	2.5
C.	Discard 300 mL normal saline	2.5
D.	Add this 10 mL medicine with the 200 mL normal saline	2.5
	TOTAL	**10**

ANS: 08

Preparation of MMC for trabeculectomy surgery with the following materials:
1. Injection MMC (2 mg)
2. Gloves
3. Syringes.

Checklist

The drug is available in a vial (2 mg/mL). It is further reconstituted with normal saline (5 mL) to make 0.4 mg/mL or in 10 mL to make 0.2 mg/mL (In the above OSPE, concentration of desired MMC may not be mention in this situation but you have the option to prepare 0.4 mg/mL or 0.2 mg/mL). But sometimes a scenario may be given for trabeculectomy such as in case of: (a) neovascular glaucoma, (b) previous failed trabeculectomy or artificial filtering devices, or (c) certain secondary glaucoma's (e.g. inflammatory, post-traumatic angle recession, and iridocorneal endothelial syndrome). In these cases, you have to prepare 0.4 mg/mL.

(Courtesy: Dr Md Lutfor Rahman, Associate Professor, Neuro-ophthalmology, NIO).

ANS: 09

Fitting of BCL into the dummy's right eye.
1. Model of eye
2. Bandage contact lens
3. Novocaine eye drop
4. If there are soap and water

ANS: 10

Prepare amphotericin B for fungal corneal ulcer.

Checklist

Step 1: Mix 10 mL of sterile water in 50 mg of amphotericin B powder. This will give 5 mg/mL solution (Solution #1)

Step 2: Take 3 mL (15 mg) from solution #1 and mix 7 mL of sterile water. This will give 15 mg/10 mL, i.e. 1.5 mg/mL, i.e. 0.15%.

Caution
- Prepared solution can be used for a week
- Keep the parent solution in freeze at 4°C (in egg rack of refrigerator)
- Drops are clear yellow in color, if they turn milky then discard them
- Protect them from light.

ANS: 11

In essential blepharospasm, botulinum toxin A is injected into the:
- Medial and
- Lateral pretarsal orbicularis oculi of the upper lid and
- Lateral pretarsal orbicularis oculi of the lower lid.

And each side is given 2.5–5.0 units. Botulinum toxin A is available in 100 units and 50 units of single-use vials, so it should be diluted before use.

Preparation

100 IU is diluted with 4 mL normal saline and 50 IU is diluted with 2 mL normal saline.
So, 1 mL contains 25 IU.
So, if we want to inject 2.5 IU in each side, we have to take 0.1 mL solution in insulin syringe.

ANS: 12

Topical voriconazole eye drops 1%.
Method
Mix 20 mL Ringer's lactate to 200 mg voriconazole lyophilized powder.
Label: Voriconazole eye drops 1%, stability: 30 days at 4°C or room temperature.

Voriconazole for intrastromal injection 50 µg/0.1 mL

Method
From 1% voriconazole solution, take 1 mL, and add 19 mL Ringer's lactate to make 0.05 mg/mL (50 µg/0.1 mL).

CHAPTER 10

Procedure

INTRODUCTION

Procedure is an important part of OSPE examination, but there are lots of procedure, sometime there are two stations in examination, such as in one station you have to prepare fortified gentamicin, or intravitreal vancomycin and another station under microscope, you have to repair a corneal injury (usually goat's eye is supplied for this station, and every examinee will get a new eye).

In this chapter, we set some stations for your practice, but students are requested to do group practice for this station such as steps of trabeculectomy, recession, or resection of extraocular muscle in squint. Such as, do the surgery of 25° exotropia in right eye. In this station, examiner will see that do you know which muscle or muscles have to cut? And do you know recession or resection? Any of the procedure can be given so you have to prepare yourself in that way.

But in this station, proper wearing of the gloves will carry some marks. So if you do not know the procedure, do not worry; proper wearing of the hand gloves will carry some marks, remember one and two marks are vital in OSPE station. So, not to be nervous, keep cool and be patience.

OSPE: 01. Do the retinoscopy of this simulated patient and draw your findings in supplied papers.
OSPE: 02. Do the refraction of this simulated patient.
OSPE: 03. Do the indirect gonioscopy in right eye.
OSPE: 04. Measure the intraocular pressure (IOP) with the tonometer.
OSPE: 05. Procedure of indirect ophthalmoscopy.
OSPE: 06. Performing anterior chamber (AC) paracentesis and discard waste product in proper container.
OSPE: 07. Construct a 6 mm scleral tunnel on the supplied eyeball.
OSPE: 08. Positioning of the patient and examination of cornea with slit lamp.
OSPE: 09. Visual acuity recording.
OSPE: 10. Steps of removal of superficial corneal foreign body (FB) with the help of slit-lamp biomicroscope.
OSPE: 11. Measurement of anterior-posterior displacement of globe.
OSPE: 12. Do the Schirmer's test I (Schirmer's without anesthetics).

OSPE: 13. Do the Schirmer's test II.
OSPE: 14. Examine the patient with direct ophthalmoscopy.
OSPE: 15. Hand wash.
OSPE: 16. Do the prism's cover test of this simulated patient who is suffering from exotropia of right eye?
OSPE: 17. Corneal scraping.
OSPE: 18. A 45-year-old school teacher having −2.50 D myopia in both eyes and using the same specs for last 20 years comfortably. Now, she came to you for difficulties in reading. Do retinoscopy from 2/3 meter distance and prescribe the spectacle.
OSPE: 19. *Construct triangular sclera flap (3 × 3 mm) for trabeculectomy (fornix based) by supplied instruments.*
OSPE: 20. *Procedure of posterior subtenon injection.*

OSPE: 01
Do the retinoscopy of this simulated patient and draw your findings in supplied papers.
- In this OSPE, it has two parts one is the procedure that you have to do in front of the observer, and the other part you have to draw the figure of your retinoscopy findings (remember your patient is SP, whatever is his refractive status you think he is emmetropic and draw your figure according to your working distance).

Checklist
A. Rapport building 0.25
B. Look at the target point 0.50
C. Adjusting the retinoscopy by focusing on the screen or wall 1.0
D. Fixed the desire distance 0.50
E. Fix the trial frame 0.25
F. Pick up the desired lens from the trial set (+1.0 for 1 m distance, and +1.50 Dsph for 2/3 meter distance) 1.0
G. See the movement of the light both in horizontal and vertical meridians 1.0
H. Keep in place of all the material used 0.25
I. Thanks' to the patient 0.25
TOTAL ***5.0***

Drawing of the retinoscopy findings:

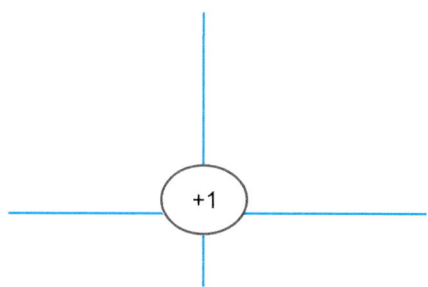

Working distance is 1 m, if working distance is 2/3 meter, then writes +1.50 instead of +1.0.

OSPE: 02
Do the refraction of this simulated patient.
- This station is more or less similar to above one, but instead of draw the retinoscopy finding, you should do ocular motility test, cover test, and measure the interpupillary distance (IPD).

Checklist
A. Rapport building 0.25
B. Look at the target point 0.50
C. Adjusting the retinoscopy by focusing on the screen or wall 1.0
D. Fixed the desire distance 0.50
E. Fix the trial frame 0.25
F. Pick up the desired lens from the trial set (+1.0 for 1 m distance, and +1.50 for 2/3 meter distance) 1.0
G. See the movement of the light both in horizontal and vertical meridians 1.0
H. Keep in place of all the material used 0.25
I. Give addition if SP is above 40 years old 1.0
J. See the ocular motility in both eyes 2.0
K. Do the cover-uncover test 1.0
L. Measure IPD 1.0
M. Thanks' to the patient 0.25
TOTAL 10.0

OSPE: 03
Do the indirect gonioscopy in right eye.

Checklist
A. Rapport building 0.25
B. The patient and the examiner must be positioned in a comfortable fashion 1.0
C. A drop of topical anesthetic is then applied to the conjunctiva of both eyes 1.0
D. Contact gel is placed in the concave part of the lens 1.0
E. The patient is then asked to open both eyes and look upward 1.0
F. The examiner can then pull down slightly on the lower lid and places the lens on the surface of the eye 2.0
G. The patient is then asked to look straight ahead 0.5
H. Start with the inferior angle 1.0
I. Continue identifying all angle structures in all four quadrants 2.0
J. Thanks' to the patient 0.25
TOTAL 10

OSPE: 04
Measure the IOP with the tonometer.

Checklist
1. Rapport building ....
2. Instill the local anesthetic drops ....

3. Pull down the lower fornix and insert the fluorescein strip ....
4. Wash out the excess fluorescein..
5. Check the calibration of the dial and set it into "1" ....
6. To measure the IOP in the right eye, the slit beam is shining on to the tonometer head from the patient's right side..
7. Use the blue filter ....
8. The blue light should be in maximum intensity and wide ....
9. Ask the patient to look straight ahead at your ear (your left ear for his right eye) ....
10. With the help of your thumb, hold up the patient upper eyelid but not to press over the globe ....
11. Direct the blue light from the slit lamp onto the prism head ....
12. Make sure that the tonometer head is perpendicular to the eye ....
13. Move the tonometer forward slowly until the prism rests gently on the center of the patient's cornea ....
14. With the other hand, turn the calibrated dial on the tonometer clockwise until the two fluorescein semi-circles in the prism head are seen to meet and form a horizontal "S" shape..
15. Note the reading on the dial and record it in the notes ....
16. Withdraw the prism from the corneal surface and wipe its tip ....
17. Repeat the procedure for the other eye ....
18. Wipe the prism with a clean, dry swab and replace it in the receptacle containing the disinfectant..
19. Thanks' to the patient ....

OSPE: 05
Procedure of indirect ophthalmoscopy.

Checklist
A. Rapport building..
B. Adjustment of the ophthalmoscope ....
C. Adjust headband crown...
D. Adjust the pupillary distance ....
E. Check illumination intensity. Check for a proper elevation/position. Check can be done by extending arm or by looking at a wall ....
F. Apply filter if desired..
G. Positioning the patient—Patient should be in a supine position..
H. Patient should be looking directly up, initially (primary position)..
I. Examiner should initially stand to the side of the patient, leaning over the patient ....
J. Insert handheld lens approximately 2 inches away from patient's eye, moving it closer or farther away to focus and refine the view ....
K. Examiner swivels his view around to view different parts of the retina, by tilting the head and walking around the patient ....
L. The doctor instructs the patient to look at various extremes of their vision ....
M. Thanks to the patient...

OSPE: 06
Performing AC paracentesis and discard waste product in proper container (red, green, and yellow).

Checklist

		Done
1.	Wearing of the gloves	1.0
2.	Adjustment of operating microscope	
	(a) Light on	0.25
	(b) Height	0.25
	(c) IPD	0.25
3.	Install anesthetic drop in the eye	0.50
4.	Cotton-tipped applicator soaked with anesthetic agent	0.50
5.	Hold the tipped at the insertion of medial rectus muscle	0.5
6.	Placed an eyelid speculum	0.5
7.	Under the microscope, fixate the eye with the help of St Martin forceps at the insertion of medial rectus muscle	1.0
8.	Enter the needle in AC	
	(a) Enter the 30 gauge (or supplied) needle into AC through temporal limbus	1.0
	(b) Bevel end of the needle pointing up and parallel with iris	0.5
	(c) Keep the needle tip over the mid-periphery of the iris and avoid to touch iris or lens throughout the procedure	0.5
9.	Withdraw fluid from AC until you can observe that it shallows slightly	0.5
10.	Withdraw the needle from AC	0.5
11.	Off the microscope switch	0.25
	– Discard end product: Plastic syringe and gloves: **Green**	1.0
	– Needle/sharp instrument: **Red**	
	– Goat's eye: **Yellow**	
12.	Maintain chronology of the procedure	1.0

OSPE: 07
Construct a 6 mm scleral tunnel on the supplied eyeball.

Checklist

Points *Done*

1.	Instill surface anesthetic drop	1.0
2.	Adjust operating microscope (light, IPD, and magnification)	1.5
3.	Wear surgical gloves	0.5
4.	Peritomy	1.0
5.	Measurement by caliper (6 mm)	0.5
6.	Incision (with 15° knife)	1.0
7.	Making a scleral tunnel (with crescent knife)	3.0
8.	Place instruments in right place	0.5
9.	Chronology maintain	1.0
TOTAL		***10***

OSPE: 08

Positioning of the patient and examination of cornea with slit lamp.

Checklist

		Done
A.	Rapport building	0.5
B.	Positioning of the patient on slit lamp	1.0
C.	Examination with diffuse illumination	1.5
D.	Examination with direct focal illumination	1.5
E.	Examination with oblique beam	1.5
F.	Examination with retroillumination	1.5
G.	Detection of cells/flare by 1 × 1 mm light	2.0
H.	Thanks to the patient	0.25
Total		*10*

OSPE: 09

Visual acuity recording.

Checklist

		Done
A.	Rapport building	0.5
B.	Recording of unaided vision of R/E for distance	1.0
C.	Recording of unaided vision of R/E with pinhole	1.0
D.	Recording of unaided vision of L/E for distance	1.0
E.	Recording of unaided vision of L/E with pinhole	1.0
F.	Recording of unaided vision of R/E for near	1.0
G.	Recording of unaided vision of L/E for near	1.0
H.	Recording of aided vision of R/E for distance	1.0
I.	Recording of aided vision of L/E for distance	1.0
J.	Recording of aided vision of R/E for near	1.0
K.	Thanks' to the patient	0.5
TOTAL		*10*

OSPE: 10

Steps of removal of superficial corneal with the help of slit-lamp biomicroscope.

Checklist

		Done
A.	Rapport building	0.5
B.	Application of topical anesthesia	2.0
C.	Positioning of the patient on slit lamp	2.0
D.	Removal of FB with sterile swab stick/FB spud/26 G needle	3.0
E.	Application of eye pad with ointment	2.0
F.	Thanks' to the patient	0.5
TOTAL		*10*

OSPE: 11
Measurement of anterior-posterior displacement of globe.
Checklist
A. Rapport building 0.5
B. Patient setup 1.0
C. Examinee position 1.0
D. Instrument placement 2.0
E. Bar reading adjustment 2.0
F. Occlusion of patient's one eye 1.5
G. Measurement of patient's both eyes 1.5
H. Thanks' to the patient 0.5
TOTAL *10*

OSPE: 12
Do the Schirmer's test I (Schirmer's without anesthetics).
Checklist
A. Seat the patient in a dimmed room with the back of the head stabilize against the header of the examining chair.
B. Remove any excess moisture from the patient's eyelid margin with a facial tissue or cotton-tipped applicator. Do not instill any eye drops into the eye before the test.
C. Fold a packaged, sterile filter paper strip at the indentation mark. To avoid contaminating the sterile strips, bend the round wick end of the test strips at the notch 120° before opening the pouch.
D. Open the pouch and remove a strip. Use the strip with the angled end for the right eye. Grasp the strip by the nonwick end to avoid contaminating the wick end with your fingertips.
E. Ask the patient to look up. Draw the lower lid gently downward, checking to make sure that the lid margin has been adequately dried with a cotton-tipped applicator. By convention, the strip with one corner cut off is used for the right eye.

(Ref: Wilson FM. Practical Ophthalmology: A Manual for Beginning Residents, 4th edition. United States: American Academy of Ophthalmology; 1996. p. 210).

OSPE: 13
Do the Schirmer's test II.
Checklist
A. Rapport building 0.25
B. Explain the procedure and take consent 1.50
C. Creating environment for test 0.50
D. Installation of surface anesthesia 1.50
E. Wiping the pre-existing tear 1.50
F. Placement of the Schirmer strip 1.50
G. Stimulation through the nostrils for 2 minutes with swab sticks 1.50
H. Take reading after a total of 5 minutes 1.50
I. Thanks' to the patient 0.25
TOTAL *10*

How to read results of the Schirmer test?
1. *Normal*: It is more than or equal to 15 mm wetting of the paper after 5 minutes.
2. *Mild*: It is 14–9 mm wetting of the paper after 5 minutes.
3. *Moderate*: It is 8–4 mm wetting of the paper after 5 minutes.
4. *Severe*: It is less than 4 mm wetting of the paper after 5 minutes.

OSPE: 14

Examine the patient with direct ophthalmoscopy.

Checklist
A. Rapport building 0.5
B. Explain the procedure 2.0
C. Fixation of target 1.0
D. Start ophthalmoscopy from one arm's length of distance that gradually moves forward 1.0
E. Procedure to see the central fundus 2.5
F. Procedure to see the peripheral fundus 2.5
G. Thanks' to the patient 0.5
TOTAL 10

OSPE: 15

Hand wash.

Checklist
A. Total duration of hand wash 2.0
B. Materials used in hand wash (soap, betadine, and hibiscrub) 2.0
C. Wash up to elbow 2.0
D. Direction of flow of water 2.0
E. Importance of hand wash and how to dry and hold up hands 2.0
TOTAL 10

OSPE: 16

Do the prism's cover test of this simulated patient who is suffering from exotropia of right eye?

Checklist

Done
1. Greetings 0.25
2. Look for any abnormal head posture 0.5
3. Shine a torchlight into the patient's eye from about 0.5 m away and observe the corneal reflexes for any tropia 1
4. Perform a cover test
   For near (33 cm) 0.5
   6 m 0.5
5. Perform an alternate cover test
   For near (33 cm) 0.5
   6 m 0.5
6. Perform the prism cover test
   For near (33 cm), prism will be placed in front of the R/E apex temporally 1.5
   6 m prism will be placed in front of the R/E apex temporally 1.5

7. Perform an alternate cover test by moving the occluder from one eye to another 1.5
8. Observe the movement of the eye behind the prism as it takes up fixation. Increase the prism strength until there is no movement seen in the deviating eye when the other eye is covered 1.5
9. Thanks' to the patient 0.25
TOTAL **10**

NB: When testing for near, you may need the patient to hold the fixating target to allow you free hand to perform the prism cover test.

OSPE: 17

A patient with corneal ulcer getting moxifloxacin eye drop but not improving, you have decided to corneal scraping.

A. Topical anesthetic is instilled
B. Scrapings are taken either with a disposable scalpel blade (e.g. No. 11 or Bard Parker), the bent tip of a larger diameter (e.g. 20- or 21-gauge) hypodermic needle, or a sterile spatula (e.g. Kimura)
C. Loose mucus and necrotic tissue should be removed from the surface of the ulcer prior to scraping
D. The margins and base (except if very thin) of the lesion are scraped
E. A thin smear is placed on one or two glass slides for microscopy, including Gram stain
F. A surface is provided on one side of one end of the slide (conventionally "up") for pencil labeling
G. The sample is allowed to dry in air at room temperature for several minutes and then placed in a slide carrier
H. Rescraping is performed for each medium and samples are plated onto culture media
I. Routinely, blood, chocolate, and Sabouraud media are used initially and the samples are placed in an incubator until transported to the laboratory.

OSPE: 18

A 45-year-old school teacher having −2.50 D myopia in both eyes and using the same specs for last 20 years comfortably. Now, she came to you for difficulties in reading. Do retinoscopy from 2/3 meter distance and prescribe the spectacle.

Checklist

Points   *Marks*
1. Greeting 0.25
2. Visual acuity
   2a. Unaided 0.5
   2b. Pinhole 0.5
   2c. With existing specs 0.5
3. Setting trial frame 0.5
4. Occlude one eye 0.5
5. Check retinoscopy 0.5
6. Retinoscopy with −1.00 DS lens
   6a. Horizontal meridian 1.0
   6b. Vertical meridian 1.0

7. Subjective tests
   (a) Distance with −2.50 DS 1.0
   (b) Near with add +1.50 DS 1.0
8. Ocular motility 1.0
9. Papillary reaction 1.0
10. Proper placing of used instruments 0.5
11. Thanks to the patient 0.25
TOTAL *10*

OSPE: 19

Construct triangular sclera flap (3 × 3 mm) for trabeculectomy (fornix based) by supplied instruments.

Checklist

Steps *Marks*

A. Wearing of the gloves 1.0
B. Microscope adjustment 0.5
C. Make conjunctival flap from upper limbus toward fornix 2.0
D. Clear episcleral tissue 1.0
E. Outline proposed flap (5 × 5 mm) with slide calipers and make incision half of the scleral thickness 1.5
F. Dissect sclera flap from apex to base 1.5
G. Cut full thickness (3 × 3 mm) sclera from the prepare base 1.5
H. Turn off microscope switch 0.5
I. Dispose disposable 0.5
TOTAL *10*

OSPE: 20

Procedure of posterior subtenon injection.

A. A topical anesthetic such as tetracaine (amethocaine) is instilled.
B. A small cotton pledget impregnated with tetracaine, lidocaine (lignocaine) 2% gel, or an alternative is placed into the superior fornix at the site of injection for 2 minutes.
C. The vial containing the steroid is shaken, 1 mL steroid (triamcinolone acetonide, methylprednisolone acetate, or 40 mg/mL) is drawn up into a 2-mL syringe and the drawing-up needle is replaced with a 25-gauge, 5/8 inch (16 mm) needle.
D. The patient is asked to look in the direction opposite to the superotemporal injection site.
E. The bulbar conjunctiva is penetrated with the tip of the needle, bevel toward the globe, and slightly on the bulbar side of the fornix.
F. The needle is slowly inserted posteriorly, following the contour of the globe, keeping it as close to the globe as possible.
G. In order not to penetrate the globe accidentally, wide side-to-side motions are made as the needle is being inserted and the limbus is watched; movement of the limbus means that the sclera has been engaged.
H. When the needle has been advanced to the hub, the plunger is slightly withdrawn and, if no blood enters the syringe, the full 1 mL is slowly injected.

CHAPTER 11

Examination Procedures

QUESTIONS

OSPE: 01. Show the examination of levator palpebrae superioris (LPS) muscle in this simulated patient of congenital ptosis.
OSPE: 02. A young patient comes to you with complain of uniocular sudden loss of vision. How will you examine the patient with given instruments (pen torch, Snellen chart, Ishihara chart, and ophthalmoscope)?
OSPE: 03. 5th cranial nerve examination.
OSPE: 04. Cranial nerve examination (3rd and 6th).
OSPE: 05. Cranial nerve examination (3rd, 4th, 6th, 5th, and 7th).
OSPE: 06. Examine the simulating patient of keratoconus with the supplied instruments (pen torch, ophthalmoscope, and retinoscope) and mention two signs with pen torch, one sign with ophthalmoscope, and one sign with retinoscope.
OSPE: 07. Protocol of examination of proptosis.
OSPE: 08. Examine a case of ptosis with running commentary.
OSPE: 09. Measuring of interpupillary distance (IPD).
OSPE: 10. Performing the cover and uncover test.
OSPE: 11. Pupillary light reflex.
OSPE: 12. Examine the patient of proptosis.
OSPE: 13. Schiotz tonometry.
OSPE: 14. Color fundus photography.
OSPE: 15. General examination of the patient.
OSPE: 16. Confrontation test.

ANSWERS

ANS: 01

Checklist

A.	Rapport building	0.5
B.	Ask to look at primary position	0.5
C.	Ask to look at extreme downgaze	1.5
D.	Hold a transparent scale marking upper lid margin	1.5
E.	Press thumb on eyebrows	1.0
F.	Ask for look at upgaze	1.5
G.	Fix scale	1.5
H.	Ask the position	1.5
I.	Thanks' to the patient	0.5
	TOTAL	***10***

ANS: 02

Checklist

A.	Rapport building	0.5
B.	Visual acuity	2.0
C.	Pupillary light reaction	
	(a) Direct	1.5
	(b) Consensual	1.5
D.	Color vision	2.0
E.	Fundus examination	2.0
F.	Thanks' to the patient	0.5
	TOTAL	***10***

ANS: 03

Checklist

A.	Rapport building	0.5
B.	Sensation of ophthalmic division of 5th nerve (fine touch)	1.5
C.	Sensation of ophthalmic division of 5th nerve (pain)	1.5
D.	Sensation of maxillary division of 5th nerve (fine touch)	1.5
E.	Sensation of maxillary division of 5th nerve (pain)	1.5
F.	Sensation of mandibular division of 5th nerve (fine touch)	1.0
G.	Sensation of mandibular division of 5th nerve (pain)	1.0
H.	Muscles of mastication (motor function of 5th nerve)	1.0
I.	Thanks' to the patient	0.5
	TOTAL	***10***

ANS: 04

Checklist

A.	Rapport building	0.5
B.	Positioning of the patient	1.0

Examination Procedures 193

C. Observation of primary gaze 2.0
D. Dextroversion 1.0
E. Dextroelevation 1.0
F. Dextrodepression 1.0
G. Levoversion 1.0
H. Levoelevation 1.0
I. Levodepression 1.0
J. Thanks' to the patient 0.5
 TOTAL *10*

ANS: 05

Checklist
A. Rapport building 0.5
B. Examination of 3rd cranial nerve 1.5
C. Examination of 4th cranial nerve 1.5
D. Examination of 6th cranial nerve 1.5
E. Sensation of ophthalmic division of 5th cranial nerve (fine touch and pain) 1.0
F. Sensation of maxillary division of 5th cranial nerve (fine touch and pain) 1.0
G. Muscles of mastication (motor function of 5th cranial nerve) 1.0
H. Examination of 7th cranial nerve 1.5
I. Thanks' to the patient 0.5
 TOTAL *10*

ANS: 06

Checklist
A. Rapport building 0.5
B. Rizzuti's reflex by torch 2.0
C. Munson sign by torch 2.0
D. Oil drop reflex by ophthalmoscope 3.0
E. Scissors reflex by retinoscope 2.0
F. Thanks' to the patient 0.5
 TOTAL *10*
Or if slit lamp has given:
A. Rapport building 0.25
B. Positioning of patient 0.25
C. Positioning of slit lamp 0.5
D. Munson sign (by looking down and holding the upper lids) 2.0
E. Diffuse illumination (see hydropic scar and Vogt's striae) 2.0
F. Oblique illumination (corneal thinning/steepening) 2.0
G. Fleischer ring (using cobalt blue filter) 3.0
 TOTAL *10*

ANS: 07

Checklist
A. Introduction and greetings.

By inspection
B. Look for facial symmetry
C. Any head/face tilt
D. Overall inspection of the face/neck (for thyroid)
E. Tremor of the hand (say the patient outstretches both hands and put a paper over the dorsum of the hand to see fine tremor).

Inspection with torch
F. Hirschberg's reflex
G. Inside the nose and mouth
H. Pupil [direct, consensual, relative afferent pupillary defect (RAPD), and anisocoria].

By palpation
I. Measure the anterior-posterior displacement of the globe
J. Lateral displacement
K. Feel the orbital rim
L. Insinuation
M. Palpate thyroid
N. Palpate cervical lymph nodes
O. Extraocular muscle (EOM) (if limitation, then duction should be performed)
P. Lid lag
Q. Retropulsation with palm of hand
R. Skin temperature
S. Pulse rate
T. Bruit with bell over globe/carotid.

ANS: 08

Checklist
A. Greetings 0.25
B. Inspecting the following points .... 0.5 × 4 .... 2.0
   i. Head posture
   ii. Brow elevation
   iii. Palpebral fissure
   iv. Presence or absence of lid crease
C. Pupillary examination
   i. Direct
   ii. Consensual.
D. Ocular motility 1.5
E. The palpebral fissure—the distance between the upper and lower eyelids in vertical alignment with the center of the pupil 1.0
F. The marginal reflex distance-1 (MRD-1) 1.0
G. Levator function 1.0
H. Corneal reflex with cotton 1.0
I. Bell's phenomena 0.5
J. Marcus Gunn jaw-winking phenomena 0.5
K. Thanks' to the patient 0.25
TOTAL ***10***

ANS: 09

A. Ask patient to fixate a distance target.
B. Facing the patient at an arm's length distance, position yourself just below the patient's gaze. Align your eyes with the patient's eyes as the patient maintains distance fixation over your hand.
C. Rest the millimeter ruler lightly across the bridge of the patient's nose.
D. Close your right eye and use your left eye to line up the zero point of the ruler with the temporal limbus of the patient's right eye.
E. Keep the ruler steady. Close your left eye and open your right eye.
F. Read the measurement that aligns with the nasal limbus of the patient's left eye.
G. Repeat the above sequence to confirm a reproducible reading.
H. Near IPD is measured in a similar way by having the patient stare at your nose instead of the distance target.

(Ref: Wilson FM. Practical Ophthalmology: A Manual for Beginning Residents, 4th edition. United States: American Academy of Ophthalmology; 1996. p. 210).

ANS: 10

A. Have the patient look at a distance fixation target, and position yourself directly opposite to the patient, within arm length (remember, level of both will be the same and you have to sit in front of the patient in such a manner that will not obstruct the patient distance vision).
B. Swiftly cover the fixating eye with an occluder or your hand, and observe the other eye for any movement. Carefully note down it direction.
C. Uncover the eye and allow about 3 seconds for both eyes to be uncovered.
D. Swiftly cover the other eye and observe its fellow for any movement.
E. Ensure that the patient is maintaining fixation on the same point as established for step 1.
F. After an interval of about a second, uncover the eye and observe it for any movement.
G. Note results but do not record them until other cover test is completed.
H. Repeat the test for near, using a near fixation point.
I. Repeat the distance and near tests using the patient's habitual refractive correction, if applicable.

(Ref: Wilson FM. Practical Ophthalmology: A Manual for Beginning Residents, 4th edition. United States: American Academy of Ophthalmology; 1996. p. 210).

ANS: 11

Checklist
1. Greetings and consent
2. Covering of one eye
3. Direction of light and elicit direct light reflex
4. Elicit consensual light reflex
5. Elicit RAPD

ANS: 12

Checklist
1. Greetings and consent
2. Inspection

3. Insinuation
4. Palpation
5. Reducibility
6. Auscultation
7. Valsalva maneuver
8. Examination of oral and nasal cavity
9. Cervical lymph node examination
10. Ask for consent

ANS: 13

Checklist
1. Greetings and consent
2. Positioning of the patient
3. Instillation of S/A
4. Preparing the instrument
5. Placing properly on eye not holding the lids
6. First with 5 g
7. Then with 10 g
8. Interpretation of measurement
9. Put back instrument properly
10. Thanks' to the patient

ANS: 14

Checklist
1. Identification of eye
2. Media
3. Disk color
4. Disk margin
5. Disk blood vessels
6. Cup-to-disk (CD) ratio
7. Neuroretinal rim (NRR)
8. Distribution of major blood vessels
9. Peripheral fundus
10. Macula

ANS: 15

Checklist
1. Greetings and consent
2. Standing on which side of the patient
3. Temperature
4. Pulse, BP
5. Anemia, jaundice, and edema
6. Heart, lung
7. Cervical lymph nodes

8. Neck veins
9. Thyroid
10. Liver, spleen, and kidney

ANS: 16

Checklist
1. Greetings and consent
2. Positioning of patient and examinee
3. Covering of patient's and examinee's eyes
4. Asking the patient to look at the uncovered eye and carrying out the procedure on one side
5. Repeat the procedure on the other side

CHAPTER 12

History Taking

QUESTIONS

Followings are the examples of history taking:

OSPE: 01. This 40-year male suffering from double vision, please take the relevant history.
OSPE: 02. History taking of red eye with discharge.
OSPE: 03. History taking of retinitis pigmentosa (RP).
OSPE: 04. A parent came to you along with his son 3-year-old with the complaints of visual problem and squint. Please take the relevant history.
OSPE: 05. Take the relevant history from the parent for his child of 2-year-old suffering from unilateral cataract.
OSPE: 06. History taking of primary open-angle glaucoma (POAG).
OSPE: 07. History taking of headache.
OSPE: 08. Recurrent uveitis.
OSPE: 09. A patient came to you with sudden onset of nystagmus, take the relevant history.
OSPE: 10. *"I woke up this morning and got a huge shock when I looked in my bathroom mirror, one-half of my face was drooping! I immediately panicked and called an ambulance!" This is the statement of a 65-year-old lady who meets you in emergency room (ER). Take the relevant history from the patient.*
OSPE: 11. A patient came to you with corneal opacity. What history should you take from that patient, mention with explanation for the relevant histories?
OSPE: 12. This 40-year male suffering from double vision, please take the relevant history.
OSPE: 13. History taking of ptosis.
OSPE: 14. A 60-year-old patient complaints of sudden dimness of vision in his right eye for last 2 days. The patient gave history of cataract surgery in that eye 7 days back. He is neither diabetic nor hypertensive.

ANSWERS

ANS: 01
Checklist

		Done
1.	Rapport building	0.25
2.	Whether double vision is monocular or binocular	1.5
3.	Direction of double vision, whether the diplopia is horizontal, vertical, or torsional	1.0
4.	Ask the patient in which direction of gaze the diplopia is worse—right, left, up, down, right and up, right and down, left and up, left and down, or distance or near	1.0
5.	Ask for diurnal variability and fatigability of diplopia	1.0
6.	Detailed history about: .... 0.25 × 6	1.5

    (a) Mode of onset
    (b) Duration of onset
    (c) Associated pain
    (d) History of strabismus in childhood
    (e) History of trauma
    (f) Neurological symptoms such as dysphagia or weakness

7.	Detailed history about: .... 0.5 × 5	2.5

    (a) Hypertension
    (b) Diabetes
    (c) Cerebrovascular disease
    (d) Cardiac atherosclerotic disease
    (e) Multiple sclerosis

8.	History of smoking and alcohol intake should be elicited	1.0
9.	Thanks' to the patient	0.25
TOTAL		***10***

ANS: 02
Checklist

1.	Rapport building	0.25
2.	Consent	1.0
3.	Occupation of the patient	1.5
4.	History of trauma	1.0
5.	Duration of symptom	1.5
6.	If there is diminution of vision	1.5
7.	Pain	1.0
8.	Photophobia	1.0
9.	Stickiness of lids in the morning	1.0
10.	Thanks' to the patient	0.25
TOTAL		***10***

ANS: 03
Checklist
1. Greetings and self-introduction 0.25
2. What is the duration of dimness of vision? 1
3. Is the dimness of vision slowly progressive? 1
4. Was it started with night vision problem? 1
5. Family history of RP. If yes, where they examine? 1
6. History of consanguine marriage of a parent 1
7. History of drug intake 0.50
8. History of trauma 0.50
9. History of hearing disorder, ataxia, nystagmus 0.75
10. History of mental retardation (you cannot ask the patient, are you mentally retarded)? But, if his guardian is at there, you can ask it to the guardian. Otherwise you can ask the patient in which class she/he reads? And you can calculate, is it correct according to his/her age? 1
11. History of heart disease 0.50
12. History of hypogenitalism, obesity, and polydactyl 0.75
13. History of diarrhea and skeletal deformity 0.50
14. Thanks to the patient 0.25
TOTAL 10

ANS: 04
Checklist
(Remember this is an open question, type of squint has not mentioned. So, your question will be according to the general question of squint. No need to try to elicit the type of squint.)
A. *Questions regarding squint*:
   i. Unilateral or altering or intermittent.
   ii. Any abnormal head posture, or movements.
   iii. When the squint is more noticeable?
   iv. Is it related to fatigue or illness?
   v. Is there symptom of any diplopia?
   vi. Mention precipitating factors like trauma and febrile episode before onset of squint.
B. *To assess low vision*:
   i. How and when was low vision noticed?
   ii. Does the child hold toys/books close to face?
   iii. Does she/he watch TV very closely?
   iv. Does he respond to visual stimuli? Visual response in unfamiliar surroundings.
C. *Birth and medical history:*
   i. Gestational age
   ii. Significant antenatal history
   iii. Maternal infection, any drugs taken during pregnancy
   iv. History of any other handicap
   v. Any untoward event during delivery

vi. Birth trauma, forceps, birth asphyxia
vii. Birth weight of the child
viii. History of being kept in incubator
ix. History of oxygenation
x. Is the child thriving well?
xi. Developmental milestone, both physical and mental
xii. Any associated systemic problem
xiii. Other associated neurological problems like cerebral palsy, epilepsy, mental retardation, and craniofacial anomalies.

D. *Family history:*
   i. Consanguinity
   ii. Similar problem in other siblings
   iii. History of any inherited eye or systemic condition.

(*Source*: Nethralaya S. Clinical Practice Pattern in Ophthalmology, 2nd edition. New Delhi: Jaypee Brothers Medical Publishers (P) Ltd.; 2012. p. 302.)

ANS: 05

Take the relevant history from the parent for his child of 2-year old, suffering from unilateral cataract.

Checklist

A. *General history:*
   i. When was white reflex noted?
   ii. Congenital cataract in the family—sibling history.
   iii. Trauma/child abuse.
   iv. Behavioral pattern of child at home.
   v. Visual status ambulation in familiar and unfamiliar surroundings.
   vi. School performance, especially reading (if the child more than 3–4 years old and school going).

B. *Birth history:*
   i. History and degree of consanguinity
   ii. Maternal infection, especially first trimester of pregnancy
   iii. Gestational age
   iv. Birth weight
   v. Birth trauma, untoward event during delivery
   vi. Supplemental oxygen therapy or being kept in incubator
   vii. Developmental milestone
   viii. Feeding/digestive behavior
   ix. Developmental milestone.

ANS: 06

History taking of primary open-angle glaucoma (POAG).

Checklist

1. Is there any family member suffering from glaucoma?
2. Profession of patient.

3. Is there frequent change of presbyopic glass?
4. Is there any visual problem?
5. Have you ever been used antiallergic eye drop?
6. Using any systemic or topical medication for other reason.
7. H/O asthma, DM, HTN.
8. History of trauma.
9. Any frontal headache.
10. Have you ever measure of your IOP by your eye doctor?
11. Is there any problem during driving?
12. In advanced stage, visual field is constricted, so asked him can he see periphery clearly, such as when he is in prayer can see the surroundings.
13. It is not a curable disease.

ANS: 07

Checklist
A. *Under demographic history*:
   i. Age
   ii. *Gender*: Menstruation history, any hormone use
   iii. Occupation
   iv. Social history
   v. Stressors (alcohol and drugs, sleep, eating, and exercise habit)
B. Past history
C. Systemic illness
D. Family history of headache:
   i. Migraine (40–60% in first-degree relatives).
E. *Under heading of characteristic of headache:*
   i. Onset
      (How long has the HA been presented)
   ii. Nature
      (Episodic versus continuous)
   iii. Frequency
      (Per week, per month, per year)
   iv. Duration
      (Minutes, hours, days, etc.)
   v. Severity
      (Pain scale or documentation of loss of normal functioning)
   vi. Character of pain
      (Stabbing, squeezing, pulsatile)
   vii. Location
      (Unilateral, bilateral, frontotemporal, occipital)

viii. Radiation aura
(Specify what type)
ix. Aggravating factors
(Photophobia, physical exertion)
x. Alleviating factors
(Medications used, sleep, position change, etc.)
xi. Associated nausea or vomiting
xii. Recent head injury or concussion.

ANS: 08

Checklist:
A. *Demography*:
   i. Age
   ii. Gender (no need to ask)
   iii. Race
   iv. Residence
   v. Occupation
B. *Ocular history*:
   i. Laterality
   ii. Primary symptoms
   iii. Duration
   iv. Onset
   v. Severity
   vi. Course
   vii. Associated findings
C. *Systemic history*:
   i. All systemic problems
   ii. Associated other diseases
D. *Treatment history*:
   i. A detail history on dosage of medicines that patient is already taking.
   ii. Response to treatment
   iii. Treatment of complications
   iv. Compliance of patient
E. *Others*:
   i. History of trauma
   ii. History of surgery.

ANS: 09

Checklist
1. Age of onset of the nystagmus
2. Whether it is constant or intermittent

3. The presence of any aggravating or alleviating factors *(e.g. head position)*
4. Presence or absence of vertigo, oscillopsia *(an illusory motion of the seen world)*, and sensation of disequilibrium (it suggests a lesion of the vestibular system)
5. Deafness or tinnitus is present with peripheral lesions of the vestibular system
6. Presence of diplopia, particularly in certain positions of gaze: patients with internuclear ophthalmoplegia (INO) may report diplopia only on lateral gaze or intermittent blurring of vision.
7. Ask questions regarding the presence of any associated symptoms, such as symptoms related to demyelinating disease (e.g. a history of loss of vision, eye pain, or numbness or weakness of the extremities)
8. Symptoms related to cerebrovascular accident (e.g. hemiplegic), and predispositions to thiamine deficiency (e.g. alcoholism, bariatric surgery)
9. Medications such as anticonvulsants and lithium may be associated with nystagmus.

ANS: 10

Checklist
A. History of presenting complaint:
   i. Which side did you notice the facial weakness on?
   ii. At what time did you first notice the facial weakness?
   iii. Do you have normal facial sensation?
   iv. Is there any visual disturbance?
   v. Are you able to eat or drink or swallow normally?
   vi. Is her speech normal? – Dysarthria?/Expressive or receptive dysphasia?
   vii. Do you have any weakness or sensory disturbance elsewhere?
   viii. Do you have any dizziness or balance problems?
B. Screen for any evidence of confusion—*ensure the patient is orientated in time/place/person.*
C. Is there any history of head trauma?
D. Is there any history of loss of consciousness?
E. Is there any recent history of illness?
F. Has the patient ever experienced anything similar in the past?
G. Past medical history:
   i. Previous similar episodes
   ii. History of stroke or transient ischemic attack (TIA)
   iii. Other neurological conditions
H. Systemic illness:
   i. Thromboembolic disease
   ii. Cardiovascular risk factors
   iii. Hypertension
   iv. Diabetes
   v. Hypercholesterolemia
   vi. Smoking

ANS: 11

Checklist
1. History of onset: Age of onset. If early onset best possible treatment could not help because of amblyopia.
2. History of trauma: If so, there may be cataract, retain foreign body in presence trauma. And B-scan should be done before surgery.
3. History of associated pain, redness, watering, discharge to exclude any corneal ulcer, aphakic/pseudophakic bullous keratopathy
4. History of past surgeries
5. History of associated frequent change of glass keratoconus
6. History of associated systemic problem—hyperlipidemia/hypercalcemia.

(*Source*: Nethralaya S. Clinical practice pattern in ophthalmology, 2nd edition. New Delhi: Jaypee Brothers Medical Publishers (P) Ltd.; 2012. p. 124.)

ANS: 12
1. Rapport building
2. Duration
3. Onset: Sudden/gradual
4. Diurnal variation
5. History of trauma
6. Drug history
7. Is it in primary gaze?
8. More in near or distance gaze
9. Any systematic diseases? Diabetes mellitus (DM), hypertension (HTN), etc.
10. General condition of body
11. History of fever
12. Thanks' to patient

ANS: 13
1. History of onset
2. Alleviating or aggravating factors
3. Family history of ptosis
4. Whether increasing, decreasing, or constant since time of manifestation
5. Association with:
    i. Jaw movement
    ii. Abnormal head posture
    iii. Abnormal ocular movement
6. History of:
    i. Trauma or previous surgery
    ii. Poisoning
    iii. Use of steroid drops
    iv. Any reaction with anesthesia
    v. Bleeding tendency
7. Previous photograph.

ANS: 14

Sl. No.		Done
1.	Greetings!	0.5
2.	Associated with pain and redness	1
3.	Visual acuity immediately after surgery	1
4.	Any complications during surgery	1
5.	Used eye drops according to instruction	1
6.	Any history of trauma	2
7.	History regarding exogenous source of infections like use of contaminated eye drops	1
8.	Query about endogenous source of infection like oral, nasal, or ear infections or others	1
9.	Any previous eye diseases like glaucoma	1
10.	Thanks	0.5
	TOTAL	***10***

CHAPTER

Counseling

13

QUESTIONS

OSPE: 01. Counsel your patient who is suffering from keratoconus.
OSPE: 02. Your patient needs fundus fluorescein angiography (FFA); counsel the patient.
OSPE: 03. A patient incidentally diagnosed as a case of glaucoma. Let him counsel.
OSPE: 04. Counsel a pregnant woman about the management who has severe nonproliferative diabetic retinopathy (NPDR) in her right eye and high-risk proliferative diabetic retinopathy in left eye.
OSPE: 05. Counsel a diabetic patient who needs cataract surgery.
OSPE: 06. Counsel a patient who needs dacryocystorhinostomy surgery.
OSPE: 07. A 60-year-old man came to you for cataract surgery. On examination with slit-lamp biomicroscopy, you got pseudoexfoliation. Let him counsel.
OSPE: 08. Counsel the parents of a child for examination under anaesthesia.
OSPE: 09. Breaking of bad news and counseling the parents of a child with retinoblastoma.
OSPE: 10. Counsel the parents of a child who may need cycloplegic refractive correction (with Atropine 1% eye drop).
OSPE: 11. A 20-year-old girl dissatisfied with her vision and spectacles using $-7ds-5dcx35^0$ in her right eye and $-5ds-3dcx90^0$ in her left eye came to you for LASIK. Her central corneal thickness (CCT) is 420 μm in right eye and 448 μm in left eye and her topography was as below. Counsel her regarding management.

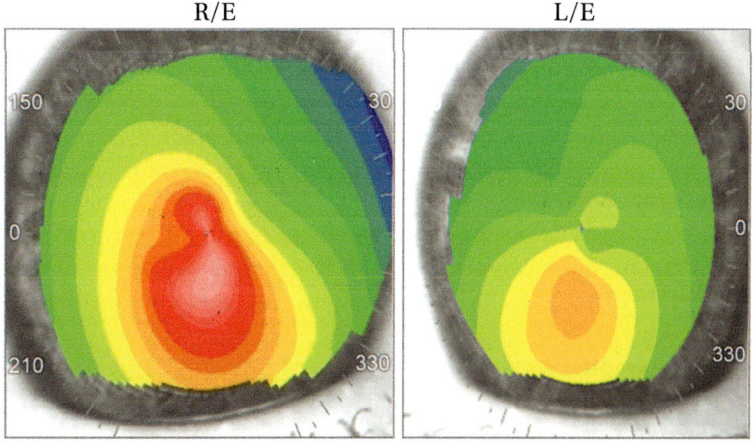

OSPE: 12. Child with unilateral cataract (Counsel the parent).
OSPE: 13. A patient came to you with acute anterior uveitis with posterior synechiae which is not releasing with maximum medication. Now you have decided to give subconjunctival injection (0.5 mL) of mydricaine. Now you have to motivate the patient.
OSPE: 14. A 70-year-old lady came to you with sudden development of floaters. After examination, you came to a conclusion that it is a natural aging process. Now you have to counsel her that it is innocuous.

or

A 65-year-old patient comes into the ED saying that he thinks "the jelly" in his eye has "peeled off again". He says he has been seeing flashes of light as well as blobs and cobwebs floating in front of his right eye. He experienced the same thing about a year ago in his other eye. His visual acuity is similar in both eyes.
OSPE: 15. A 25-year-old lady is suffering from Vogt-Koyanagi-Harada (VKH) for 2 years. It was relapsed for 2 times after withdrawal of oral steroid within 1 month. Now you have decided to give her immunomodulating drugs, either azathioprine or cyclophosphamide. Counsel the patient.
OSPE: 16. An 18-year-old boy diagnosed as keratoconus. He used rigid gas permeability (RGP) lens but his condition is deteriorating day by day. Now you decided to do corneal crosslinking (CXL). Counsel the patient.
OSPE: 17. A 55-year-old man is in service, came to you with the complaints of progressive dimness of vision of right eye for last 2 years. On examination, you found that he is suffering from grade 3 age-related cataract (right eye) and visual acuity is 6/60. Left eye is aphakic and his best corrected visual acuity (BCVA) of left eye is 6/12 N6. Now you have to counsel him regarding his treatment plan.
OSPE: 18. A 37-year-old software engineer complains of persistent redness, foreign body sensation, and intolerance to light and air for the last 6 months. Counsel the patient regarding diagnosis and treatment of his condition.
OSPE: 19. Motivate a person for eye donation.
OSPE: 20. Grief counsel at hospital for eye donation.
OSPE: 21. Counsel a patient for intravitreal injection of bevacizumab (Avastin) in diabetic macular edema.
OSPE: 22. Counsel the parents for their kids who are suffering from vernal keratoconjunctivitis.
OSPE: 23. Counsel the parents for probing of 1.5-year-old child.
OSPE: 24. A 70-year-old woman came to you with bilateral senile mature cataract with proliferative diabetic retinopathy. Let her counsel for cataract surgery.
OSPE: 25. Counsel the mother of a 1-year-old baby for ptosis correction which covers the visual axis.
OSPE: 26. A 33-year-old lady, using spectacles since childhood, came to you by hearing the news that miracles can be done with laser, which will make her life easy and she will get rid of her glass. So, you did some pre-Lasik investigations, and results are as follows:
- Topography:
  Topography shows that most of the color in the center of the cornea is hot color.

Topography also shows: Sim K1 in right eye is 43.50; Sim K2 is 50.50
Sim k1 in left eye is 45.00; Sim K2 is 48.0.
- Applanation tonometry:
Right eye 15 mm Hg; left eye 9 mm Hg
- C: D ratio is:
0.7 in right eye and 0.4 in left eye
- Schirmer test:
2: 5 mm in B/E
  – Now, you have to counsel the lady about her desires.

OSPE: 27. A 25-year-old young male patient had painful blind eye (NPL) (which relives after taking pain killer, but he needs to take pain killer 3–4 times in a week). Counsel him for evisceration.

OSPE: 28. Counseling of high myopia.

OSPE: 29. Counseling about Lasik.

OSPE: 30. Counsel for keratoplasty for corneal opacity.

OSPE: 31. Counsel about amblyopia.

OSPE: 32. A 30-year-old patient of known case of Retinitis pigmentosa (RP). Now counsel the patient regarding treatment and future plan.

OSPE: 33. A 70-year-old man came to you for follow-up visit. He is a known case of Primary open angle glaucoma (POAG) for last 10 years. He develops cataract. He is also hypertensive and diabetic. Let him counsel.

OSPE: 34. A 72-year-old woman with hypertension and type 2 diabetes mellitus came to you for a scheduled ocular examination, though her last complete eye examination was more than 5 years ago. She states that she has never worn glasses and is happy with over-the-counter reading glasses for reading fine print.
She states that everyone in her family has "healthy" eyes and no one wears glasses. On examination, you find that her visual acuity of right eye 6/9 and visual acuity of left eye 6/12. Not improved with pin hole, on direct ophthalmoscopy you find she is suffering from background diabetic retinopathy. Now you have to counsel the patient regarding her ocular condition and regular follow-up.

OSPE: 35. A patient with corneal ulcer is getting moxifloxacin eye drop but not improving, you have decided to do corneal scraping. Now you have to motivate the patient.

ANSWERS

ANS: 01
Checklist
A. Greetings and self-introduction 0.25
B. Tell about the disease process
   (a) Cause is unknown 0.50
   (b) May be familial 0.50
   (c) If other family members have any eye problem consult with eye doctor 0.50
   (d) It usually progresses with age 0.50
   (e) Choose profession according to vision 0.50
C. Tell about treatment modalities
   (a) Spectacles may not be sufficient 0.50
   (b) You can go for 3CxR 0.50
   (c) Tell about advantage and limitation of RGP 1.00
   (d) Cost of RGP lens 0.50
   (e) Hi brid C.L 0.50
   (f) Intracorneal Intacs or Ferrara ring implant with femtosecond laser 0.50
   (g) Keratoplasty(Deep anterior lamellar keratoplasty) 0.50
D. Tell about prognosis
   (a) It is a lifelong disease 0.50
   (b) Regular follow-up 0.50
   (c) If there is any problem consult your doctor immediately, such as pain and photophobia 1.00
E. Advice ....
   (a) Not to rub your eye 0.5
   (b) Not to use any ocular drop without consulting your eye doctor 0.5
   (c) Thanks to patient 0.25
TOTAL **10**

ANS: 02
1. Greetings 0.25
2. Explanation of procedure:
   (a) Inj. Sodium fluoride 1.50
   (b) Taking of picture 1.50
3. Prerequisites:
   (a) Dilated pupil 1.00
   (b) Renal function test 1.00
   (c) Any hypersensitivity of fluoride 0.50
4. Possible side effects: 1.00
   (a) Nausea/vomiting 1.00
   (b) Yellow urine 1.00
   (c) Anaphylaxis/syncope 0.50
   (d) Talk about cost 0.50
Thanks 0.25
TOTAL **10**

ANS: 03

1. Greetings 0.25
2. Give idea of POAG 2.00
3. Rx Medical 1.50
4. Rx Surgical 1.50
5. Complications of surgery 1.00
6. Fate if untreated 1.00
7. Regular follow-up 1.00
8. It is a lifelong disease like diabetes mellitus/hypertension 1.00
9. Advice 0.50
10. Thanks 0.25
TOTAL 10

ANS: 04

1. Greetings 0.5
2. Explain about the disease process 1.0
3. Management
   i. Strict control of blood glucose, blood pressure, renal function, anemia 2.0
   ii. Mention the modalities of Rx of diabetic retinopathy 1.0
   iii. Limitations of antivascular endothelial growth factor in pregnancy 1.0
   iv. Both eyes should be treated with PRP 2.0
   v. Mode of delivery must be elective cesarian section 1.0
   vi. Inform about adverse effects and cost 1.0
4. Thanks 0.5
TOTAL 10

Explanation: Pregnancy itself is a risk factor for progression of diabetic retinopathy, so it is aggressively treated by laser. Another important thing is that trial of normal vaginal delivery might lead to vitreous hemorrhage during bearing down effect so mode of delivery should be elective caesarian section.

ANS: 05

1. Greetings and self-introduction 0.25
2. Explain the disease
   (a) It is an aging process (DM accentuated aging process) 0.50
   (b) Only surgery is the choice 1.00
3. Options of management of the disease
   (a) SICS 1.00
   (b) Phaco 1.00
4. Need of operation at this stage (advantage and disadvantage)
   (a) Phaco will be easier at this stage and no need of L/A only topical is sufficient 0.50
   (b) If it becomes mature, we will go for SICS and it needs L/A 0.50
   (c) Procedure and complication (among all endophthalmitis is the devastating) 1.00
   (d) We have to take some extra precautions for diabetics, such as you should contact your physician that you are going for cataract surgery and he will adjust your diabetic medicine if she/he thinks so 1.00

5. Diabetic patient has more chance to develop complications 0.50
6. In spite of uneventful surgery, you may not regain full vision if there is any lesion caused by diabetics in your retina or optic nerve 1.00
7. Abide by some rules after surgery for 10–14 days in case of phaco and about 1 month for SICS (any 3) .... 0.5 × 3 .... 1.5
   (a) Not to use water in your eyes
   (b) Use dark black sunglass
   (c) Not to lean forward during prayer or for any reason
   (d) Regular follow-up
8. Thanks to patient 0.25
   TOTAL ***10***

ANS: 06
1. Greetings and self-introduction 0.25
2. Explain the disease
   (a) Describe the tear passage 1
   (b) Recurrent infection caused the block 1
   (c) If not treated, there will be recurrent conjunctivitis, corneal ulcer 1
3. Options of management of the disease
   (a) DCR 1
   (b) Endolaser DCR 1
   (c) DCT 1
4. Need of operation at this stage (advantage and disadvantage)
   Procedure and complications
   (a) It is a bypass operation 1
   (b) Need to cut the bones 1
   (c) Success is not guaranteed 1
5. Feedback from the patient 0.5
6. Thanks to patient 0.25
   TOTAL ***10***

You may also add these points during DCR counseling if time permits:
- If not treated: Abscess, cellulitis, cavernous sinus thrombosis, and meningitis
- If not treated: Burst abscess and fistula formation
- Some investigations prior surgery: For diagnosis and to see any contraindication
- For detection of site of obstruction
- Need for intubation or not
- Presence of other diseases: Diabetes mellitus, hypertension, bleeding disorder, sinus disease, and atrophic rhinitis.

ANS: 07
1. Greetings and self-introduction 0.5
2. Give idea of PXF 2.0
3. Treatment option 1.0
4. Complication during surgery
   (a) Poor dilatation 1.0

(b) PC rent 1.0
(c) Zonular dehiscence.. 1.0
5. Complication after surgery
   (a) Raised IOP 1.0
   (b) Uveitis 1.0
   (c) Poor vision 1.0
6. Thanks' to the patient 0.5
TOTAL 10

ANS: 08
Checklist
A. Greeting... 0.25
B. Explain purpose of the procedure... 1.50
C. Explain the procedure 1.50
D. Explain the benefit of the procedure 1.50
E. Explain the risks.. 1.50
F. Ask if the parents understood the counseling (feedback)...................... 1.50
G. Any query from the parents.. 1.0
H. Ask for consent... 1.0
I. Thanks 0.25
TOTAL 10

ANS 09
1. Greetings 0.25
2. Inform about the nature of the disease.. 2.0
3. Though it is cancer but not life-threatening or even vision can be save if treated properly 2.0
4. Genetic counseling 1.5
5. It is a treatment of multidiscipline so you may need to contact with pediatric, oncologist radiotherapist, etc 1.0
6. Regular follow-up is the vital part of the treatment 1.0
7. Approximate cost of the treatment 1.0
8. Feedback 1.0
9. Thanks' to the patient 0.25
TOTAL 10

ANS: 10
1. Greetings to the parents 0.25
2. Explain the refractive error... 1.0
3. Explain the option of treatment 1.0
4. Explain what if not treated 1.0
5. Explain cycloplegic refraction... 1.0
6. Explain how to apply cycloplegic... 1.0
7. Explain side effect of cycloplegic and precaution.................................. 1.5
8. Care and use of spectacles... 0.75
9. Any query from the parents.. 0.75

10. Regular follow-up	0.75
11. Ensure the use of spectacle	0.75
12. Thanks	0.25
TOTAL	**10**

If time permit you add following points in your counseling:
Side effects of atropine
Dosages of Atropine

ANS: 11

1. Greetings	0.5
2. Describe the disease process and diagnosis	2.0
3. Tell her Lasik is contraindicated	1.0
4. Treatment options and limitations	
A. RGP contact lens	1.0
B. Keratoplasty	1.0
C. Intacts implants	1.0
D. Corneal collagen cross-linkage with Riboflavin	1.0
5. Prognosis and follow-up	2.0
6. Thanks	0.50
TOTAL	**10**

ANS: 12

1. Greetings and self-introduction	0.25
2. Surgery is mandatory	1.0
3. If child is below 1 year, no IOL and if more than 1 year, IOL have to be implant	1.5
4. Risk of surgery	1.0
5. Risk of anesthesia	1.0
6. If surgery is not done recently, what will be the problem?	1.0
7. What will be the problem, if Aphakia? Occlusion therapy	1.0
8. What will be the problem if pseudophakia?	1.0
9. What is the advantage of aphakia/pseudophakia?	2.0
10. Thanks to parent	0.25
TOTAL	**10**

(Ref: Clinical Practice Patterns in Ophthalmology: Sankara Nethralaya, 2nd edition. p. 73.)

ANS: 13

1. Greetings	0.25
2. Explain about synechiae	
A. It is the adhesion of iris with lens with proteinous exudates	1.0
B. The injection will not be given inside your eyeball, it will be given just beneath the conjunctiva	1.0
C. It is the complication of your disease	1.0
D. It will obstruct your normal fluid (aqueous) drain inside the eye	1.0
E. So there will be initially raised IOP	1.0
F. That will cause severe pain	1.0
G. Lastly, vision will be gone and eyeball will be soft and small	0.5

3. Explain about the injection
   A. It is the cocktail of injection atropine, adrenaline and lignocaine or procaine 1
   B. It is the most effective drug to release synechiae 1
   C. Though it is a combination of drugs, it has some side effects, i.e. tachycardia, hypotension 0.5
   D. May induce tachycardia and hypertension; more chances of side effects if you are suffering from cardiovascular disease 0.5
4. Thanks 0.25

TOTAL 10

ANS: 14

1. Rapport building 0.25
2. Explain what is floater?
   There is a gel-like substance in eye, sometimes part of the gel becomes liquefied and these cast tiny shadows on the retina. These are floaters 2.0
3. Explain why it occurs?
   It occurs usually in old age and sometimes in early age in diabetic patient 2.0
4. What is the fate of the floaters?
   In most cases, floaters are part of the natural aging process and simply an annoyance. They can be distracting at first, but eventually tend to "settle" at the bottom of the eye, becoming less bothersome. They usually settle below the line of sight and do not go away completely 2.0
5. Is there any treatment of floaters?
   No treatment is recommended 1.5
6. When it needs treatment?
   On rare occasions, floaters can be so dense and numerous that they significantly affect vision. In these cases, vitrectomy may be needed 1.0
7. What are the risks of vitrectomy?
   This operation carries significant risks to sight because of possible complications, which include retinal detachment, retinal tears, and cataract. Most eye surgeons are reluctant to recommend this surgery unless the floaters seriously interfere with vision 1.0
8. Thanks to the patient 0.25

TOTAL 10

ANS: 15

1. Greetings and introduction 0.25
2. Give idea about drugs
   (a) Immunosuppressive drug 1.0
   (b) It may continue over 1 year 0.5
   (c) Expensive 0.5
3. Before starting
   (a) Must consult with expert physician or internist 0.5
   (b) Ensure absence of any infection 0.5
   (c) Ensure absence of hematological or hepatological abnormality 0.5
   (d) Written informed consent 0.5

4. Give idea about the side effect/complication of the drugs
   (a) Nausea 0.5
   (b) Vomiting 0.5
   (c) Nephrotoxicity 0.5
   (d) Hepatotoxity 0.5
5. Give idea why you have chosen the drug
   (a) Steroid-dependent case 1.0
   (b) Steroid-related complications 0.5
6. Regular follow-up must at 4–6 weeks interval with
   (a) Complete blood count 0.5
   (b) Liver function test 0.5
   (c) Renal function test 0.5
7. Feedback 0.5
8. Thanks 0.25
   TOTAL 10

ANS: 16

1. Greetings and introduction 0.25
2. Mention Rx options of keratoconus other than RGP
   (a) CXL 1.0
   (b) Intracorneal ring implant 0.5
   (c) Keratoplasty 0.5
3. Explain why you choose CXL
   (a) Halts progression of the disease 1.0
   (b) Sometimes reverse it 0.5
4. Preoperative investigation
   (a) Corneal topography 1.0
   (b) Corneal pachymetry 0.5
5. Explain procedure
   (a) Apply anesthetic drop 0.50
   (b) Remove epithelium 0.50
   (c) Apply riboflavin 0.1% drop 0.50
   (d) Apply UV-A for 30 mins 0.50
6. Postoperative Rx
   (a) BCL for 3–7 days for epithelization 0.5
   (b) Antibiotic drop 4 times daily for 7 days 0.5
   (c) Steroid eye drop 4 times tapering over 2 months start after re-epithelization 0.25
7. Postoperative follow up
   (a) Every day for first 2–3 days 0.50
8. Complication
   (a) Irritation 0.5
   (b) Corneal edema 0.25
   (c) Corneal haze 0.25
   (d) Dry eye 0.5
   (e) Corneal scarring 0.5

9. Cost expensive	0.5
10. Thanks	0.25
TOTAL	***10***

ANS: 17

Done

1. Greetings 0.25
2. Explanation of cataract surgery and also complications 1.5
3. If we do phaco surgery, then you will face some problems
    (a) Left eye will be inactive 1.0
    (b) If you use the current glass there will be double vision 1.0
4. You have few options for left eye (L/E)
    (a) Secondary implant of IOL in anterior chamber 1.0
    (b) Secondary implant of IOL by scleral fixation 1.0
    (c) You can use contact lens in L/E 1.0
5. If you do not agree to take hassle for L/E, we can do
    (a) R/E will be also aphakia 1.0
    (b) If aphakia, we need this sort of glass in R/E also 0.5
    (c) For the glass the image size will be bigger 0.5
    (d) Weight of the glass can make you unhappy 0.5
6. Any feedback from patient 0.5
7. Thanks' to patient 0.25
TOTAL ***10***

ANS: 18

Points to be noted   *Done*

1. Greetings 0.25
2. Mention the diagnosis 2.0
3. Explain the disease 2.0
4. Counsel the treatment regarding
    A. Need for frequent use of artificial tears 1.0
    B. To give some break instead of continuous use of computers 0.5
    C. To blink frequently while using computers 0.5
    D. To avoid direct contact with air cooling system 0.5
    E. To adjust the monitor position 0.5
    F. To use large font instead of small font 0.5
    G. Not to use very bright screen with poor contrast 0.5
    H. Adequate seating arrangement 0.5
    I. Use LCD (Liquid-Crystal Display) monitor instead of CRT (Cathode-Ray Tube) monitor 0.25
    J. There will no direct light over the screen 0.25
    K. Feedback from the patient 0.5
5. Greetings/thanks 0.25
TOTAL ***10***

ANS: 19

1. Greetings 0.25
2. Eye donation is donating one's eye after his/her death 1.5
3. Only corneal blind people are benefited from donated eye 1.5
   Anyone can donate eyes irrespective of
   Age 0.5
   Gender 0.5
   Blood group 0.5
4. The cornea should be removed as early as possible after death (6 h) 1.0
5. Eyes of donated person can save vision of two corneal blind person 1.0
6. Donated eye is not for sale 1.0
7. Help regarding registration for eye donor 1.0
8. The donor name will be remembered with respect by the recipient and their family forever 1.0
9. Thanks 0.25
   TOTAL *10*

ANS: 20

1. Process involved in obtaining consent for eye donation
   A. Introduction: Counselor introduces himself/herself 0.5
   B. Expresses of sympathy 0.5
2. Talk about the facts of eye donation
   A. No disfigurement 0.5
   B. Takes only 30 minutes 0.5
   C. No delay in funeral arrangements 0.5
   D. Confidentiality about the donor and recipient 0.5
   E. Certificate of appreciation 0.5
   F. Assurance that eyes are not sold 0.5
   G. Express gratitude for listening patiently 0.5
   H. Provide pamphlet and phone number for further details/contact 0.5
3. Steps in obtaining consent
   A. Understanding and sharing the grief 0.5
   B. Learn as much information as possible from the family 0.5
   C. Understand the situation of grief such as sudden death, younger patient, head of the family or terminally ill patient 0.5
   D. Get consent within the hospital 0.5
   E. Explain the process of eye donation, and the functions of the eye bank
   Allow the final decision making to the family 0.5
4. Points to be emphasized during counseling
   A. Benefit to two blind individuals 0.5
   B. Absence of mutilation 0.5
   C. Cornea is the only part used 0.5
   D. No delay in funeral ceremony 0.5
   E. You are working as a grief counselor let be motivate the family for eye donation ...0.5
   TOTAL *10*

ANS: 21

1. Rapport building 0.25
2. Your disease needs some intervention with injection 1.00
3. It reduces edema by inhibition of new vessels 1.00
4. It costs about 10,000 taka (120 usd) per injection 1.00
5. You need more than one usually once in a month for consecutive 3 months 0.50
6. It has got some risk 1.00
7. Bleeding (Subconjunctival, vitreous hemorrhage) 1.00
8. Retinal tear/detachment 1.00
9. Infection (Endophthalmitis) 1.00
10. Loss of vision (from any of above) 0.50
11. Need for surgery (to address some of the complications above) 0.50
12. Thanks 0.25

ANS: 22

1. Rapport building 0.25
2. Idea about VKC: One type of recurrent bilateral allergic conjunctivitis 1.5
3. Time of attack: Seasonal—late spring and summer personal 1.5
4. Treatment option
   Topical
   Mast cell stabilizer 0.25
   Steroid 0.5
   Oral: Anti-histamine 0.25
   Intralesional: Subtarsal steroid injection 0.5
5. Complication of treatment
   Drowsiness: antihistamine 0.25
   ↑ IOP: Steroid 1.0
6. Complications if treatment not taken
   Corneal vascularization 0.5
   Corneal scar 0.5
   Corneal ulcer perforation 0.25
7. Prognosis
   95% usually disappear at late teens 1.0
   5% develop atopic conjunctivitis 0.5
8. Advice:
   Avoidance of allergens 0.25
   Cool compression 0.25
   Lid hygiene and treatment of blepharitis 0.25
   Do not rub the eye 0.25
9. Thanks to the patient 0.25
TOTAL *10*

ANS: 23
1. Greetings 0.25
2. Explain about type of disease at present condition
   (a) Obstruction of NLD 1.0
   (b) Spontaneous resolution occurs in over 95% of cases within 1st year 1.0
   (c) Not resulted in their baby 0.5
3. What are the options of treatment?
   (a) Massage over the sac region 1.0
   (b) Probing 1.0
   (c) DCR 0.5
   (d) Silastic tubing with or without balloon 0.5
   (e) Endoscopic procedure 0.25
4. To tell parent that probing is needed for this child 0.5
5. To describe probing to the patient 1.0
   Passage of a fine metallic tube via the canalicular system and NLD 0.5
6. When it is done?
   (a) Delayed until the age of 12–24 months 1.0
7. Type of anesthesia required? General anesthesia (G/A)
   (a) Investigation for G/A and hazard of G/A 0.5
8. Take written consent 0.5
9. Asking about any query 025
10. Thanks to the patient 0.25

ANS: 24
1. Rapport building 0.25
2. Explain vision after cataract surgery is guarded and its importance for surgery 1
3. Your problem is not only cataract; retina is also diseased so after cataract surgery your vision will not be fully regained 1
4. After all you have do cataract surgery, because sometime cataract can cause some other ocular problem, such as sudden raise of IOP, and it's an ocular emergency 1
5. Cosmetically white spot in pupillary area is not accepted and it will increase day by day, so need surgery 0.50
6. Why cataract surgery is needed?
   (a) There is problem in retina and usually it does not fully cure so after cataract surgery one may not regain full vision 1
   (b) In spite of that, we have to do cataract surgery because due to haziness of ocular media we can't see retina properly, so before retinal management we have to clear your cataract 2
   (c) In retinal treatment, you may need intravitreal injection and laser treatment sometimes surgery may be needed, but due to cataract we can't it 1
   (d) So cataract surgery has to be done before retinal treatment 1
7. In spite of routine investigation of cataract, we have to do B-scan ultrasonography 1
8. Thanks 0.25
TOTAL ***10***

ANS: 25

1. Greetings 0.25
2. Explain the disease 1.0
3. Complication/outcome of the disease 1.0
4. Management options 1.0
5. Explain the procedure 1.0
6. Explain the benefit 1.0
7. Explain the risks 1.0
8. Explain the chance of amblyopia 1.0
9. Ask if the patient understood the counseling 1.0
10. Any query from the patient 1.0
11. Ask for consent 0.5
12. Thanks 0.25
TOTAL 10

ANS: 26

A. Greetings and self-introduction 0.25
B. Tell about her topography 3.0
   Cornea shows thinner in the apical portion so LASIK may not be done
   Below 450 µm thickness is contraindicated.
C. Tell about the applanation tonometer 1.5
   IOP change is significant (difference between 2 eyes)
   During the insertion of suction cup IOP may increase above 65 mm Hg so there may be chance of vision reduction
D. C : D ratio is significant 1.0
   So, you may be a patient of POAG
   To diagnose the POAG we should do VFA and OCT
   POAG is a silent killer of vision.
E. You are suffering from dry eye, LASIK will also increase dryness 1.0
F. You can use RGP contact lens 1.0
   Tell her about the advantage and disadvantage of RGP lens as well as cost 1.0
G. Other option is clear lens extraction 1.0
H. Thanks to the patient 0.25

ANS: 27

A. Rapport building 0.5
B. Explain his present condition
   B1. Pain killer is not the solution, it is for temporary relief 1.0
   B2. Pain killer has lots of side effects including gastric ulcer and kidney problem 0.5
   B3. NPL eye is a dead eye and no chance to regain vision 1.0
   B4. So removal of the eye is the best solution 1.0
C. Brief about the surgical procedure 1.5
D. Though it is evisceration so cosmetic purpose will be well-maintained and prosthesis will move with eye movement 1.0
E. State about possible risk 1.0

F. If untreated, chance of phthisis bulbi 1.0
G. Ask for feedback 0.5
H. Discuss with family and friends 0.5
I. Thanks to the patient 0.5
TOTAL **10**

ANS: 28 and 29

A. Rapport building 0.5
B. Following points should be told about myopia
    B1. It is a congenital problem 0.5
    B2. Explain him, what is myopia? 1.0
C. Treatment options:
    C1. Spectacle 1.0
    C2. Contact lens 0.5
    C3. Lasik 0.5
    About Lasik
    C3a. It cannot be done before 18 years 0.5
    C3b. Usually after Lasik you do not need glass, but sometimes there is some residual myopia, and may need glass for clear vision 0.5
    C3c. After age of 40 you may need near correction 0.5
    C3d. Lasik has got some disadvantages, such as, dry eyes, halos, etc. 0.5
D. You should wear the spectacle whole day except during sleep, shower, etc. 0.5
E. We shall examine your fundus whether it is simple or pathological myopia 0.5
F. If simple myopia, usually power will not deteriorate after 20 years of age 0.5
G. If pathological myopia, usually power will not be fixed and may increase lifelong 0.5
H. Advise
    H1. Try to avoid excessive near work, such as prolonged computer/smart phone use .. 0.5
    H2. Follow-up according to your doctor instruction 0.5
    H3. Try to avoid eye trauma, and to play where chance of trauma is more 0.5
I. Thanks to the patient 0.5
TOTAL **10**
F. Advise postoperative
- Do not let the eye come in contact with water for a few days 0.25
- Use dark black sunglass for few days 0.25

    Ask for feedback 0.50
    Thanks 0.25
TOTAL **10**

ANS: 30

A. Rapport building 0.25
B. Tell about keratoplasty: It is an operation where your unhealthy cornea is replaced by donor cornea 2.00
C. Why keratoplasty is needed? Cornea is a transparent structure, but your cornea has become opaque, so it has to be replace if you like to see with this eye 1.50

Counseling

D.	Does it need any tissue matching? No, cornea is an avascular structure no need of blood grouping	0.50
	tissue matching	0.50
E.	Any healthy cornea can be transplanted	0.25
F.	Before surgery you need to do some investigations: such as	
	IOP measurement	0.50
	B-scan ultrasonography	0.50
G.	You may need use of eye drop more than year	0.50
H.	There is chance of some complications:	
	Graft failure	1.00
	Raised IOP	0.50
	Uveitis	0.25
I.	You may need frequent follow-up visit	0.50
J.	Any feedback	0.50
K.	Thanks	0.25
TOTAL		**10**

ANS: 31

A.	Rapport building	0.25
B.	What is amblyopia? In the absence of an organic lesion, a difference in best corrected VA of two Snellen lines or more is indicative of amblyopia	1.5
C.	The child has no major problem in the eye	1.0
D.	It is due to the eye was not properly used and it became lazy	1.0
E.	Though the boy is 7-year old, still there is a chance to improve	1.0
F.	It was hard to correct if he is more than 12 years of age	0.5
G.	Child should wear the spectacle whole day	0.5
H.	The child needs occlusion therapy	1.5
I.	What is occlusion therapy? The child will close the better eye every day for 2–3 hours regularly, it can be done by patching the good eye	1.0
J.	You have to monitor that the child should close his eye honestly	0.5
K.	He may need patching up to 10 years of his age	0.25
L.	You need regular follow-up according to your doctor instruction	0.25
M.	Any feedback	0.5
N.	Thanks	0.25
TOTAL		**10**

ANS: 32

1.	Rapport building	0.25
2.	Prescribe glass if it will improve any vision	1
3.	Give idea about low vision aids	1
4.	Advise field expander	1
5.	RP may be associated with posterior polar cataract, advise surgery if there any chance of vision improvement	1
6.	Treatment of CMO with tablet acetazolamide	1

7. Advise ocular examination of other family member 1
8. Address other associated systemic problems 1
9. Genetic counseling 1
10. Rehabilitation 1
11. Information regarding any new scientific development 0.5
12. Thanks 0.25
TOTAL 10

ANS: 33
1. Greetings 0.25
2. About hypertension
   (a) How long you are suffering from hypertension? 1.0
   (b) Is it well-controlled or not? 0.5
   (c) Are you taking any medicine for hypertension? 0.5
   (d) Can you mention the name? 0.5
   (e) If blood thinner is included, you have to discontinue it before surgery 1.0
3. About DM
   (a) How long you are suffering from DM? 0.5
   (b) Are you taking any medicine for DM? 0.5
   (c) Before surgery, your blood sugar not be more than 10 Mmol/L 1.0
   (d) Can you mention the name? 0.5
4. About glaucoma
   Have you any idea about glaucoma? 1.0
   It causes permanent loss of vision 1.0
5. About cataract
   Your cataract needs surgery 0.5
   But we are not sure how much your vision will improve due to glaucoma and DM 1.0
6. Have you any query? You have time to take decision 0.5
7. Thanks 0.25
TOTAL 10

ANS: 34
1. Greetings 0.25
2. State present situation
3. Visual acuity is not 6/6 1
4. Diabetic change is there 1
5. There is 50% chance to develop DR within 10 year, and 90% chance to develop DR within 30 years (If diabetes is well control) 1
6. State the risk of DR
   (a) Vitreous hemorrhage 1
   (b) RD 1
   (c) CMO 1

Counseling

7. Importance of diabetes control, and regular follow-up though she seems there is no problem 1
    If she is satisfied, continue the over the counter glass 0.5
    Avoid the risk factors .... 0.0 .... 25 x 8 .... 2.0
    Control of diabetes
    Hypertension
    Nephropathy
    Hyperlipidemia
    Smoking
    Cataract surgery
    Obesity
    Anemia
    Thanks 0.25
TOTAL *10*

ANS: 35
1. Greetings 0.5
2. We need your consent 1.0
3. Tell why scarping? 3.0
4. It is a painless procedure, or minimum pain 1.0
5. Stop all antibiotics for 12 hours 1.0
6. Final report will get after 72 hours 1.0
7. Start antibiotic/antifungal according to Gram stain and KOH 2.0
8. Thanks 0.5
TOTAL *10*

CHAPTER 14

Radiology

QUESTIONS

Ophthalmologists are not very familiar with radiology of orbit, paranasal sinuses (PNS), and brain, but these are very important for diagnostic point of view; so before starting the chapter, I introduce some important landmarks of computed tomography (CT) and magnetic resonance imaging (MRI) scans.

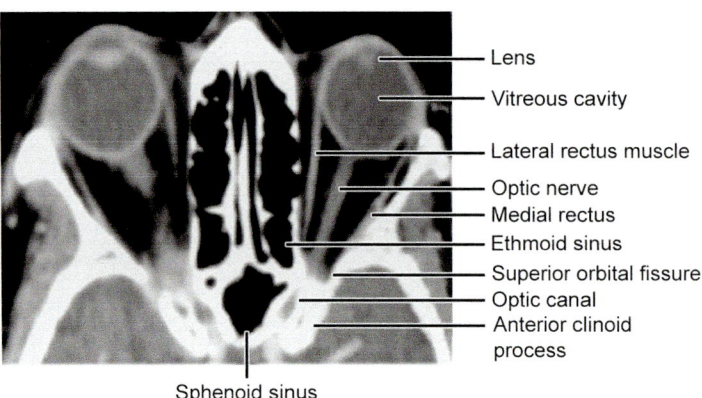

Axial CT scan at midlevel of orbit showing important structures.

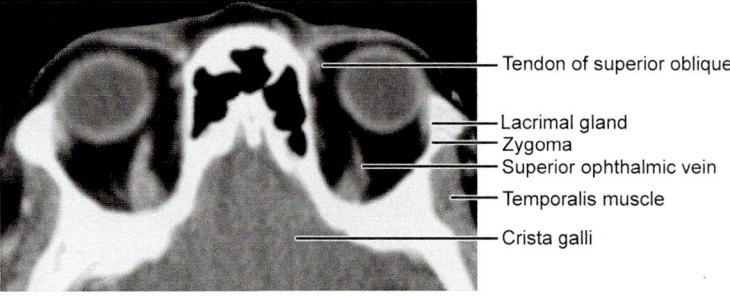

Axial CT scan at upper level of orbit showing important structures.

Radiology

The MRI findings in T1-weighted, T2-weighted, and fat suppressor mode:

	T1-weighted	T2-weighted	Fat suppressed
Bone cortex	No signal	No signal	No signal
Bone marrow	Bright	Bright	Dark
Fat	Very bright	Bright	Very dark
Muscle	Gray	Gray	Gray
Aqueous/vitreous	Dark	Bright	Dark
Lens	Gray	Gray	Gray
Sclera	Gray	Gray	Gray
Cerebrospinal fluid (CSF)	Dark	Bright	Dark
Blood vessels	No signal	No signal	No signal
Air	No signal	No signal	No signal

OSPE: 01

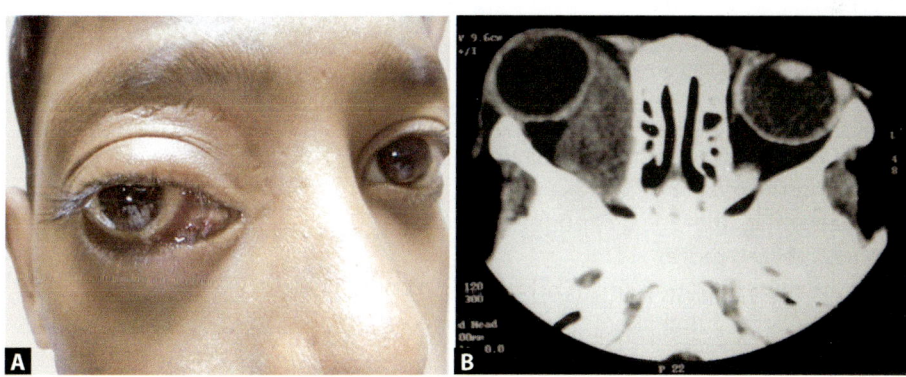

(Image Courtesy: Dr Muztaba Nuruddin, CEITC)

A. What are the MRI findings at here?
B. What is the name of the growth?
C. What type of disease is this?
D. What is its appearance and what is the most common site in ocular tissue?
E. Sometimes, it is filled with blood that may regress with time. What is the name of it?

OSPE: 02

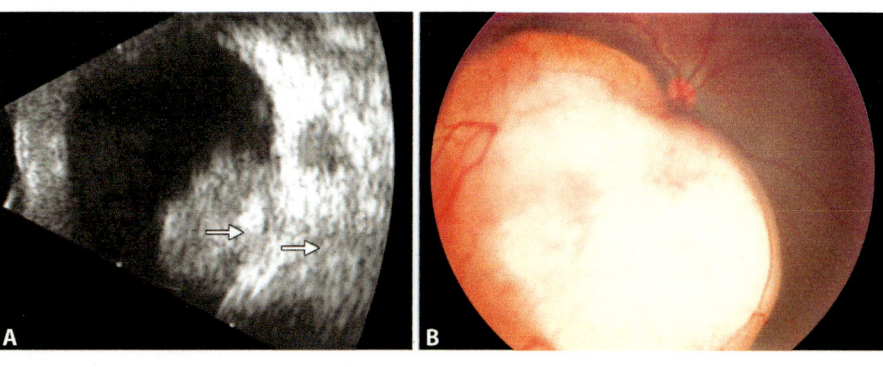

This is the fundus picture of a child 2-year-old.
A. What is the name of both the pictures?
B. What shows in both images?
C. What is your diagnosis?
D. What are the presenting symptoms? Mention 3.

OSPE: 03

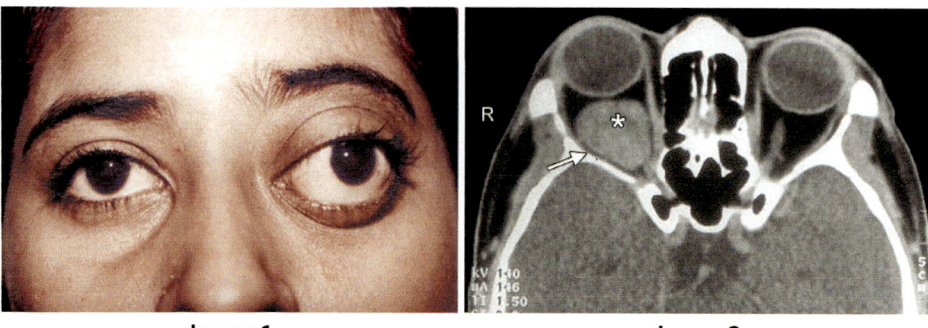

Image 1   Image 2

(*Image Courtesy: Dr Muztaba Nuruddin, CEITC*)

A. What are the positive findings in image 1, and image 2?
B. What is your diagnosis?
C. Which age and gender most commonly involved?
D. When it increased more?
E. What is the most common site in orbit?
F. What are the differential diagnoses?

OSPE: 04

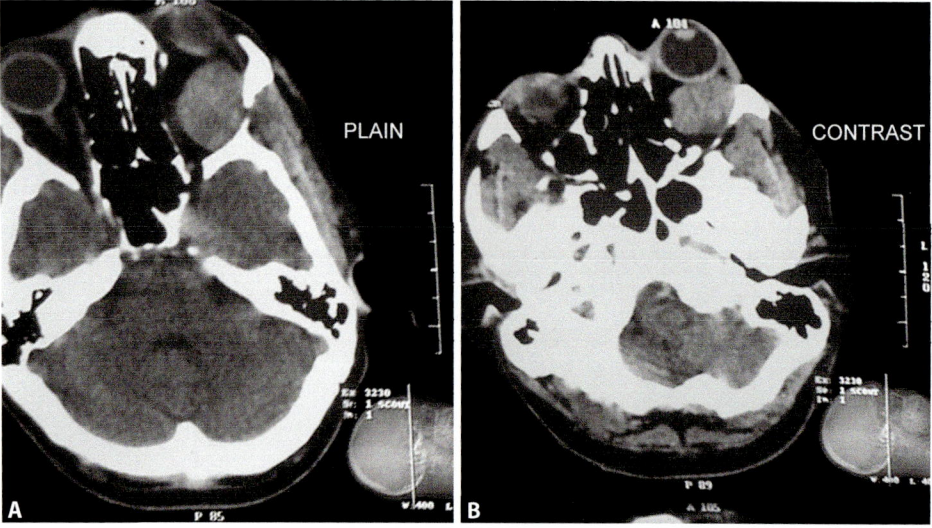

(*Image Courtesy: Dr Muztaba Nuruddin, CEITC*)

A. What does the CT scan show?
B. What is the provisional diagnosis?
C. Write three differential diagnoses.
D. What additional parts of the history and examination are especially pertinent regarding this patient's presentation? (2 history and 3 examination)

OSPE: 05

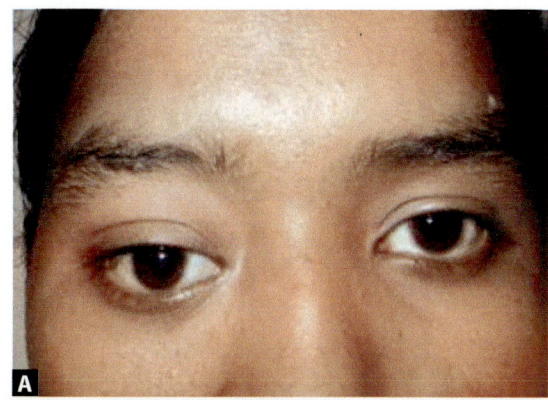

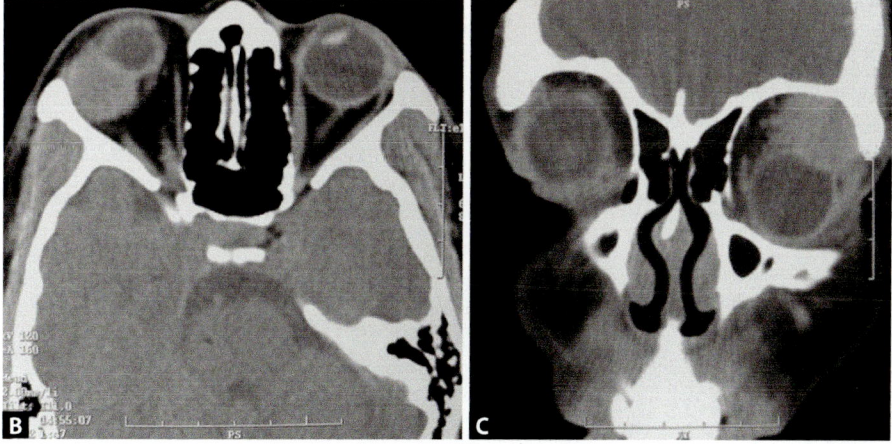

(Image Courtesy: Dr Muztaba Nuruddin, CEITC)

This 20-year-old-lady came to your chamber with the complaints of forward bulging of the right eye. On examination, you got it is a non-axial proptosis of the right eyeball. On palpation a hard, non-reducible mass in the right superotemporal orbit. There was neither tenderness nor any sign of inflammation. The mass was not pulsatile.

The CT scan was done. Answer the following questions:

A. What is the view of the two CT scans?
B. What is positive finding in CT scan?
C. What is your diagnosis?
D. From CT scan, can you comment is it a malignant or benign condition?

OSPE: 06

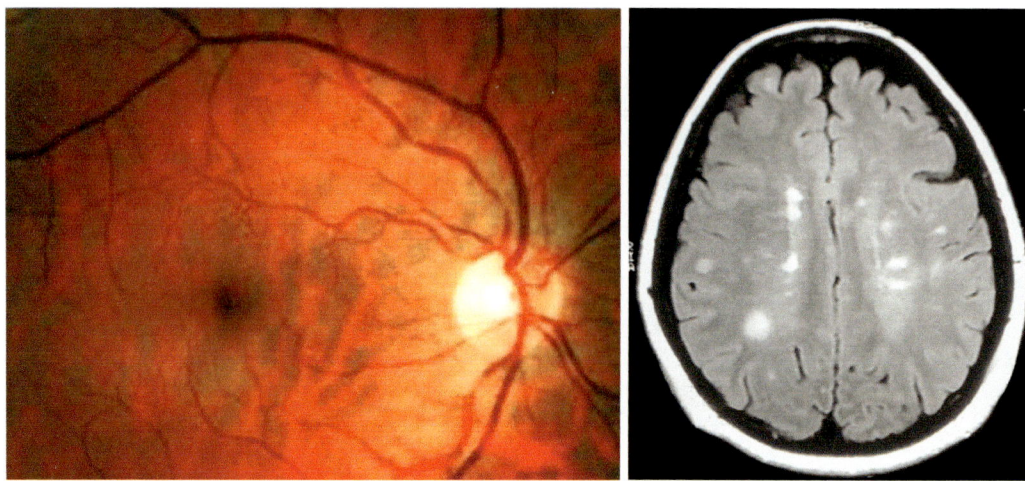

Image 1 **Image 2**

These two images are taken from the same patient.
A. What is the name of the image 1 and image 2?
B. What shows in image 1 and image 2?
C. What is your probable diagnosis?
D. Do you think it's first attack or recurrent?

OSPE: 07

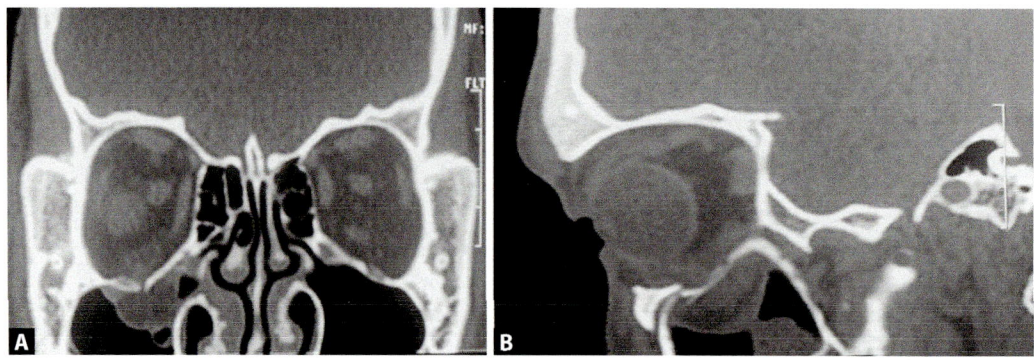

(Image Courtesy: Dr Soma Rani Roy, CEITC)

These two images of CT scan have taken from a patient.
A. What are the view at here?
B. Mention one positive finding in the image A.
C. What is your diagnosis?
D. What signs you may get?

OSPE: 08

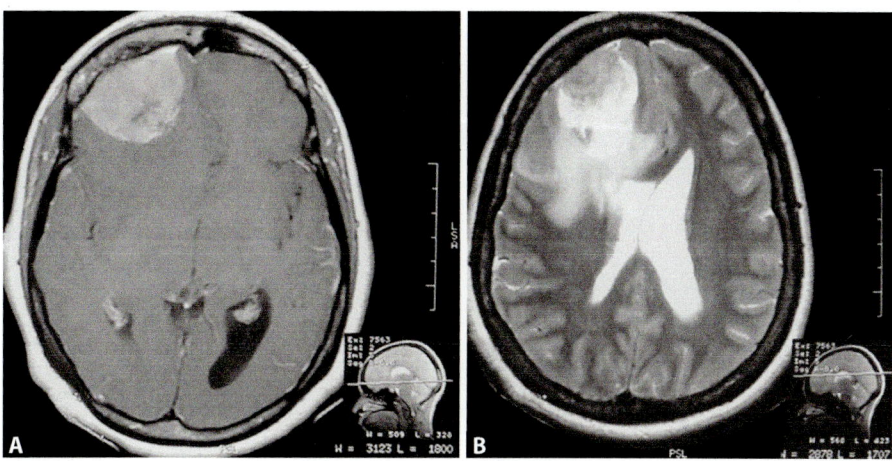

(Image Courtesy: Dr Soma Rani Roy, CEITC)

These two images are taken from a patient who is suffering from severe headache and vomiting for last 2 months.
A. Which one is T1 weighted and T2 weighted images?
B. What are the positive findings?
C. What is your provisional diagnosis?
D. What it indicates—severe headache and vomiting?

OSPE: 09

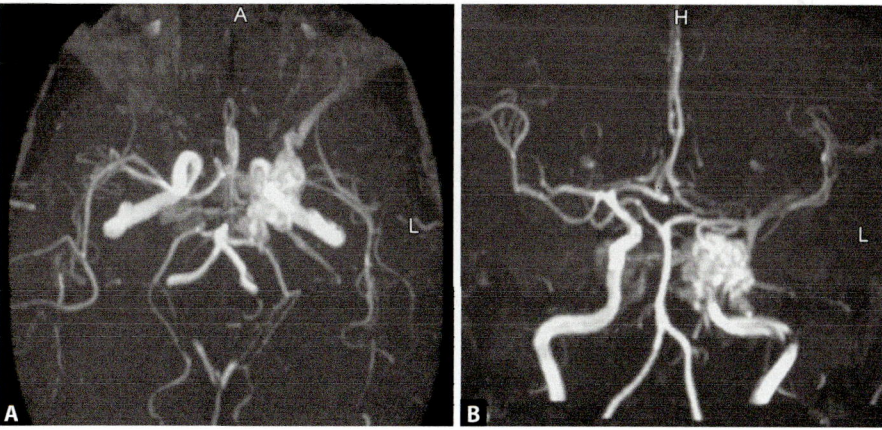

These two images taken from a 24-year-old-man, who came to you eight hours after trauma.
A. What is the name of the images?
B. What is the positive finding?
C. What is provisional diagnosis?
D. What may be the cause? Mention 2.

OSPE: 10

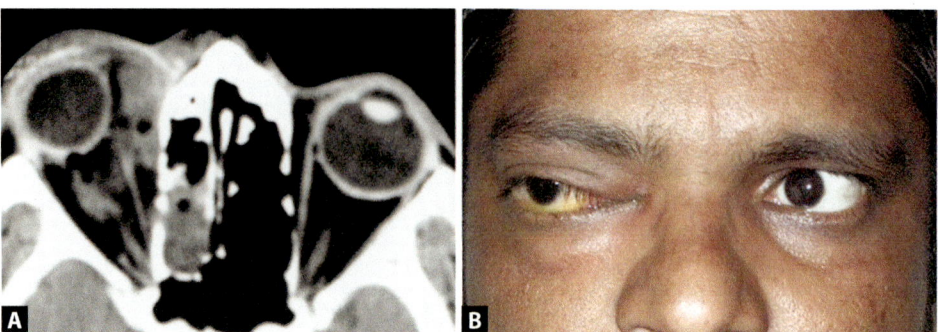

The patient is suffering from uncontrolled diabetes and toothache (upper jaw) for last 3 days, and suddenly he develops proptosis, chemosis, restricted ocular movement, periocular edema and erythema.
A. What is your diagnosis?
B. What are the positive findings in CT scan?
C. What are the differential diagnoses? Mention 2.
D. Write down the one important treatment.

OSPE: 11

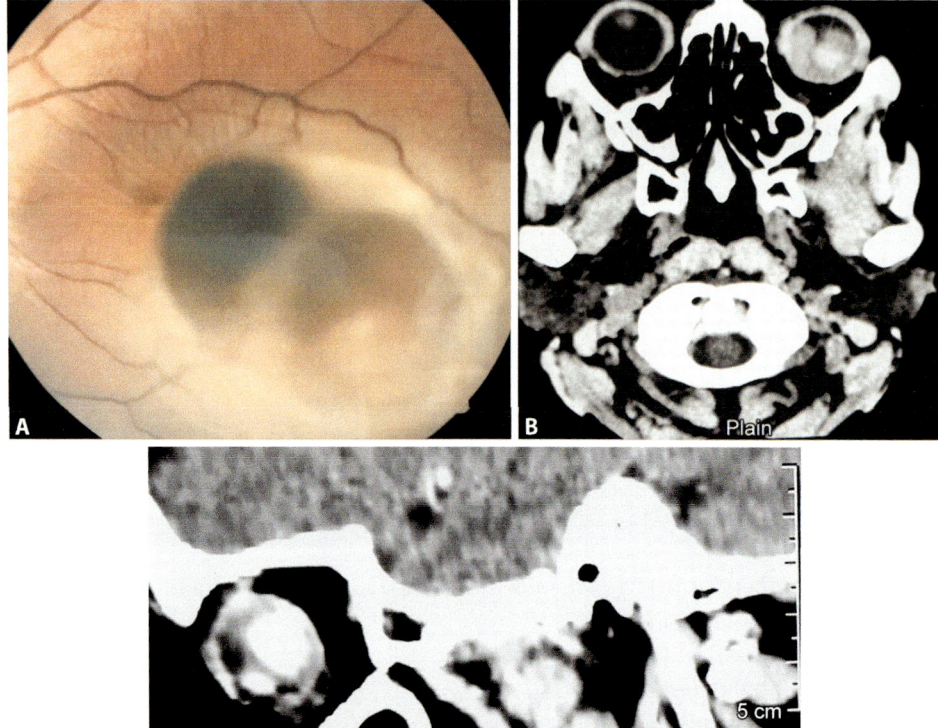

(Image Courtesy: Dr Soma Rani Roy, CEITC)

These three images have taken from the same patient. But, the fundus photograph was taken 1 year before the CT scan. Between these two CT scan, one is plain scan and the other has taken after contrast injection.
A. Why the lesion in color fundus photography is smaller than the CT lesion?
B. Which CT scan is plain and which one is with contrast?
C. What are the positive findings in both CT scans?
D. What is your provisional diagnosis?
E. How will you confirm your diagnosis?

OSPE: 12

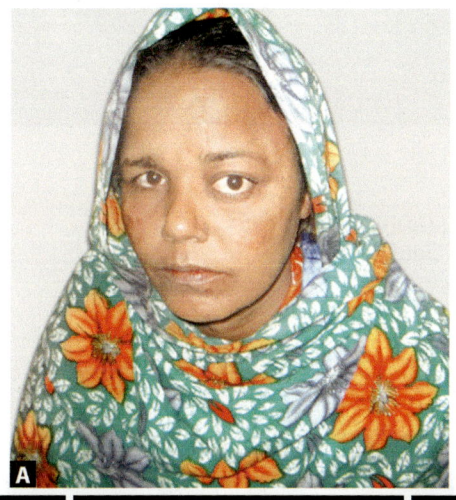
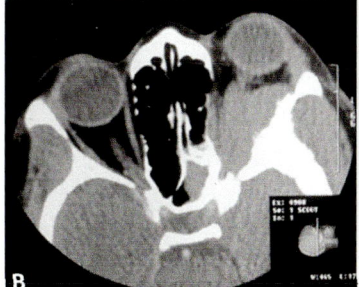
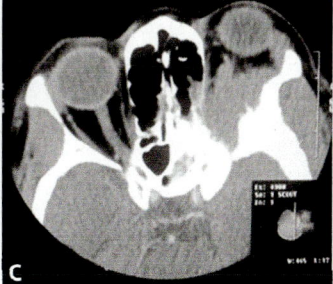
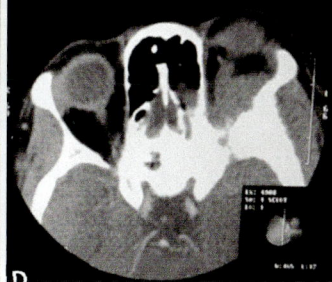

(Image Courtesy: Dr Soma Rani Roy, CEITC)

This middle-aged woman presented with left-sided proptosis and temporal fullness. Her CT scan is given here:
A. What is the positive finding in CT scan?
B. What is your provisional diagnosis?
C. From where it arises?
D. When they impair visual field?

OSPE: 13

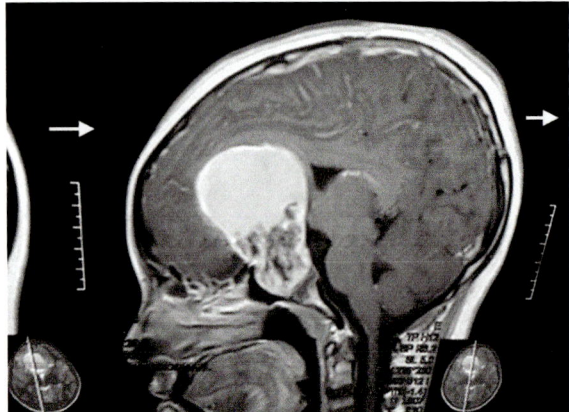

A. What is the diagnosis?
B. From where it arises?
C. Which age group most commonly involve?
D. What is the early visual field defect?
E. What are the symptoms?

OSPE: 14

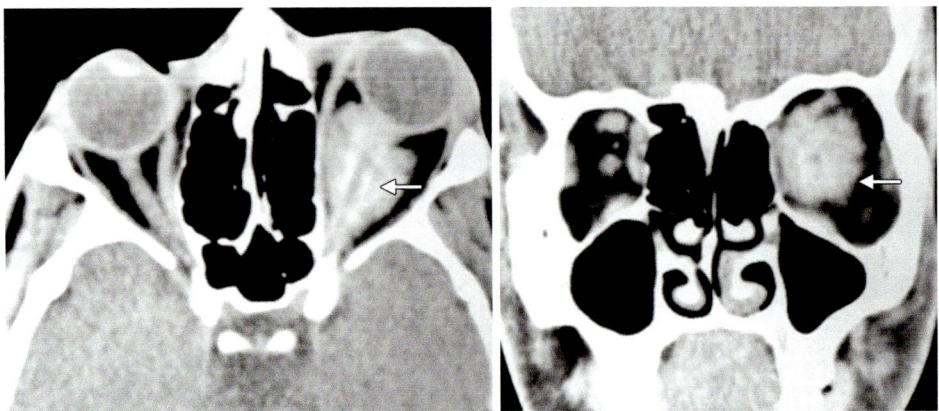

Image 1   Image 2

Orbital CT of a 48 year-old woman with slowly progressive proptosis in the left eye over the past 8 months. Image 1 CT with contrast and image 2 is plain CT.
A. What are your positive findings in both CT scans?
B. What is your probable diagnosis?
C. Mention three differential diagnoses.

OSPE: 15

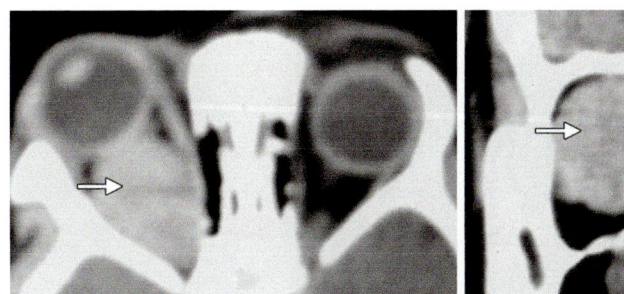
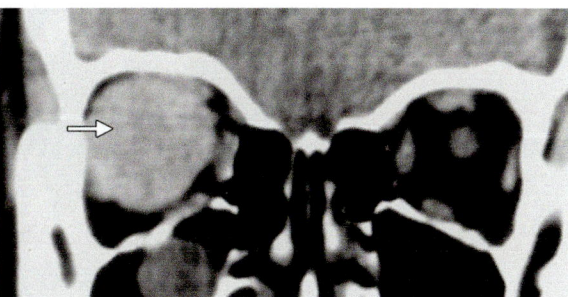

Image 1   Image 2

This is the CT scan of a 5-year-old boy came to you with temporal and inferior displacement of the globe, who is also suffering from neurofibromatosis type 1.
A. Which one is axial and coronal scan?
B. What is the positive finding in image 1? Mention 1.
C. What are the positive and negative findings in image 2? Mention 2.
D. What is your provisional diagnosis?
E. Mention one differential diagnosis.

OSPE: 16

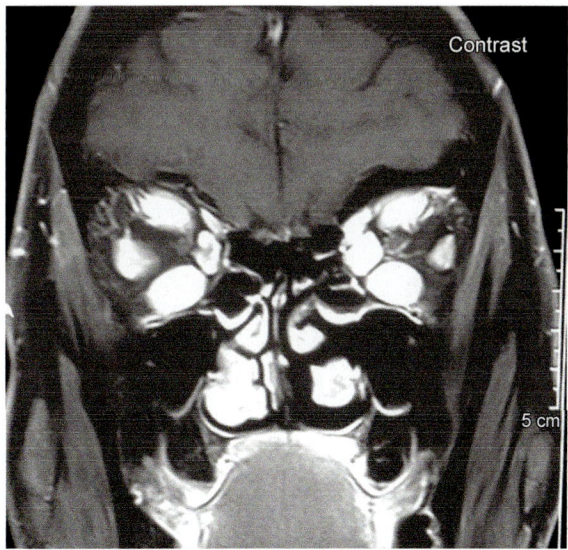

(Image Courtesy: Dr Soma Rani Roy, CEITC)

This is the MRI of a 65-year-old woman with unilateral proptosis.
A. What is the orientation of the MRI?
B. What abnormalities are shown?
C. What is the most likely diagnosis?
D. What abnormalities may occur during ocular motility test?

OSPE: 17

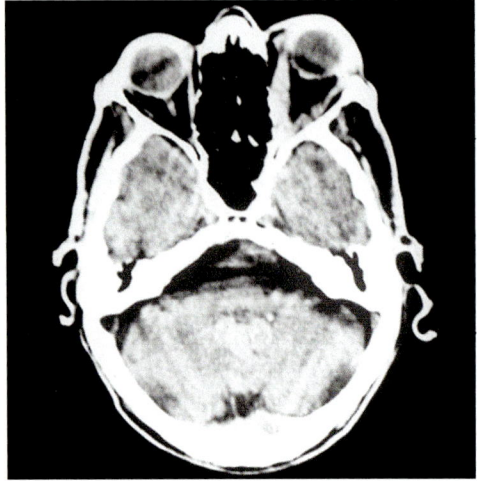

(Image Courtesy: Dr Soma Rani Roy, CEITC)

A lady 30-year-old came to you with the complaints of acute ocular and periocular redness, swelling and pain. This is the image of her CT scan.
A. What is the view of the CT scan?
B. What is the positive finding?
C. What is your provisional diagnosis?
D. Mention one differential diagnosis.
E. How will you differentiate your D/D from provisional diagnosis from the CT scan?

OSPE: 18

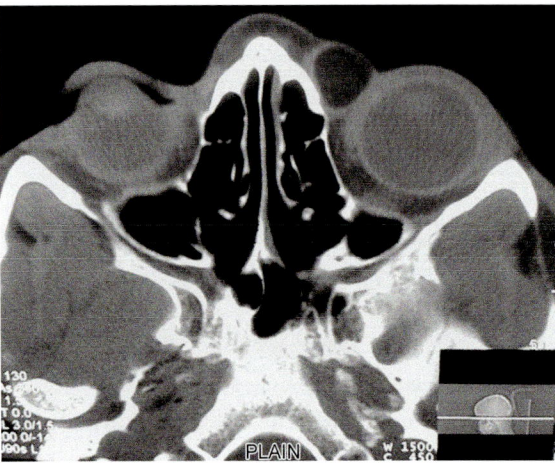

A. What is the view of the CT scan?
B. What is the positive finding?
C. What is your diagnosis?
D. How it presents usually?

OSPE: 19

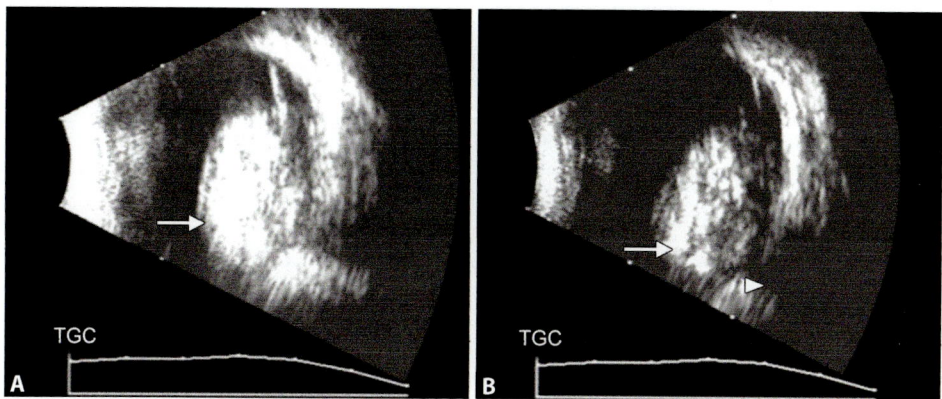

These are the B scan of a boy of two years old. Mother of the child complains that the baby is suffering from strabismus and poor vision. On ophthalmoscope, media was not so clear and B scan ultrasonography was done.

A. What does the B scan ultrasonography see?
B. What is your diagnosis?
C. What other radiological investigation you will do? And why?
D. What is the most common presentation of this disease?

OSPE: 20

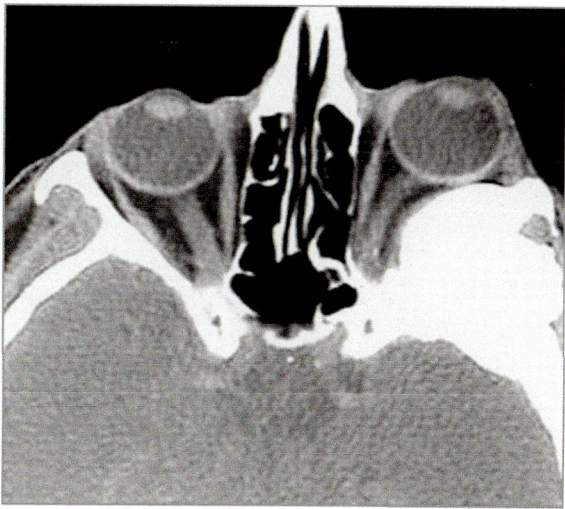

This 70-year-old man suffered from progressive left exophthalmos. His CT scan is shown as above:

A. What does the CT scan show?
B. What is the most likely diagnosis?
C. What are the advantages of CT scan over MRI in orbital imaging?

OSPE: 21

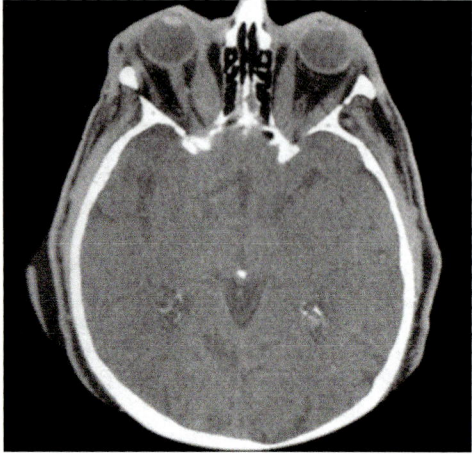

This is the MRI of brain and orbit of a female 40-year-old and suffering from thyroid eye diseases.
A. What is the positive finding in the MRI?
B. Mention one differential diagnosis.
C. What is the reason of no pain during ocular movement?
D. How will you differentiate it from idiopathic orbital inflammatory disease (IOID)?

OSPE: 22

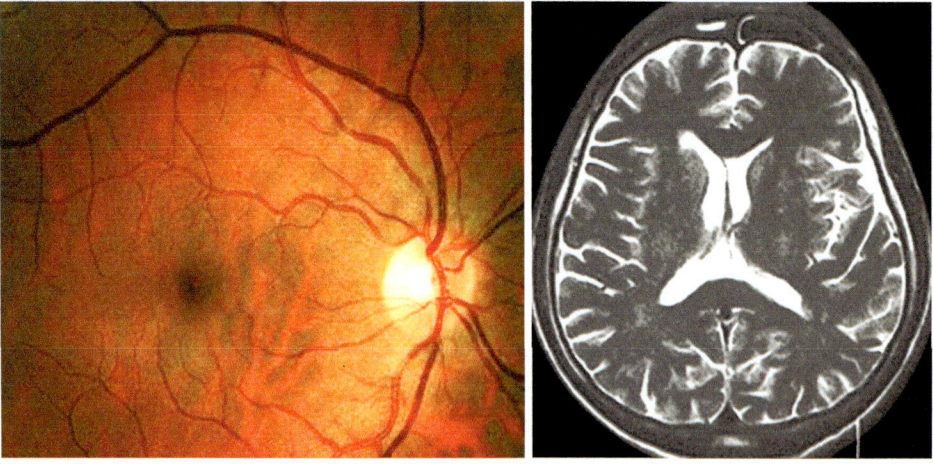

Image 1   Image 2

These two images are from same patient. Image 1, color fundus photo and image 2, MRI of the brain.
A. What is the positive finding in image 1 and image 2? Mention one for each.
B. What is the diagnosis?
C. What are the symptoms? Mention three afferent symptoms and three efferent symptoms.

ANSWERS

OSPE: 01. Lymphangioma
OSPE: 02. Retinoblastoma
OSPE: 03. Cavernous hemangioma
OSPE: 04. Optic nerve sheath meningioma
OSPE: 05. Lacrimal gland pleomorphic
OSPE: 06. Multiple sclerosis
OSPE: 07. Orbital floor fracture
OSPE: 08. Meningioma in right frontal region
OSPE: 09. Carotid cavernous fistula
OSPE: 10. Orbital cellulitis
OSPE: 11. Choroidal melanoma
OSPE: 12. Sphenoid wing meningioma
OSPE: 13. Craniopharyngioma
OSPE: 14. Optic nerve sheath meningioma
OSPE: 15. Optic nerve glioma
OSPE: 16. Thyroid eye disease
OSPE: 17. Idiopathic orbital inflammatory disease (IOID)
OSPE: 18. Orbital dermoid
OSPE: 19. Retinoblastoma
OSPE: 20. Sphenoid wing meningioma
OSPE: 21. Thyroid ophthalmopathy
OSPE: 22. Multiple sclerosis

ANS: 01

A. 1.0×3 .... 3.0
   (a) Homogenous lesion with cystic component
   (b) Calcification within the lesion
   (c) Minimal or no displacement or compression of adjacent structures
B. Lymphangioma 3.0
C. Hamartomatous vascular tumor 1.0
D. It looks like soft bluish masses. It is most commonly seen in the upper nasal quadrant...1
   + 1 .... 2.0
E. Chocolate cysts 1.0
TOTAL **10**

ANS: 02

A. Image 1: B-scan ultrasonography. Image 2: Color fundus photo .... 0.5 + 0.5 .... 1.0
B. (a) The B-scan shows a high reflective mass with calcification (arrow) 1.5
   (b) CFP shows large endophytic mass extending below and temporal to the disc shows large endophytic mass extending below and temporal to the disk 1.5
C. Retinoblastoma 3.0

D. (a) Leukocoria (white pupillary reflex) is the most common presentation 1.5
   (b) Strabismus is the second most common presentation 1.0
   (c) Painful red eye with secondary glaucoma 0.5
   (d) Poor vision 0.5
TOTAL 10

ANS: 03

A. (a) In image: 1, there is proptosis in left eye.. 1.5
   (b) In MRI, a well-circumscribed mass in intraconal space........................... 1.5
B. Cavernous hemangioma.. 2.5
C. Middle-aged female 1.0
D. Growth may be accelerated by pregnancy 1.0
E. Lateral part of the muscle cone just behind the globe................................... 1.0
F. .... 0.5 × 3 .... 1.5
   (a) Optic nerve sheath meningioma
   (b) Schwannoma
   (c) Lymphoma
TOTAL 10

ANS: 04

A. .... 1.5 × 2 .... 3.0
   (a) CT scan shows oval, well circumscribed, intraconal lesion, isodense, or slightly hyperdense to muscle
   (b) Mild contrast enhancement due to low vascular flow
B. Cavernous hemangioma (These tumors are the most common benign orbital tumors in adults)... 2.5
C. D/D
   (a) Optic nerve sheath meningioma.. 1.0
   (b) Schwannoma 0.5
   (c) Lymphoma.. 0.5
D. History of:......................(Any 2)....................... 2 × 0.5 .... 1.0
   (a) Pain
   (b) Double vision
   (c) Episodes of amaurosis
   Examination of: ....(Any 3)....................3 × 0.5 .... 1.5
   (a) Visual acuity
   (b) Color vision
   (c) Ocular motility
   (d) Visual fields, and
   (e) Exophthalmometry
TOTAL 10

Radiology

ANS: 05
A. Image A: axial; and image B: coronal sections of the CT scan 3
B. Fairly well-defined orbital mass in the area of lacrimal gland 2
C. Right lacrimal gland tumor is the most probably a pleomorphic 2
D. Yes. The mass was indenting over the globe. No bony erosion could be seen. 3
TOTAL 10

ANS: 06
A. Color fundus photo and MRI of the brain 3.0
B. Figure A: Temporal pallor of the optic disk. Figure B: T1-weighted axial MR image showing characteristic periventricular plaques..3.0
C. Multiple sclerosis 1.5
D. Recurrent attack. Because temporal pallor of the disk indicates previous attack..........2.5
TOTAL 10

ANS: 07
A. Image 1: Coronal and Image 2: Sagittal 3
B. CT shows—tear-drop appearance in coronal cut 2
C. Orbital floor fracture 2
D. Infraorbital nerve anesthesia involving the:..3
  - Lower lid
  - Cheek
  - Side of nose
  - Upper lip
  - Upper teeth and gums

Total...10

ANS: 08
A. Figure A is T1-weighted and Figure 2 is T2-weighted images 3
B. (a) A fairly large well-defined extra-axial area is noted in the frontal lobe showing iso intense in T1 and hyperintense in T2 2
  (b) Mass effect is evident by compression to frontal lobe of right lateral ventricle and mid line shift toward left 2
C. Meningioma in right frontal region 2
D. Raised intracranial pressure (ICP)..1
TOTAL 10

ANS: 09
A. Magnetic resonance angiogram (MRA)..2
B. (a) Dilatation of left superior ophthalmic vein, and 2
  (b) Engorgement of the cavernous sinuses 2
C. Carotid cavernous fistula...2
D. (a) After trauma..1
  (b) Secondary to a ruptured aneurysm of the cavernous ICA..1
TOTAL 10

ANS: 10

A. Orbital cellulitis 3
B. (a) Axial view of CT scan showing diffuse shadow with heterogeneous density, and ... 1
   (b) Lucent pockets of gas formation, extraconal and intraconal 1
   (c) The ethmoid sinuses are opacified 1
C. (a) Orbital hematoma after trauma 1
   (b) Hemorrhage into an orbital lymphangioma 1
D. Broad spectrum I/V antibiotic 2
TOTAL **10**

ANS: 11

A. The CFP was taken 1 year earlier than CT scan 2
B. Upper one is plain, and the lower one is with contrast 2
C. CT-shows almost whole globe is occupied by lesion in axial cut and in sagittal section with contrast, the lesion is well visualized and took the contrast with surrounding exudates ... 2
D. Choroidal melanoma 2
E. By histopathology 2
TOTAL **10**

ANS: 12

A. Retrobulbar isointense mass lesion with sphenoid bone thickening 3
B. Sphenoid wing meningioma 3
C. Arachnoid meningeal epithelial cells 2
D. Tumors near the sella or optic nerve can cause visual field defects 2
TOTAL **10**

ANS: 13

A. Craniopharyngioma 3
B. Arising from vestigial remnants of the Rathke pouch along the pituitary stalk 2
C. Children 1
D. Inferotemporal fields 1
E. (a) Dwarfism 1
   (b) Delayed sexual development, and 1
   (c) Obesity 1
TOTAL **10**

ANS: 14

A. Answer a and b for image 2, c, d and e for image 1
   (a) A solid tumor around the optic nerve 2.0
   (b) Fluffy and indistinct margins (blue arrow) 1.0
   (c) Calcification, "tram-track" appearance and contrast enhancement (yellow arrow) ..
   .... 2.0
   (d) The hypodense spot in the center of the lesion is the optic nerve 1.0
   (e) The hyperdense spots along the optic nerve are due to calcification 1.0

Radiology 243

   B. Optic nerve sheath meningioma...2.0
   C. Any three:
      (a) Optic nerve glioma...1.0
      (b) Metastatic disease 0.5
      (c) Leukemic infiltration 0.5
      (d) Neurosarcoidosis..0.5
   TOTAL 10

ANS: 15

A. Image 1 is axial and image 2 is coronal..2.0
B. (a) The axial section of CT scan shows spindle-shaped tumor of the optic nerve with very distinct margins..2.0
C. (a) The coronal section shows a large intraconal tumor 1.0
   (b) The optic nerve is not seen separately (arrows) 1.0
   (c) The margins are well made-out...0.5
   (d) There is no evidence of calcification 0.5
D. Optic nerve glioma 2.0
E. Optic nerve meningioma 1.0
TOTAL 10

ANS: 16

A. Coronal section 2.5
B. Enlargement of the muscles in both eyes especially the inferior rectus..............2.5
C. Thyroid eye disease..2.5
D. Any of the following abnormalities may occur:
   (a) Lid lag 1.5
   (b) Restricted eye movement in all directions especially up gaze 1.0
TOTAL 10

ANS: 17

A. Axial view..2
B. Enlargement of medial rectus muscle involving the tendon................................2
C. Idiopathic orbital inflammatory disease (IOID) 2
D. Thyroid eye diseases...2
E. In IOID, CT scan shows involvement of tendon but in thyroid eye disease tendon is spare 2
TOTAL 10

ANS: 18

A. Axial plane..2
B. CT Both in soft tissue and bony window showing circumscribed lesion in superonasal orbit 3
C. Orbital dermoid 3
D. It usually presents as a painless subcutaneous mass 2
TOTAL 10

ANS: 19

A. (a) B scan images show high reflectivity and large amounts of calcification 2
   (b) The calcification and shadowing (arrowhead) are better made out in the second image taken at reduced gain 2
B. Retinoblastoma 2
C. (a) MRI scan—to see the extension through optic nerve 1
   (b) CT scan to see the bony extension 1
D. White pupillary reflex/leukocoria 2
TOTAL 10

ANS: 20

A. Hyperostosis of the left lateral portion of the sphenoid with left proptosis 2.0
B. Sphenoid wing meningioma 3.0
C. (a) Better bony definition than MRI, especially in detecting orbital fractures and bony metastasis 1.5
   (b) Detecting metallic foreign body within the orbit or globe (contraindicated in MRI) 1.5
   (c) Shorter running time than MRI 1.0
   (d) Less expensive than MRI 1.0
TOTAL 10

ANS: 21

A. Enlargement of muscle belly 3
B. IOID 2
C. Due to sparing of the tendon 3
D. In IOID, there is involvement of tendon 2
TOTAL 10

ANS: 22

A. Temporal pallor. Plaques in the periventricular area .... 1.5 + 1.5 .... 3.0
B. Multiple sclerosis 3.0
C. Symptoms:
   Afferent symptoms:
   (a) Optic neuritis 1.0
   (b) Loss of visual acuity 1.0
   (c) Color vision and color sensitivity are affected 0.5
   Efferent symptoms .... 0.5 × 3 .... 1.5
   (a) Diplopia
   (b) Oscillopsia
   (c) Nystagmus
TOTAL 10

Miscellaneous

CHAPTER 15

QUESTIONS

OSPE: 01

Referral note, a patient, who is suffering from cataract came for surgery but uncontrolled diabetes, refer the patient to endocrinologist with a referral note.

OSPE: 02

A 20-year-old girl having uneventful dacryocystorhinostomy (DCR) surgery under L/A right side of the eye. Prepare a discharge certificate for the patient.

OSPE: 03

A 60-year-old male patient having uneventful phacoemulsification with posterior chamber (PC)-intraocular lens (IOL) implantation under topical anesthesia in his right eye. Prepare a discharge certificate for the patient.

OSPE: 04

Give a list of what instruments and device you keep ready in a FFA room for schedule and tackle the emergency?

OSPE: 05

A 55-year-old male, came to you with the complaints of sudden loss of vision in both eyes for 4 days. He gave history of DM for 22 years, hypertension for 15 years, and he had cataract surgery in both eyes for 12 years before.

On examination:
- VAR: 6/60. VAL: Counting finger 2 ft not improve with pinhole
- Pupillary reaction was sluggish in right eye but reacting and regular in left eye
- There was green-yellow defect in both eyes
- Intraocular pressure (IOP) was 12 mm of Hg in both eyes
- *Magnetic resonance imaging (MRI)*: Shows nothing abnormality.

His color fundus photo of both eyes and Humphrey visual field of both eyes were supplied here.

Answer the following questions:
A. What is the positive finding in both fundus pictures? Mention one each.
B. What is the positive finding in both VFA?
C. What is your diagnosis?

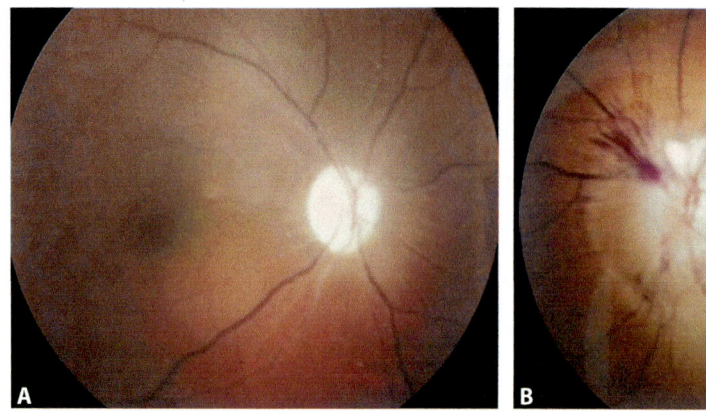

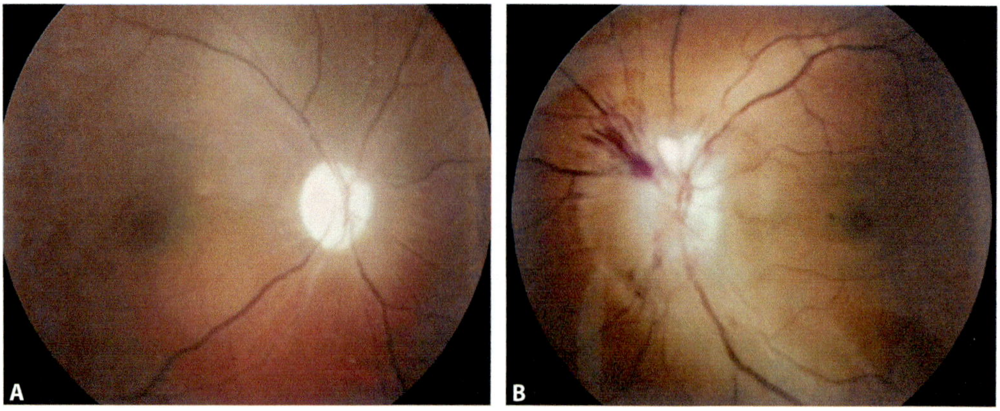

A | **B**

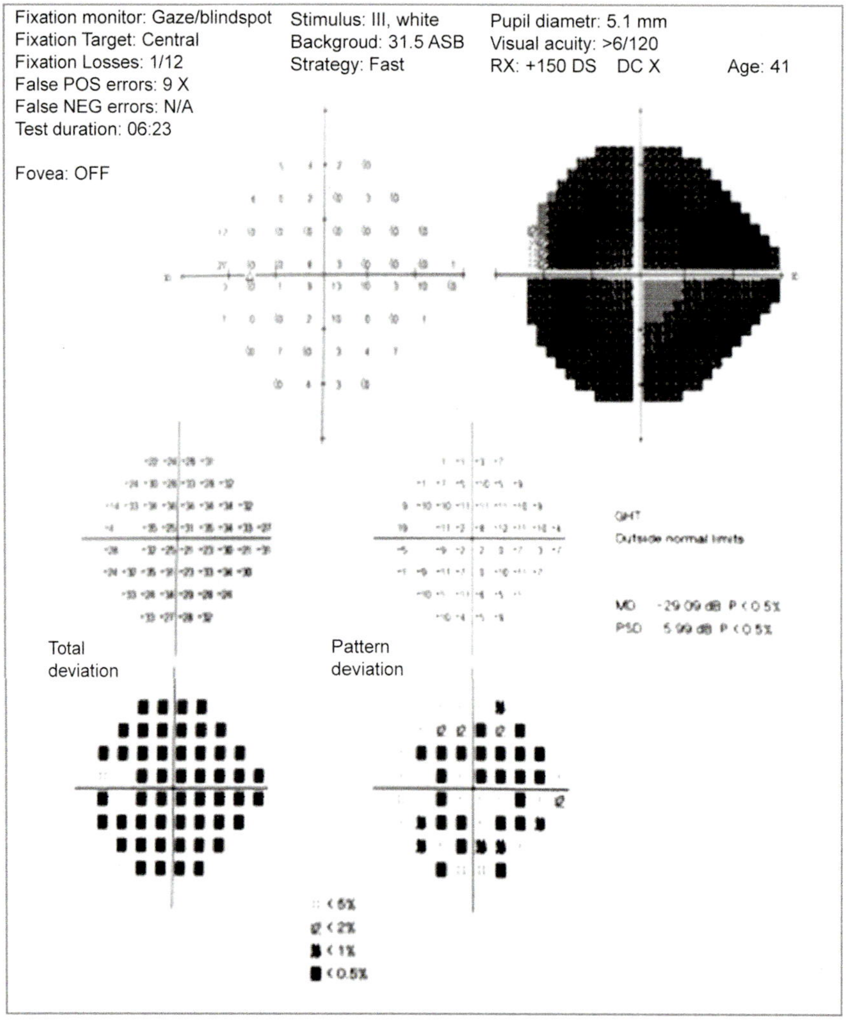

```
Fixation monitor: Gaze/blindspot    Stimulus: III, white          Pupil diameter: 5.1 mm
Fixation Target: Central            Background: 31.5 ASB          Visual acuity: >6/120
Fixation Losses: 1/12               Strategy: Fast                RX: +1.50 DS   DC X           Age: 41
False POS errors: 9 X
False NEG errors: N/A
Test duration: 06:23

Fovea: OFF
```

Total deviation

Pattern deviation

GHT: Outside normal limits

MD −29.09 dB P < 0.5%
PSD 5.99 dB P < 0.5%

< 5%
< 2%
< 1%
< 0.5%

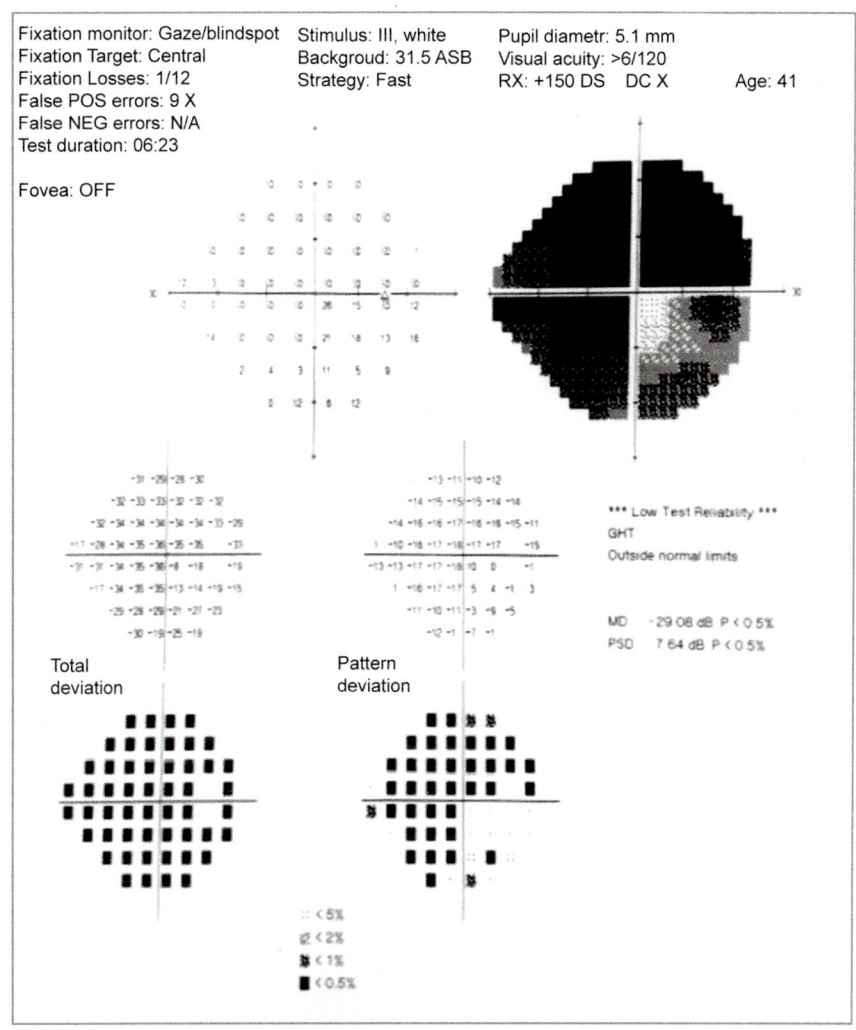

OSPE: 06

These three images have been taken from the same patient. The patient was asymptomatic on routine eye examination "bunch of grapes" found in the retina (Fig A). Fluorescein angiography (FA) was done, "B" and "C" is the FA of "A" and it shows delayed filling of the vascular lesions in the venous phase (B) followed by bright staining of the plasma component within the vascular lesions in the later phase of angiogram (C).

A. What is your diagnosis?
B. What type of diseases is this?
C. Why "bunch of grapes" are there?
D. It is usually asymptomatic but when it becomes symptomatic?

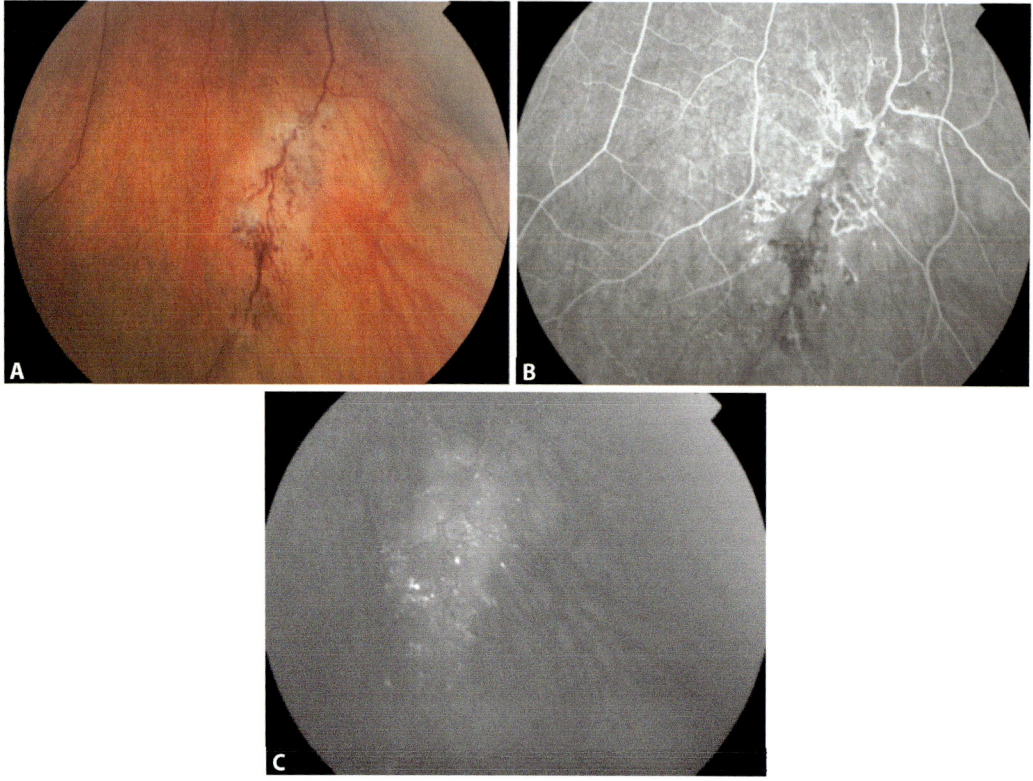

OSPE: 07

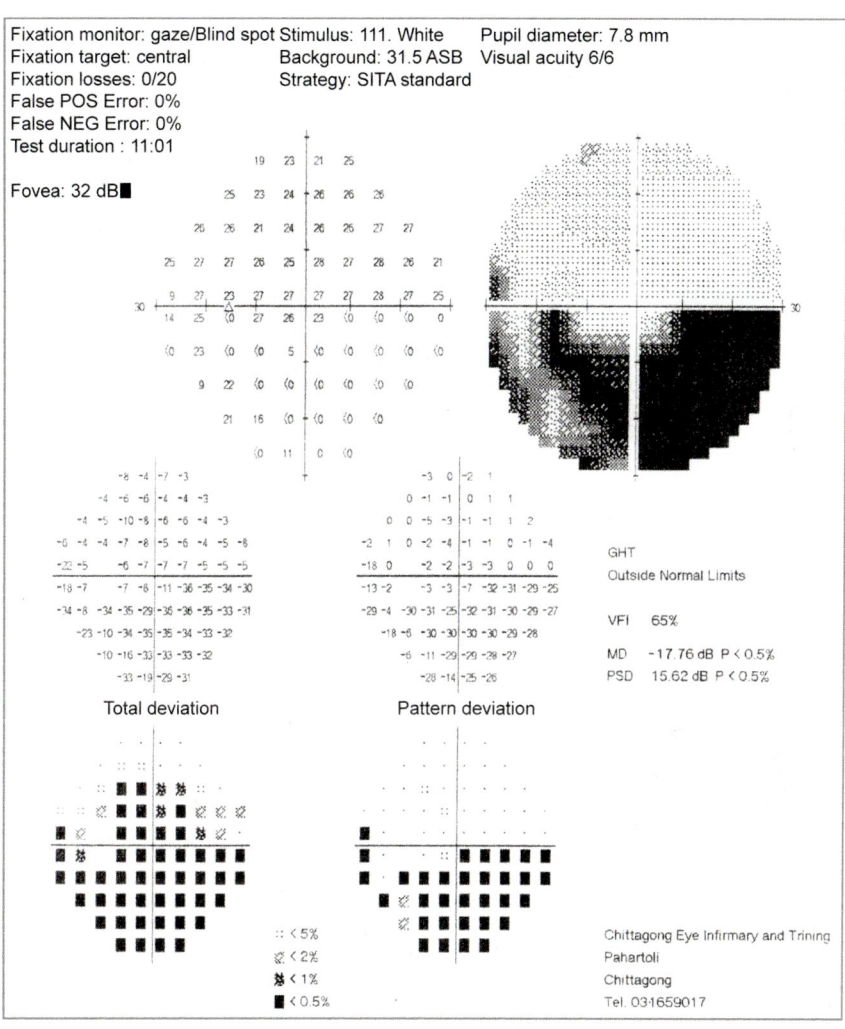

A. What is the name of the test?
B. What stands for SITA?
C. Is the test reliable?
D. What indicates the gray scale?
E. What shows the pattern deviation?
F. What is your probable diagnosis?
G. What are the D/Ds?

OSPE: 08

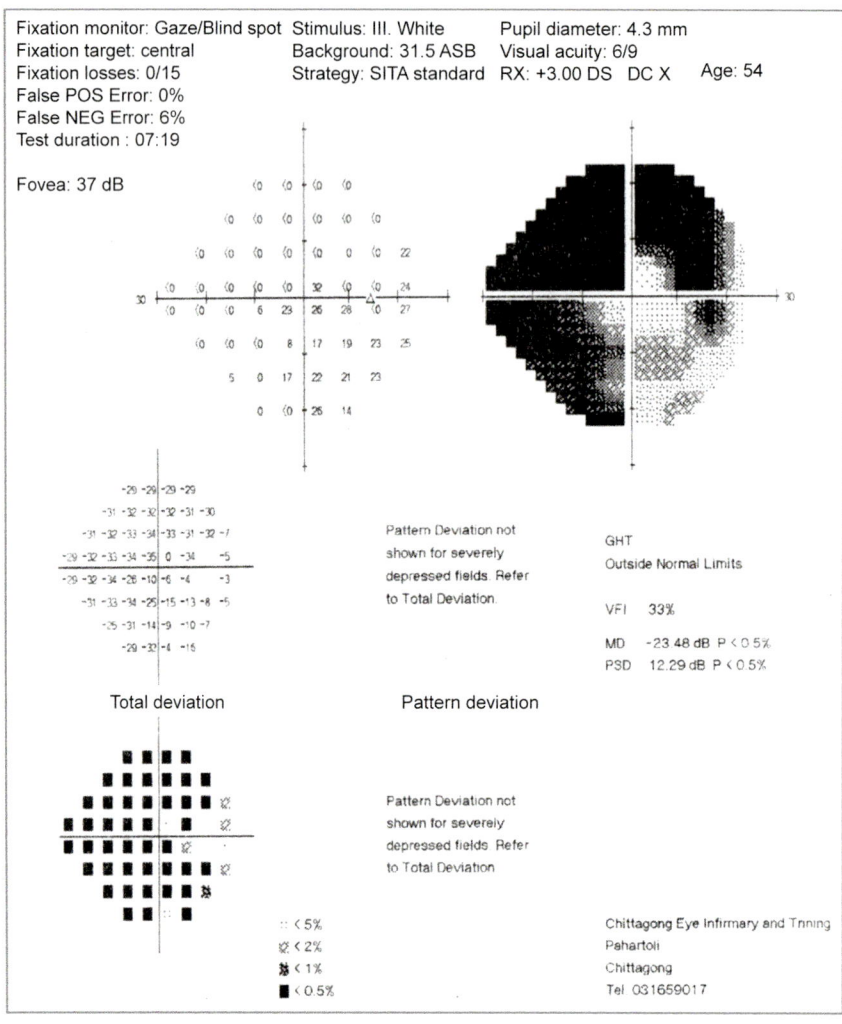

A. What is the name of the test?
B. Is the field test reliable? Why?
C. What stands for SITA?
D. What indicates the gray scale at here?
E. The test is done in which pattern?
F. What is your probable diagnosis?
G. What are the D/Ds?

OSPE: 09

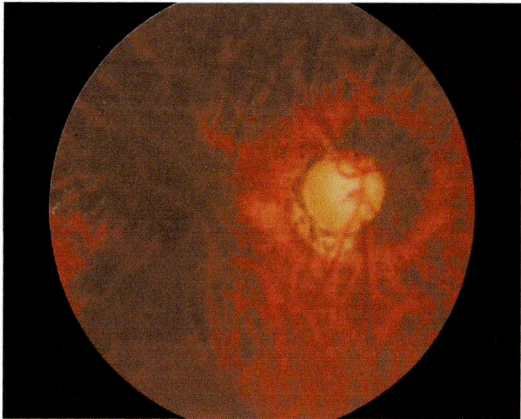

A. What is the name of the tracing paper?
B. Write three positive findings.
C. What is your diagnosis?
D. What is the D/D?

OSPE: 10

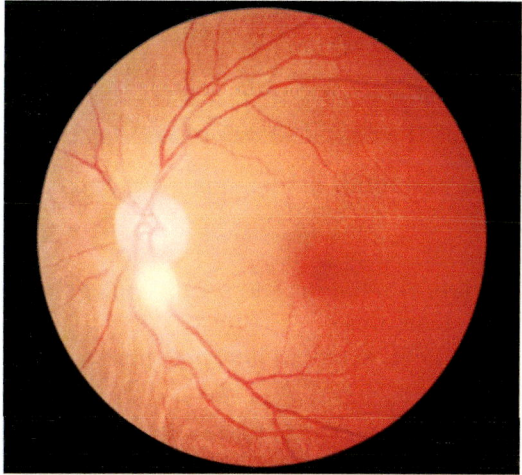

(Courtesy: Green Eye Hospital, Dhanmondi, Dhaka)

A. What is the white area around the disk?
B. Does it usually create any symptoms?
C. What change you may get in visual field?
D. Can it disappear? If yes, when?

OSPE: 11 (Same photo: 6)

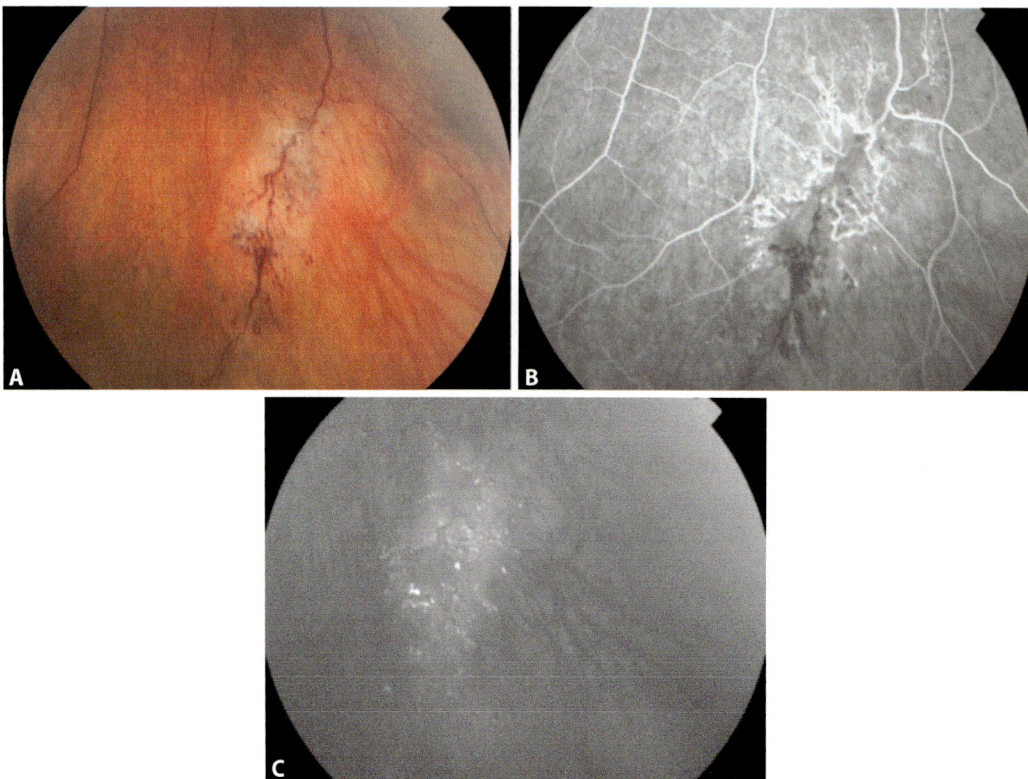

Color photograph of retinal cavernous hemangioma (A) and corresponding fluorescein angiogram (B and C).

Answer the following questions:
A. What are the positive findings in fundus fluorescein angiography (FFA)?
B. Mention two differential diagnoses.
C. What type of diseases is retinal cavernous hemangioma?

OSPE: 12

Write down the retinoscope findings of the following glass from 67 cm distance.
OD: –0.75 Dsph/–0.75 Dcyl 180
OS: Plano/–1.00 Dcyl 180.

OSPE: 13

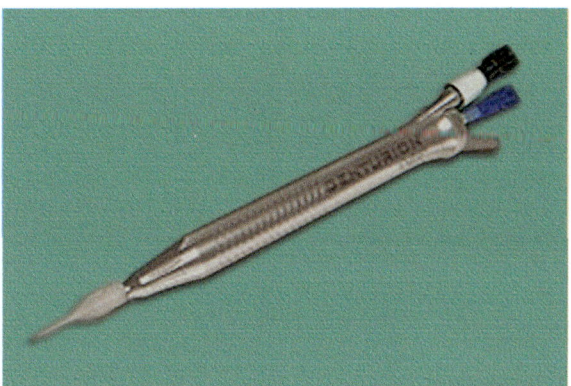

A. Identify the instrument. Who invented it?
B. What is the function of the sleeve that covers the tip of the internal tube?
C. Name three important parameters that have to present during surgery.

OSPE: 14

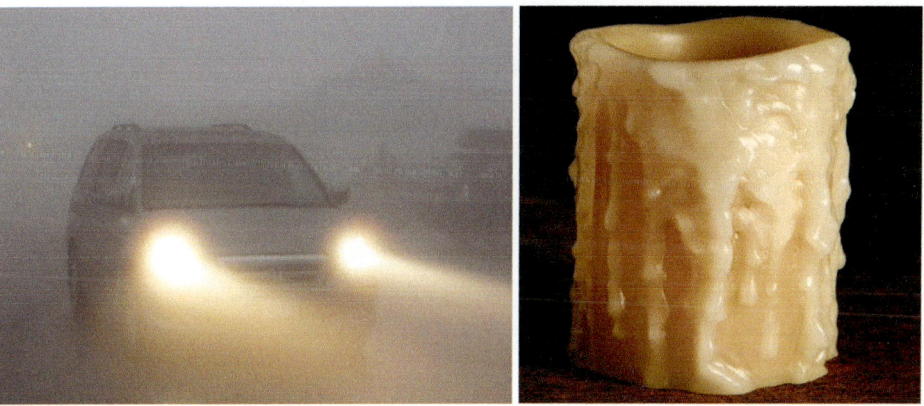

Fig. 1   Fig. 2

These two pictures represent two systemic diseases which usually involve ocular tissue.
A. Mention the name of the diseases.
B. What they called?
C. Both the diseases involve different structures of the eyeball but when you get these pictures?
D. In Figure 1, is it active or chronic stage?
E. Why vision loss is there (Fig. 1)? Mention two.

OSPE: 15

These three pictures indicate postoperative complication of cataract surgery. What are the names and why they occur?

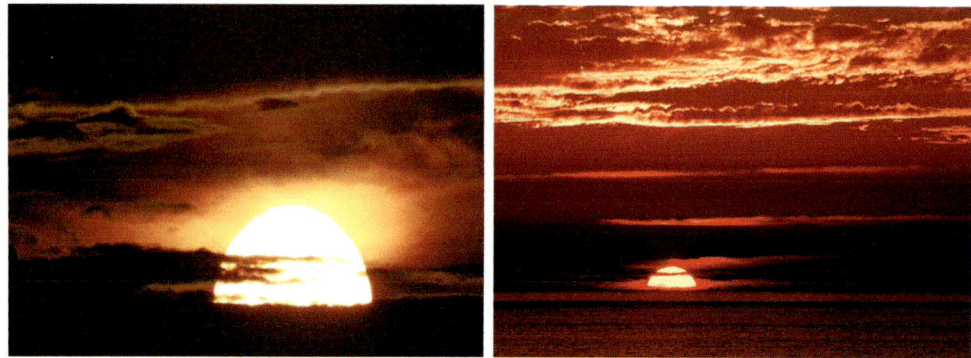

Fig. 1　　　　　　　　　　　　　　　　　Fig. 2

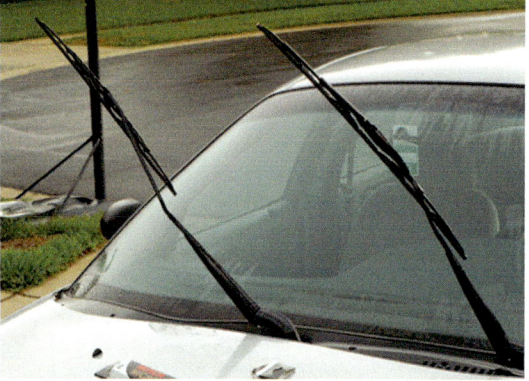

Fig. 3

OSPE: 16

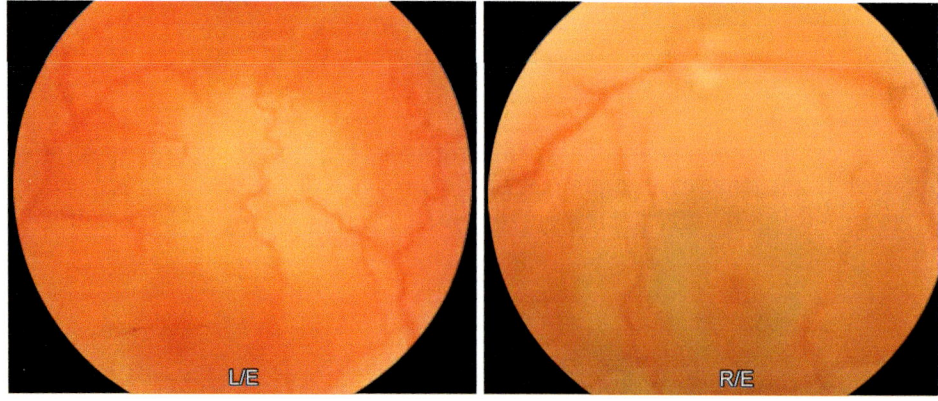

This is the image of a preterm baby (both eyes).
A. What is the image called?
B. What are the positive findings?
C. What is the diagnosis?
D. What is the treatment?

OSPE: 17

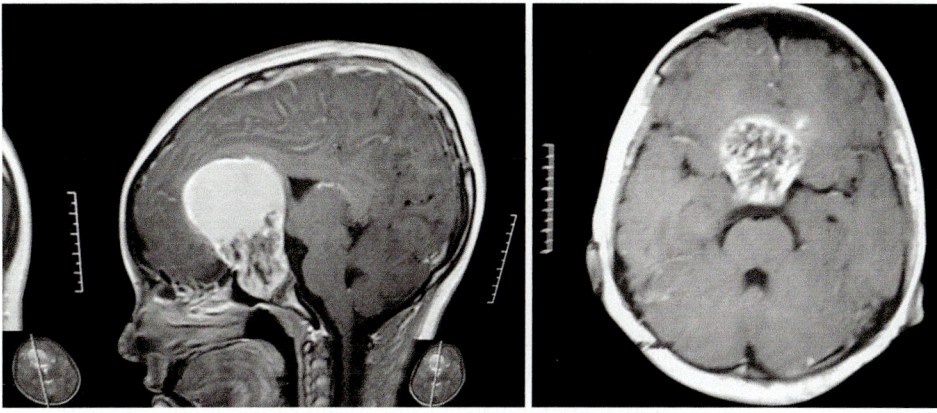

Image 1   Image 2

(Courtesy: Dr Bidoura Tanim, Assistant Professor, Department of Radiology, NIO)

A. What is view of the image 1 and image 2?
B. Is these plain view or postcontrast view?
C. What are the positive findings in these images?
D. What is your probable diagnosis?

OSPE: 18
Measures tear film breakup time:
(supplied materials: Fluorescein strip, slit lamp)

OSPE: 19
Applying pressure patches and shields with following materials:
Eye pad, eye shield, scissors, adhesive tape, and alcohol pad.

ANSWERS

ANS: 01
Referral note:
A patient, who is suffering from cataract came for surgery but uncontrolled diabetes, refer the patient to diabetologist with a referral note.

Date and time: 29/04/2018
Time: 8:30 AM

To,
Assistant/Associate Professor
Department of Endocrinology
Dhaka Medical College, Dhaka

Dear Sir,
With due respect,

I am the undersigned, like to inform you that patient Mr X, 67 years old, hailing from Manikganj suffering from bilateral senile mature cataract (B/E). He is also a patient of diabetes mellitus (DM) last 20 years, at present his blood sugar [2 hours after breakfast (ABF)] is 15 mmol/dL in spite of taking insulin regularly. He needs cataract surgery but uncontrolled diabetes is contraindicated for his surgery.

So, I will be obliged if your kind enough to give your valuable opinion regarding his diabetes control.

Thank you
Signature
Name of doctor
Designation
Institute and Department.

Marking Scheme

A.	Date and time	1
B.	Addressing: Professor/Associate Professor/Assistant Professor	1
C.	Dear Sir	1
	Content:	
D.	Patient identification	1
E.	From where	1
F.	Patient findings	1
G.	What we want	1
H.	Thank you	1
I.	Name and designation	1
J.	Signature	1
	TOTAL	**10**

ANS: 02

	Parameters	Marks
Identification of the patient	Name	0.5
	Age	0.25
	Gender	0.25
	Address	0.5
	Mobile number	0.25
Operation note	Date and time	0.25
	Name of surgery	0.25
	Indication of surgery	0.25
	Name of anesthesia	0.5
	Name of surgeon	0.5
Postoperative findings	Condition of incision area	0.5
	Any discharge	0.5
	Conjunctiva, eyelid, and cornea	0.5
Postoperative treatment	Systemic antibiotic	1.0
	Systemic analgesic	0.5
	Antiulcerant	0.25
	Topical antibiotic	0.5
Advice	No water to eye	0.5
	Use dark glass	0.25
	Regular use of medicine	0.25
	Any problem come to doctor	0.25
	Follow-up	0.25
Identification of certificate preparatory	Signature with date	0.25
	Name of the doctor with designation	0.5
	Seal of the department	0.5
TOTAL		**10**

ANS: 03

	Parameters	Marks
Identification of the patient	Name	0.5
	Age	0.25
	Gender	0.25
	Address	0.5
	Mobile number	0.25
Operation note	Date and time	0.5
	Name of surgery	0.5
	Name of anesthesia	0.5
	Name of surgeon	0.5
Postoperative findings	Visual acuity	1.0
	Anterior segment	1.0
	Posterior segment	0.5
Postoperative treatment	Topical antibiotic	0.5
	Topical steroid	0.5
Advice	No water to eye	0.25
	Use dark glass	0.25
	Regular use of medicine	0.25
	Any problem come to doctor	0.25
	Follow-up	0.25
Identification of certificate preparatory	Signature with date	0.5
	Name of the doctor with designation	0.5
	Seal of the department	0.5
TOTAL		**10**

ANS: 04

1. Emesis basin
2. Oxygen
3. Sphygmomanometer and stethoscope
4. Couch for patient to lie down
5. Ice pack
6. Tourniquet
7. Disposable needles
8. Disposable syringes
9. Intravenous (IV) set and scalp vein set
10. Airway devices
11. Ambu bag

12. Inj Adrenaline
13. Inj atropine
14. Inj Anti histamine
15. Inj Steroid
16. Inj Deriphylline
17. Inj Dextrose saline.

ANS: 05

A. Upper: Shows optic atrophy 1.5
   Lower: Shows disk swelling 1.5
B. Right eye: Gross field defect 2.0
   Left eye: Tubular field defect 2.0
C. Pseudo-Foster Kennedy syndrome 3.0
TOTAL *10*

ANS: 06

A. Cavernous hemangioma
B. Rare unilateral congenital hamartoma
C. Clusters of saccular aneurysms resembling a "bunch of grapes"
D. Vitreous hemorrhage.

ANS: 07

A. This is the Humphrey visual field analyzer (HVFA) of central 30-2 threshold test of left eye 0.5
B. The field is reliable because the fixation loss, false positive, and false-negative errors are within normal limits 2.0
C. The strategy used is Swedish Interactive Threshold Algorithm (SITA) standard format 1.0
D. The gray scale reading indicates darker tone occupying whole inferior field and only sparing central field 2.0
E. Pattern deviation shows scotoma occupying whole inferior field and only sparing central field 1.5
F. Glaucoma 2.0
G. Superior branch retinal vein occlusion (BRVO), superior branch retinal artery occlusion (BRAO) .... 0.5 × 2 .... 1.0
TOTAL *10*

ANS: 08

A. This is the HVFA of central test of left eye 0.50
B. The field is reliable because the fixation loss, false positive, and false-negative errors are within normal limits 2.0
C. Swedish Interactive Threshold Algorithm standard format 1.0
D. The gray scale reading indicates darker tone occupying whole superior and inferior field only sparing central and inferotemporal field 2.0
E. The test is done in 24 – 2 .... 0.5

F. Advanced glaucoma [primary open-angle glaucoma (POAG)] 1.0
G. .... 1 × 3 .... 3.0
    (a) Advanced retinitis pigmentosa (RP)
    (b) After panretinal photocoagulation (PRP)
    (c) Central retinal artery occlusion (CRAO) with patent cilioretinal artery.
TOTAL **10**

ANS: 09
A. This is the color fundus photograph (CFP) of right eye 1.0
B. .... 1.5 × 3 .... 4.5
    (a) Showing almost total cupping and absence of neuroretinal rim
    (b) Bayoneting sign is present (superior)
    (c) Peripapillary atrophy.
C. Diagnosis: Advanced glaucoma 3.0
D. Coloboma of the disk 1.5
TOTAL **10**

ANS: 10
A. Medullated nerve fiber 2.5
B. No 2.5
C. There will be scotoma opposite to the nerve 2.5
D. Yes, in optic atrophy or demyelinated diseases 2.5
TOTAL **10**

ANS: 11
A. Fundus fluorescein angiography shows delayed filling of the cavernous vascular lesions in the venous phase (B) followed by bright staining of the plasma component within the vascular lesions in the later phase of angiogram (C).
B. Retinal capillary hemangioma and Coats' disease.
C. Congenital vascular hamartomas.

ANS: 12

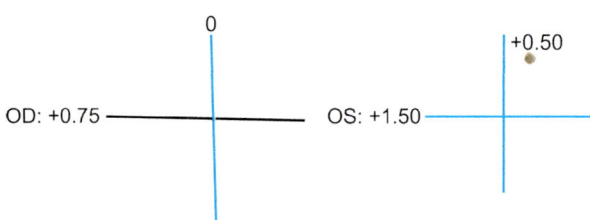

ANS: 13
A. Phaco handpiece 1
    Charles David Kelman 1
B. It protects the cornea, iris from transmitted heat energy by the probe 2
C. (a) Power 2

Miscellaneous 261

    (b) Vacuum 2
    (c) Flow rate 2
TOTAL **10**

ANS: 14

A. Ocular toxoplasmosis and sarcoidosis .... 2 + 2 4
B. Fog in the light and candle wax dripping .... 1 + 1 2
C. When uveal tissue involve 1
D. Active 1
E. Any two .... 2 × 1 2
    (a) Macular inflammatory lesions/edema
    (b) Optic nerve involvement
    (c) Vascular occlusion.
TOTAL **10**

ANS: 15

Fig. 1
Sunrise syndrome: 1
    Most commonly occurs due to the misplacement of the superior haptic in the ciliary sulcus, while the inferior one is placed into the capsular bag that allows the IOL to subluxated superiorly 3
Fig. 2
Sunset syndrome: 1
    May result from undetected anterior capsule rupture extending inferiorly allowing the inferior haptic of PC-IOL to escape through the defects 3
Fig. 3
Windshield wiper syndrome: When the overall size of the IOL is smaller, it moves horizontally 2
TOTAL **10**

ANS: 16

A. Color fundus photo 1.0
B. Dilated and torture vessels 4.0
C. Retinopathy of prematurity (ROP)/AROP 3.0
D. Laser/antivascular endothelial growth factor (anti-VEGF) 2.0
TOTAL **10**

ANS: 17

A. This is the MRI of brain sagittal and axial views 2
B. Postcontrast scan 2
C. (a) A large suprasellar mass with intrasellar extension 1
    (b) The mass enhanced strongly with some signal void areas inside representing calcifications 1
    (c) Optic chiasm is compressed by the lesion 1
D. The lesion is craniopharyngioma 3
TOTAL **10**

ANS: 18

A. Pull the lower lid and touches the fluorescein strip into the lower palpebral conjunctiva (do not use fluorescein drop because it will increase the tear volume) 2.0
B. Positioning of the patient into slit lamp .... 0.5 × 5 .... 2.5
    (a) Chin rest
    (b) Forehead fixed into the band
    (c) Canthal marking adjusted
    (d) Fixed slit lamp into "0"
    (e) Fixed your interpupillary distance (IPD)
C. After positioning, the patient turn on the slit-lamp switch 0.5
D. Use diffuse illumination with cobalt-blue filter 1.0
E. Ask the patient to look straight ahead and to blink... 1.5
F. While observing the eye through slit lamp, count yourself the number of seconds that elapse between the blink and the appearance of the first dry spot. The dry spot will appear blue-black (because of the dark blue illumination) when the green-stained tear film pulls away the area of breakup 1.5
G. Repeat the test one or more times for each eye, because a single measurement might be falsely high or low 1.0
   TOTAL *10*

ANS: 19

A. Apply a piece of adhesive tape, about 15 cm long, to the eye pad 2
B. Ask the patient to close both eyes 2
C. Clean the forehead and zygoma with an alcohol pad to remove the skin oils. This helps the tape stick to the skin 2
D. Fold one pad half, and position the eye pad diagonally over the closed lids of the affected eye and tape firmly, but gently, to the forehead and cheek.. 2
E. Apply a second and third piece of tape to ensure the pad lies flat 1
F. Extra protection can be given by taping a shield over the pad in the same way 1
   TOTAL *10*

Video Station

CHAPTER 16

QUESTIONS

OSPE: 01 (VDO: 01) *(VDO Courtesy: Dr Ishtiaque Anwer) 24 Sec*
A. What surgery is there going on?
B. In spite of cataract another pathology is there can you mention it?
C. What is the name of the color solution inside the eye? Why it is used?
D. What is inserting?
E. When it is indicated?

OSPE: 02 (VDO: 02) *(VDO Courtesy: Dr Ishtiaque Anwer) 20 Sec*
A. What is the name of this surgery?
B. What is the name of the white semicircular device?
C. Why it is used?
D. Mention two indications.
E. What are the advantages to use this device?

OSPE: 03 (VDO: 03) *(VDO Courtesy: Dr Ishtiaque Anwer) 29 Sec*
A. What is the name of this surgical step?
B. What specialty in this case and what is the name of this special step?
C. When this is applied?
D. What problem may arise during this process?
E. What is the name of the color solution inside the eye? Why it is used?
F. What disaster had happened in Bangladesh for this color solution?

OSPE: 04 (VDO: 04) *(VDO Courtesy: Dr Ishtiaque Anwer) 08 Sec*
A. What is the name of this step?
B. What is the purpose of this step?
C. How it performs?
D. What complication may arise during this step?

OSPE: 05 (VDO: 05) *(VDO Courtesy: Dr Ishtiaque Anwer) 31 Sec*
A. What surgery is there going on?
B. What instrument was used to mark over the lens?
C. What are the steps that can be performed with this machine?
D. What are the disadvantages of this machine? Mention 3

OSP: 06 (VDO: 06) *(VDO Courtesy: Dr Ishtiaque Anwer) 29 Sec*
A. What surgery is there going on?
B. What is the step?
C. What happened in this step?

OSPE: 07 (VDO: 07)
A. What surgery is there going on?
B. What is the step?
C. What happened in this step?

OSPE: 08 (VDO: 08) *(VDO Courtesy: Dr Ishtiaque Anwer) 21 Sec*
A. What is the name of the surgery?
B. Which layer of the cornea has ablated?
C. After ablation what is doing?
D. Burning is going on in which layer?
E. What is the fate of ablated portion?

OSPE: 09 (VDO: 09) *(VDO Courtesy: Dr Ishtiaque Anwer) 27 Sec*
A. What is the name of the step?
B. What other methods that we can perform this step?
C. Which instrument is inside the eye?
D. What complication may arise during this step?

OSPE: 10 (VDO: 10) *(VDO Courtesy: Green Eye Hospital) 45 Sec*
See the video and answer the following questions:
A. What is the name of the test?
B. What is your diagnosis?
C. What are the other tests that you can do? Mention 3.
D. How can you measure the amount of deviation?
E. What may be the expected visual acuity in both eyes?

OSPE: 11 (VDO: 11) *(VDO Courtesy: Green Eye Hospital) 16 Sec*
A. What is the name of the test?
B. What will be the interpretation of the test?
C. What is your diagnosis?
D. How can you measure the amount of deviation?
E. How can you assess postoperative diplopia at here?

OSPE: 12 (VDO: 12) *(VDO Courtesy: Green Eye Hospital) 17 Sec*
A. What is the name of the test?
B. What is your interpretation?
C. What is the next step of the test?
D. What is the direction of prism and why?
E. What will be the actual amount of deviation?

OSPE: 13 (VDO: 13) *(VDO Courtesy: Dr Ishtiaque Anwer) 30 Sec*
A. What is the name of the surgery?
B. In which direction, conjunctival incision is giving?

C. Which is the name of the inserted device?
D. When it is uses?

OSPE: 14 (VDO: 14) *(VDO Courtesy: Prof Dipak Kumar Nag) 41 Sec*
A. What is doing at the beginning of the video?
B. What is the name of white liquid given during the surgery and why?
C. What is filled inside the eye at the end of the surgery?
D. What is the name of the procedure?

OSPE: 15 (VDO: 15) *(VDO Courtesy: Prof Dipak Kumar Nag) 45 Sec*
A. What is the name of this procedure?
B. Scleral fixation suture usually given in which distance?
C. How you calculate IOL power from normal biometry in this situation?
D. Name 2 other procedures alternative of such procedure.

OSPE: 16 (VDO: 16) *(VDO Courtesy: Green Eye Hospital) 12 Sec*
A. What is the name of the diagnostic test?
B. Name 2 positive findings.
C. What is the most probable diagnosis?
D. Name 3 treatment options for such condition.
E. Name one drug contraindication in this case.

OSPE: 17 (VDO: 17) *(VDO Courtesy: Green Eye Hospital) 60 Sec*
A. What is the name of the surgery?
B. What is doing by surgeon?
C. What problem is there going on?
D. How can manage it? Mention 3 points.
E. What complications may arise? Mention 2 points.

OSPE: 18 (VDO: 18)
A. What is the indication of this surgery?
B. Name the instrument that is using for the procedure.
C. What is the name of the procedure you have seen in the video?
D. What complications may occur during the procedure?

OSPE: 19 (VDO: 19) *(VDO Courtesy: Prof Dipak Kumar Nag) 46 Sec*
The following video is a part of beginning of a vitreoretinal (VR) surgery.
A. What is trying to do by surgeon?
B. What instrument is using here?
C. What is the purpose of doing this activity?
D. What may be the most possible indication of the surgery?

OSPE: 20 (VDO: 20) *(VDO Courtesy: Prof Dipak Kumar Nag) 118 Sec*
A. What is the name of this surgery?
B. What are introducing into the eye?
C. What is their function?
D. What is their size?
E. What is the name of the plate? Describes its function.

OSPE: 21 (VDO: 21) *(VDO Courtesy: Green Eye Hospital) 49 Sec*
A. What is the name of the surgery?
B. Name the instruments are using at here.
C. What is constructed in sclera by giving incision?
D. What is the advantage of it?
E. What is the main complication of this surgery?

OSPE: 22 (VDO: 22) *(VDO Courtesy: Green Eye Hospital) 22 Sec*
This is the VDO of SICS surgery. Answer the following questions:
A. What is the name of this step?
B. What instrument is using here?
C. What complication may happen during this step? Mention 2.
D. What is the next step? And what instrument will be use?

OSPE: 23 (VDO: 23) *(VDO Courtesy: Dr Sharah Rahman) 32 Sec*
A. What is the name of the surgery?
B. Which method is using here to divide the nucleus?
C. What other methods is there to divide the nucleus?
D. Which technique is suitable for the beginner?
E. What is the problem in this technique?

OSPE: 24 (VDO: 24) *(VDO Courtesy: Prof Dipak Kumar Nag) 37 Sec*
A. What is the generic name of this medicine?
B. What is the amount (both in gm and mL) that gives intravitreal injection
C. What are the indications? Mention 3.
D. What is the name of other medicine that we can use?
E. What is the location in sclera to inject (Intravitreal) both in aphakic and phakic eye?

OSPE: 25 (VDO: 25) *(VDO Courtesy: Prof Dipak Kumar Nag) 44 Sec*
A. What is the name of the surgery?
B. What is the name of the instrument, using inside the eye?
C. What is doing by surgeon?
D. Which laser is using at here?

OSPE: 26 (VDO: 26) *(VDO Courtesy: Green Eye Hospital) 98 Sec*
A. What is the name of this surgery?
B. What steps you have seen in video? Mention 3.
C. What is the purpose of step 2 and 3?
D. What complications may happen in step 1 and 2? Mention one in each.
E. What is the next step?

OSPE: 27 (VDO: 27) *(VDO Courtesy: Dr Ishtiaque Anwer) 30 Sec*
Irrigation and aspiration are going on in this video clip: Answer following questions:
A. What is the type of I/A handpiece at here?
B. What is another type? Mention 1.
C. What materials are irrigating?
D. What materials are aspirating?
E. What complication may arise in this stage?

OSPE: 28 (VDO: 28) *(VDO Courtesy: Dr Ishtiaque Anwer) 62 Sec*
A. What surgery is going on?
B. What is the indication of this surgery?
C. What is the name of the instrument (mouse like) over the cornea?
D. What instrument is inserting into the anterior chamber?
E. What is peeling from the anterior chamber?

ANSWERS

OSPE: 01 (VDO: 01): Phacoemulsification
OSPE: 02 (VDO: 02): Capsular tension ring (CTR)
OSPE: 03 (VDO: 03): Capsulorhexis
OSPE: 04 (VDO: 04): Hydrodissection
OSPE: 05 (VDO: 05): Phacoemulsification: Femtosecond laser
OSPE: 06 (VDO: 06): Phacoemulsification: Divide the nucleus
OSPE: 07 (VDO: 07): Phacoemulsification: Sculpting of the lens
OSPE: 08 (VDO: 08): LASIK (Laser in-situ keratomileusis)
OSPE: 09 (VDO: 09): *Continuous curvilinear capsulorhexis*
OSPE: 10 (VDO: 10): Cover test
OSPE: 11 (VDO: 11): Alternate cover test
OSPE: 12 (VDO: 12): Alternate prism cover test
OSPE: 13 (VDO: 13): Trabeculectomy
OSPE: 14 (VDO: 14): Endolaser photocoagulation
OSPE: 15 (VDO: 15): Pars plana vitrectomy + scleral fixation IOL
OSPE: 16 (VDO: 16): Optical coherence tomography (OCT) macula shows serous sensory detachment of the macula/PED/CSR
OSPE: 17 (VDO: 17): Surge during phacoemulsification
OSPE: 18 (VDO: 18): Fragmatome of dropped nucleus
OSPE: 19 (VDO: 19): Put scleral buckle in RD surgery
OSPE: 20 (VDO: 20): Small-gauge vitrectomy
OSPE: 21 (VDO: 21): Manual small incision cataract surgery (MSICS)/SICS
OSPE: 22 (VDO: 22): Nucleus delivery in MSICS/SICS
OSPE: 23 (VDO: 23): Phacoemulsification with divide-and-conquer technique
OSPE: 24 (VDO: 24): Intravitreal ranibizumab
OSPE: 25 (VDO: 25): Pars plana vitrectomy
OSPE: 26 (VDO: 26): Continuous curvilinear capsulorhexis in phacoemulsification
OSPE: 27 (VDO: 27): Coaxial I/A handpiece
OSPE: 28 (VDO: 28): Goniosynechialysis

ANS: 01 (VDO: 01)

A. Phacoemulsification with posterior chamber intraocular lens implantation 2.0
B. Coloboma 2.0
C. Trypan blue 2.0
D. Iris hook 2.0
E. When the pupil cannot be dilated 2.0
TOTAL *10*

ANS: 2 (VDO: 02)

A. Phacoemulsification with posterior chamber intraocular lens implantation 2
B. Capsular tension ring (CTR) 2

C. For the stabilization of the capsular bag in the presence of weakened or compromised zonule 1
D. Pseudoexfoliation and Marfan's syndrome 2
E. Any three 3
    (a) Circular expansion and stabilization of the capsular bag
    (b) Safe IOL centration in eyes with zonular dehiscence
    (c) Prevents IOL decent ration after capsular shrinking
    (d) Reduced risk of capsular fibrosis
TOTAL 10

ANS: 3 (VDO: 03)

A. Capsulorhexis 2
B. Double capsulorhexis 2
C. When the primary capsulorhexis is smaller than the desired size 2
D. There is chance of radial tear 2
E. Trypan blue 1
F. Endophthalmitis in epidemic form 1
TOTAL 10

ANS: 4 (VDO: 04)

A. Hydrodissection 3
B. Separate the nucleus and cortex from the capsule 3
C. A blunt cannula is inserted just beneath the edge of the capsulorhexis and fluid is injected gently under the capsule 2
D. PCT 2
TOTAL 10

ANS: 5 (VDO: 05)

A. Phacoemulsification 2
B. Femtosecond laser 2
C. (a) Greater precision and integrity of incisions 1
    (b) Reduced phacoemulsification energy 1
    (c) Good refractive outcomes due to more precise capsulorhexis placement 1
D. Any three .... 1 × 3 3
    (a) Higher cost
    (b) Longer total operating time
    (c) Difficulties with technically challenging cases (e.g. small pupils).
    (d) There is a substantial learning curve
TOTAL 10

ANS: 6 (VDO: 06)

A. Phacoemulsification 4
B. Divide the nucleus 3
C. Dropped nucleus 3
TOTAL 10

ANS: 7 (VDO: 07)
A. Phacoemulsification 4
B. Sculpting of the lens 4
C. PCT 2
TOTAL 10

ANS: 8 (VDO: 08)
A. LASIK 2
B. Epithelium 2
C. Application of laser 2
D. Stroma 2
E. Reposition 2
TOTAL 10

ANS: 9 (VDO: 09)
A. *Continuous curvilinear capsulorhexis2*
B. • Can opener 2
   • Envelope technique 2
C. *Capsulorhexis forceps* *2*
D. *Radial tear* *2*
TOTAL 10

ANS: 10 (VDO: 10)
A. Cover test 2.0
B. Left convergent squint 1.5
C. .... 1 × 3 .... 3.0
   (a) Uncover test
   (b) Alternate cover test
   (c) Prism cover test
   (d) Ocular motility test
D. Alternate prism test 2.0
E. Expected to be good/equal in both eyes 1.5
TOTAL 10

ANS: 11 (VDO: 11)
A. Alternate cover test 2
B. It measures total amount of deviation—amount of deviation before and after the test ... 2
C. Alternate concomitant divergent squint 2
D. Alternate prism cover test 2
E. By placing the prism equivalent to deviation 2
TOTAL 10

ANS: 12 (VDO: 12)
A. Alternate prism cover test 2
B. Deviation is more than the amount of prism used/eyes still move to take fixation 2
C. To increase the strength of prism 2

Video Station

D. Apex is directed outwards as there is exotropia 2
E. With the amount prism when the eye will not move inwards to take fixation 2
TOTAL **10**

ANS: 13 (VDO: 13)
A. Trabeculectomy 2.5
B. Fornix based 2.5
C. Ahmed valve 2.5
D. Intractable glaucoma 2.5
TOTAL **10**

ANS: 14 (VDO: 14)
A. Endolaser photocoagulation 3
B. (a) Triamcinolone acetonide 2
   (b) To stain the residual vitreous 1
C. Air 1
D. Pars plana vitrectomy + Endolaser + Fluid air exchange 3
TOTAL **10**

ANS: 15 (VDO: 15)
A. Pars plana vitrectomy + Scleral fixation IOL 3
B. 1.5–2.0 mm from limbus 3
C. Add +0.50 D with biometric power 2
D. (a) Anterior chamber intraocular lens (ACIOL) 1
   (b) Iris claw lens 1
TOTAL **10**

ANS: 16 (VDO: 16)
A. OCT macula 2
B. (a) Serous sensory detachment of the macula 1
   (b) Pigment epithelial detachment (PED) 1
C. Central serous chorioretinopathy (CSR) 2
D. ....Any 3 .... 1 × 3 3
   (a) Observation
   (b) Focal laser
   (c) Photodynamic therapy (PDT)
   (d) AntiVEGF injection
E. Steroid 1
TOTAL **10**

ANS: 17 (VDO: 17)
A. Phacoemulsification with posterior chamber intraocular lens implantation/ phacoemulsification with PCIOL 1
B. Fragmentation of the nucleus 1
C. Surge 3

D. It can be managed by (any 3) .... 1 × 3 3
   (a) Proper tunnel construction
   (b) Reduced bottle height
   (c) Reduced flow rate
   (d) Reduced vacuum
E. Complications (any 2) .... 1 × 2 2
   (a) PCT
   (b) Dropped nucleus
   (c) Corneal endothelial decompensation
TOTAL *10*

ANS: 18 (VDO: 18)

A. Dropped nucleus 3
B. Fragmatome 2
C. Pars plana vitrectomy and lensectomy 2
D. .... 1 × 3 3
   (a) Iatrogenic retinal break
   (b) Vitreous hemorrhage
   (c) Retinal detachment
TOTAL *10*

ANS: 19 (VDO: 19)

A. Grasping the extraocular muscle 2.5
B. Muscle hook 2.5
C. To put scleral buckle/band 2.5
D. Retinal detachment 2.5
TOTAL *10*

ANS: 20 (VDO: 20)

A. Smallgauge vitrectomy 2
B. Trocar and cannula 2
C. Infusion, illumination, and working 2
D. They are 23–25 gauge 2
E. Trocar-fixation plate (pressure plate forceps) 2
TOTAL *10*

ANS: 21 (VDO: 21)

A. MSICS/SICS (manual small incision cataract surgery/small incision cataract surgery ... 2.0
B. (a) Side port entry blade/crescent knife 15 degree 1.0
   (b) Keratome 1.0
   (c) Crescent knife 1.0
   (d) Corneal forceps 1.0
C. Scleral tunnel 2.0
D. It is water-tight and no suture is need after surgery 1.0
E. Endothelial cell loss/corneal endothelial decompensation 1.0
TOTAL *10*

Video Station 273

ANS: 22 (VDO: 22)
A. Nucleus delivery 3
B. Vectis 2
C. (a) Posterior capsular rupture 1
   (b) Endothelial cell loss 1
D. Irrigation and aspiration. Simcoe double-way cannula .... 2 + 1 3
TOTAL 10

ANS: 23 (VDO: 23)
A. Phacoemulsification with posterior chamber intraocular lens implantation 2
B. Divide and conquer 2
C. (a) Phaco chop 1
   (b) Stop and chop 1
D. Divide and conquer 2
E. Higher phaco time/power because more sculpting 2
TOTAL 10

ANS: 24 (VDO: 24)
A. Ranibizumab 2
B. 0.5 mg and 0.05 mL .... 1 + 1 2
C. Any three:
   (a) Neovascular (wet) age-related macular degeneration (wAMD) 1
   (b) Macular edema following retinal vein occlusion (RVO) 1
   (c) Diabetic macular edema (DME) 1
   (d) Diabetic retinopathy (DR) 1
   (e) Myopic choroidal neovascularization (mCNV) 0.5
D. Bevacizumab 2
E. 3.5–4.0 mm posterior to the limbus (pars plana) 1
TOTAL 10

ANS: 25 (VDO: 25)
A. Pars plana vitrectomy 3
B. Intraocular forceps 2
C. Membrane peeling 2
D. Endolaser green/diode 3
TOTAL 10

ANS: 26 (VDO: 26)
A. Phacoemulsification with posterior chamber intraocular lens implantation 2
B. (a) Continuous curvilinear capsulorhexis 1
   (b) Hydrodissection 1
   (c) Hydrodelineation 1
C. Hydrodissection frees the cataract from the lens capsule, and hydrodelineation splits it into endonuclear and epinuclear sections 2
D. Radial tear in Step 1 and posterior capsular tear in Step 2 .... 1 + 1 2
E. Breaking of nucleus 1
TOTAL 10

ANS: 27 (VDO: 27)
A. Coaxial I/A handpiece 2
B. Bimanual I/A handpiece 2
C. Balanced salt solution (BSS)/Ringer lactate... 2
D. (a) Cortical matter 1
    (b) Epinucleus 1
    (c) Viscoelastic materials 1
E. PCT 1
TOTAL ***10***

ANS: 28 (VDO: 28)
A. Goniosynechialysis 2
B. Peripheral anterior synechiae 2
C. Goniolens 2
D. Microforceps 2
E. Release of peripheral iris from cornea 2
TOTAL ***10***